SOCIAL CHANGE AND HEALTH IN TANZANIA

EDITED BY

KRIS H. HEGGENHOUGEN
AND
JOE L.P. LUGALLA

SOCIAL CHANGE AND HEALTH IN TANZANIA

EDITED BY

KRIS H. HEGGENHOUGEN
AND
JOE L.P. LUGALLA

DAR ES SALAAM UNIVERSITY PRESS LTD.

Published by
Dar es Salaam University Press Ltd.
P.O. Box 35182
Dar es Salaam
TANZANIA

ISBN: 9976 60 406 8
ISBN-13: 978-9976-60-406-1

Contents

Abbreviations

AIDS	-	Acquired Immune Deficiency Syndrome
BC	-	Bacille Calmette-Guerin (Anti-tuberculosis vaccine)
CDDP	-	Control of Diarrhoeal Diseases Programme
CSDS	-	Child Survival and Development Programme
DHS	-	Demographic Health Survey
DPT	-	Diphtheria, Polio and Tetanus
EPI	-	Expanded Programme of Immunization
GDP	-	Gross Domestic Product
GOBI-FFF	-	Growth, Oral Rehydration, Breastfeeding, Immunization-Female Education, Family Planning and Food Supplements
HIV	-	Human Immunodeficiency
IMR	-	Infant Mortality Rates
IMF	-	International Monetary Fund
MCH	-	Maternal and Child Health Services
NACP	-	National AIDS Control Programme
NSC	-	National Summit for Children
NGO	-	Non-Governmental Organization
NFPP	-	National Family Planning Programme
PHC	-	Primary Health Care
SMI	-	Safe Motherhood Initiative
SAP	-	Structural Adjustment Programme
STD	-	Sexually Transmitted Diseases
TB	-	Tuberculosis
VT	-	Vertical Transmission
UNAIDS	-	United Nations Programme on HIV/AIDS
UNDP	-	United Nation Development Programme
WHO	-	World Health Organization
WSC	-	World Summit for Children
WB	-	World Bank

Notes About Contributors

Aldin Mutembei,
Lecturer, Department of Kiswahili,
University of Dar es Salaam,
Dar es Salaam, Tanzania.

Anita Sandstrom
Professor, Department of Epidemiology,
Public Health, and Clinical Medicine,
Umea University, Sweden.

Graziella Van den Bergh,
Research Fellow, Department of Women's Health and
Gender Studies,
University of Bergen,
Oslo, Norway.

Gideon Kwesigabo,
Lecturer, Department of Epidemiology and Biostatistics,
Muhimbili University College of Health Sciences,
University of Dar es Salaam,
Dar es Salaam, Tanzania.

Japhet Z. Killewo,
Associate Professor, Department of Epidemiology and Biostatistics,
Muhimbili University College of Health Sciences,
University of Dar es Salaam,
Dar es Salaam, Tanzania.

Jessie K. Mbwambo,
Assistant Lecturer, Department of Psychiatry,
Muhimbili University College of Health Sciences,
University of Dar es Salaam,
Dar es Salaam, Tanzania.

Joe L.P. Lugalla,
Professor,
Department of Anthropology,
University of New Hampshire, USA.

Knut-Inge Klepp,
Professor, Center of International Health/Center for
Health Promotion Research,
University of Bergen, Norway.

Kris Heggenhougen,
Professor, Department of International Health,
School of Public Health, Boston University,
Boston, Massachusetts, USA.

Lars Dahlgren,
Professor of Sociology,
University of Umea, Sweden.

M.L. Waziri,
Muhimbili Medical Center,
Dar es Salaam, Tanzania.

Maria Emmelin,
Lecturer, University of Umea,
Sweden.

Melkizedeck T. Leshabari,
Associate Professor, Department of Behavioral Sciences and
Director of the Institute of Public Health,
Muhimbili University College of Heath Sciences
University of Dar es Salaam,
Dar es Salaam, Tanzania.

Noah K. Ndosi,
Associate Professor, Department of Psychiatry,
Muhimbili University College of Health Sciences
University of Dar es Salaam,
Dar es Salaam, Tanzania.

Peter A. Kopoka,
Senior Lecturer, Institute of Development Studies,
University of Dar es Salaam,
Dar es Salaam, Tanzania.

Saidi H. Kapiga,
Assistant Professor, Department of Population and International Health,
Harvard School of Public Health,
Boston, Massachusetts, USA.

Sebalda Leshabari
Assistant Lecturer
Muhimbili University College of Health Sciences,
University of Dar es Salaam,
Dar es Salaam, Tanzania.

Sylvia F. Kaaya,
Senior Lecturer and Head, Department of Psychiatry,
Muhimbili University College of Health Sciences,
University of Dar es Salaam,
Dar es Salaam, Tanzania.

Willy Urassa,
Senior Lecturer, Department of Microbiology/Immunology,
Muhimbili University College of Health Sciences,
University of Dar es Salaam,
Dar es Salaam, Tanzania.

Acknowledgements

This book is a product of the commitment and labour of a variety of persons. First and foremost are the authors of the various papers that constitute the chapters of this book. The original idea of producing a book of this type began in the mid 1990s during which time the editors held discussions with most of the authors while they were research fellows of the Health and Behavior Fellowship Program for East Africa in the Department of Social Medicine at the Harvard Medical School. Most of these papers were developed, prepared, or improved upon when the authors were in this program. We are therefore thankful to the Carnegie Corporation of New York for supporting this program. We are particularly grateful to Patricia Rosenfield of Carnegie who worked with the program throughout the 1990s. It is this support that helped to bring most of the authors to Boston and also financed a variety of workshop retreats that took place in Tanzania in order to develop these papers. Since the work began in Boston, we would like to convey our sincere thanks to the academic staff of the Department of Social Medicine at the Harvard Medical School for supporting and interacting with the Carnegie Fellows while they were in Boston and also for supporting the idea of producing a book of this type.

Most of the authors of the chapters are or were members of the academic staff of the University of Dar es Salaam. We wish to acknowledge the support rendered by this institution for granting most of the authors a year's study leave to spend time at the Harvard Medical School. Without this permission and support, it is very unlikely that this book would have been written.

Most of the papers were originally reviewed by a variety of scholars before the decision was made to include them in this volume. Therefore, we also wish to show our gratitude for the work performed by these reviewers, too numerous to mention by name. Their comments were redirected to the respective paper authors, and we believe strongly that their comments have been of great help in shaping the present status of the book. Some of the papers have already been published elsewhere. We therefore wish to convey our thanks to the editors of the *Review of African Political Economy*, the *International Journal of Urban and Regional Research,* and the *Social Science and Medicine* journal for allowing us to reprint the chapters which at first appeared as articles in these journals (as noted at the end of the relevant chapters). The Social Science and Medicine group of the University of Dar es Salaam shouldered the task of paying the copyright fees to the *Social Science and Medicine* journal. For all this, we also say thank you.

The chapters in this book have been written by social scientists and people from the medical field. Some of the chapters have been co-authored by people of different disciplines. The focus of the Carnegie Fellowship Program was on the interdisciplinary collaboration between social scientists and medical practitioners in dealing with health and medical problems. This book reflects that endeavor. We therefore wish to acknowledge our thanks to all those who stood behind the program, and in particular, we wish to mention Professors Arthur Kleinman, Bryon Good, and Mary-Jo Del Vecchio-Good.

Finally, we wish to acknowledge the administrative assistance of Carolyn Stolzenberg and Stephanie Smith, both from the Department of Anthropology at the University of New Hampshire, for typing the entire manuscript and organizing the bibliography. Our sincere appreciation also go to Lisa Feldman Massey for the editorial work. Although this book is a result of the efforts of many individuals and groups, the views expressed in various chapters are those of the authors and in no way represent other people or institutions that have helped the success of this project.

Introduction

Kris Heggenhougen and Joe Lugalla

The inter-relationship between social change and health is as evident, if not more so, in Africa as in other regions of the world. One of the classical public health events in the history of disease etiology clearly shows this inter-relationship. Some 10,000 years ago, small groups of hunters and gatherers in West Africa began joining together and shifted their form of living to that of slash and burn agriculturalists. This produced enough food to allow a much larger group of people to live together in close proximity, and this, with the added introduction of animal husbandry, created large hosts of both animals and people which facilitated the introduction of malaria, which from then on became a human disease which is still plaguing large parts of Africa to this day.

Closer to our own period of time, when we discuss social change and health in Africa, we must naturally include the upheavals brought about by colonialism resulting in both short-term and long-term health effects. Any initial contact between two groups of people who have previously never interacted is bound to introduce diseases which can have devastating effects since the other group has little or no little immunity to fight off the consequences of infection. There were, of course, a whole range of social changes brought about during the colonial period which can be seen reflected in the (negative) epidemiological health and disease pattern among, especially, the local population, only a small part of which resulted directly from battles of conquest as such. But one aspect of colonialism which occurred at least in the British colonies was the plantation system in combination with the imposition of a poll (or hut) tax. The poll tax required payment in money (not easily obtainable for subsistence farmers and others outside the cash economy) and thus the men began to work for pay as migrant farmers for longer and longer periods on the plantations. Not only did this disrupt family life as it had been known up to that time, it also created an increase in the incidence and prevalence of various forms of sexually transmitted diseases since the large groups of men on the plantations naturally did not remain celibate during the extensive period of time they were away from their wives. There are those who argue that the legacy of this plantation and migrant worker situation can be viewed as at least one explanation why the HIV+ rate is much higher in African countries with such a system than in those without it. However, it must also be noted that the improvement in public health also depends in large measure on (guided) social change. Thus, while the social changes referred to above have had a negative health outcome, one of the main reasons for the whole (social) development effort (when defining development by its broadest and most encompassing and equitable social as well as economic parameters) is precisely to improve the health and welfare of the population.

Since attaining their independence in late 1950s and 1960s, African countries have been confronted with a variety of social, economic, cultural, and political changes. The forces behind these changes have been from both internal and external sources, and the impact upon people's lives in general, and upon social and economic progress in particular, has been negative in some cases, positive in others, and in many instances the impact has been both positive and negative.

In some countries, successive military coups, political instability, and lack of a clear political direction with specific development objectives followed their independence. In these countries, besides external factors (including inequitable trading relations where countries received minimum payment for the one or two commodities they had to sell), lack of political stability and constant civil strife have been responsible for the deterioration of social and economic progress and have caused massive human suffering. In such countries, the majority of people have not adequately enjoyed the expected fruits or benefits of independence. Famine, hunger, poor health, and lack of educational opportunities have been common phenomena. Although some of these countries are now stabilizing as a result of the end of the cold war, the rapid winds of so-called modernization through globalization are causing new conflicts and economic contradictions. The economic crisis is escalating in many African countries, and one of the reasons for this is the advent of the unacceptably high mortality rate of young adults at their most productive age, mostly as a result of AIDS. We can see, then, that not only is the etiology of AIDS in large measure related to social changes, as alluded to above, but the consequences of this disease (of AIDS itself) leads to further social changes/disintegration such as a pandemic of young adult deaths, the reduction of the skilled and manual labor force, and the creation of millions of orphans, to mention but three social change consequences. It is unavoidable to note that most African countries, some more than others, are in crisis — a crisis that threatens the health and social welfare of the majority of the population.

Some countries have, of course, been relatively stable since attaining their independence. But even in these countries, the attempts to introduce political improvements and development programs that would positively change what these countries inherited from colonialism have been, inadequate and have left much to be desired. In some of these countries, the external environment has always been hostile and has tended to frustrate some of the good intentions of the post-independent governments. In others, internal weaknesses associated with poor policy formulation, corruption, lack of political will, and commitment from leaders, have been a detriment to social and economic progress. Although a variety of changes have taken place in these countries in the areas of politics, economics, and social life, these changes have been disappointing in that they have had hardly any positive impact in key areas of development such as, for example, security, access to education, health, and a good standard of living for the majority of the people.

Tanzania (originally known as Tanganyika) is among those countries of sub-Saharan Africa that have enjoyed peace and political stability ever since she attained her independence in 1961. She acquired the name Tanzania after Tanganyika united with the island sultanate of Zanzibar in April of 1964. From independence to date, Tanzania has passed through different political and development periods, each driven by different political ambitions and developmental directions and each having consequences in terms of the people's health.

We can distinguish four main developmental periods that have characterized Tanzania since independence. The first period begins with independence in 1961 and ends in early 1967, which marks the beginning of Tanzania's phase of socialist policies for development. The nature of politics that dominated Tanzania during the period up to 1967, however, did not differ much from what was inherited from the colonial government. Although racial discrimination was abolished in the provision of education and heath services, the private sector, in particular religious organizations, continued to dominate in the provision of health and education. Emphasis on health provision continued to be curative rather than preventive.

In 1967, the Tanganyika African Nation Union (TANU), the only official party at that time, redefined its political ideology and developmental direction. Julius Nyerere, the then president of the Republic of Tanzania and Chairman of TANU, introduced on February 5th the well-known Arusha Declaration, which became a blueprint for the country's socialist construction. It rejected the capitalist path to development and vowed to build a socialist society based on the principles of "Ujamaa ('familyhood') and Self-Reliance." The Ujamaa policy, the focus of which was on rural development and self-reliance, also introduced the policies of nationalization. The so-called commanding heights of the economy — like banks, insurance firms, and other companies — were nationalized. The nationalization process also included schools and health institutions. This marked the beginning of the provision of free education and medical care. As far as health care was concerned, the emphasis shifted from curative to preventive and from huge investments in a few big hospitals to the construction of primary rural health care centers and rural dispensaries. In terms of health personnel training, the new focus was on training Medical Assistants and Rural Medical Aides — and somewhat later, the training also included Community Health Workers (Heggenhougen *et. al.*, 1987). The political slogan of the time was "*Mtu ni Afya*" (a human being is health). This slogan advocated the importance of a holistic preventive community approach to health rather than a curative one. During this period, emphasis was placed on consciousness raising about *Ujamaa's* philosophy and policy by the government throughout the country (Green 2001). In addition, the Arusha Declaration sought to marshal the commitment of Tanzania to building a nation based on the principles of socialism, equality and self-reliance. These principles for social change were expected to improve the health and welfare of Tanzanians.

The Ujamaa policy of Tanzania, despite its failure to create a socialist Mecca, managed to introduce human-oriented policies that emphasized the redistribution of economic resources to the rural poor. Although there is evidence that the policy was coercive and sometimes violated some of the basic principles of human rights, it created conditions which allowed the majority of people not only to easily access the basic necessities of life—like land — but also good education and health care. In the health sector, as a result of the Ujamaa policy, Tanzania managed to create an extensive network of health facilities. "An accessibility study carried out in six [of the country's 20] regions in 1979 found that 92 percent of the population was within 10 kms. and 70 percent were within 5 kms. of a health facility, and 45 percent had such a facility within their local community" (Heggenhougen, *et. al.*, 1987:27).

The third developmental phase of Tanzania began in the early 1980s and extended into the mid 1990s. This phase was mainly characterized by the growing conviction on the part of many politicians and other leaders that the country had a number of policy and development problems. It became clear that Tanzania was in a serious social and economic crisis, which had begun in the mid 1970s and had manifested itself in extensive and persistent internal and external macroeconomic imbalances. The internal disequilibrium was evident mainly in growing savings-investment gaps at a time when governmental expenditure was widening. Agricultural production declined—often as a result of farmers having to wait more than a year to be paid (if then) — leading to a shortage of foreign earnings, making it difficult for the government to import manufactured goods from abroad such as fuel and industrial spare parts. This, in turn, paralyzed the industrial sector, leading to a progressive decline in industrial capacity utilization (Lugalla, 1997). The importation of raw materials slowed, leading to a dramatic deterioration of capital stock, spare parts, and other commodities (Green, 2001). While Tanzania's long-term foreign debt was $188 million in 1970, by 1994, this had risen to $6.2 billion (ibid). Acute shortages of basic essential commodities like clothing, sugar, soap, and cooking oil resulted. Existing data also demonstrate that real agricultural output declined. The only sector that continued to expand in real terms was public administration. In brief, the fundamental political economy problem of Tanzania at this time was that material production was decreasing, but public administration was expanding. In Marxist terms, one could say that the superstructure was now becoming a fetter to the development of productive forces. As Green (2001) has argued, all of this eventuated in economic recovery negotiations with the twin Bretton Woods institutions — the International Monetary Fund (IMF) and the World Bank.

This crisis had serious consequences for the government's ability to provide basic social services such as education and health care. As far as health was concerned, its quality began to deteriorate tremendously. Shortages in medicine and essential equipment in hospitals, rural heath centers, and dispensaries became apparent. Lack of incentives; such as good living wages and a good working environment demoralized the health personnel and bred inefficiency and corruption.

In the mid-1980s, in order to deal with this crisis, the government, at the urging of the IMF and WB, adopted structural adjustment policies (SAPs), which, besides other measures, advocated the reduction of government expenditure on health and education. These policies also introduced user fees under the polite name of cost sharing. Tanzanians who had been enjoying free health services since 1967 were, in the early 1990s, subjected to paying whenever they visited a heath facility. As a result of the structural adjustment policies, the government was also forced to adopt a variety of other reform policies. The economy was liberalized, and the free market system was allowed to become the driving force of the economy. Tanzania also began privatizing all state enterprises. But even so, many private hospitals and other health care facilities were embraced by the state and received considerable donor support. The Kilimanjaro Christian Medical Center and the Bugando Medical Center — among the famous consultant and referral hospitals which were nationalized during the Ujamaa period — have now been returned to their former owners, namely the Good Samaritans/Lutheran Church and the Catholic Church respectively.

Other health reform policies included the introduction, in July 1996, of the voluntary Community Health Fund in a few districts and in the entire nation as of April 2001 (Community Health Fund Act, 2001) and the compulsory National Health Insurance Fund via an Act of Parliament, Number 8 of 1999. The government has also allowed foreign health care providers to operate in Tanzania. These range from multinational health insurance companies like AAR and Medex to Chinese teams of traditional doctors. It is too early to say whether these changes and new developments are having positive (or negative) results. However, there is strong evidence that the poor majority of the population have not fared well as far as health conditions are concerned. Existing reports reveal that enrolment rates in the Community Health Fund are not encouraging. There is also an uproar from many civil servants about the functioning of the new health insurance scheme. Unfortunately, these changes have happened at a time when inflation is rampant, many Tanzanians are being retrenched from employment, with the majority experiencing stagnation in real wages and suffering great erosion in their purchasing power.

Despite these problems, the health policy of the government of Tanzania continues to emphasize equality in the distribution of health services and views access to health services as a basic human right. Throughout the 1980s and early 1990s, much of the focus continued to be on primary health care, which emphasizes the strengthening of district management capacity, multi-sectoral collaboration, and community involvement. This goes hand in hand with the current policy of decentralization.

As mentioned earlier, one of the most challenging health problems that has confronted Tanzania during the past fifteen years has been the rapid spread of HIV/AIDS. The number of people estimated to be infected with HIV was 1,745,320 in December 1999. According to the National AIDS Control

Program (NACP), the disease is also becoming more and more noticeable even in remote rural communities. Recent studies reveal that the agricultural sector, which is the backbone of the economy, is particularly devastated since most of those dying are in the age group of fifteen to forty-five years (Lugalla and Kibassa 2002). The World Bank estimates that, because of AIDS, life expectancy in Tanzania will revert to forty-five years by the year 2010 instead of the projected fifty-six years (ibid). The World Bank also predicts that the mean age of the working population will decline from thirty-one and one-half to twenty-nine years by the year 2010, and that, overall, the younger work force will have less education, less training, and less experience (Tanzania's Daily News 25-3-1999, Lugalla and Kibassa 2002). The number of orphans was estimated to increase to 680,000 by the year 2000 (Tanzania's Daily News 25-3-1999); in 1999, it was believed that 10 percent of AIDS orphans in sub-Saharan Africa were in Tanzania (Majira News Paper 21-3-1999).

In looking at the processes of social change and development that have characterized Tanzania since her independence, there is no doubt that their impact on health policies and on people's health has been overwhelming. Major influencing factors in Tanzania's social and economic life, such as the disappearance of most of the socialist tones in Tanzania's development strategies, the impact of structural adjustment policies, the dominance of globalization and a "free" market economy are (for better or worse) creating a new Tanzania. This, as well as the rising rates of poor people who are increasingly becoming the majority, has to be contextualized, analyzed, and understood if, in this climate, Tanzania is to attain—and set in progressive motion—a valid, appropriate, and effective social development process. In so doing, Tanzania would once again re-emerge as an example of how a poor country can effectively meet the challenges of ensuring the health and welfare of its population.

The Setting of the Book

The chapters compiled in this volume endeavor to contribute to that objective. Written by social scientists and health professionals, they examine what has happened to people's health during the past forty years of Tanzania's independence. The authors discuss a variety of health issues and health problems that are dominant in Tanzania. They trace the factors behind these problems, how they affect people's health, and how the government has tried and is trying to address them. Finally, they suggest possible policy solutions that can remedy inadequacies. In order to highlight a number of key health issues and how they affect different social groups, we have divided the book into four main parts. These are "Youth and Health," "Reproductive Health and HIV/AIDS," "Mental Health," and "Poverty and the Political Economy of Health."

"Youth and Health" is concerned with the health conditions experienced by Tanzanian youth. The five chapters in this part address issues ranging from youth and development, unprotected sex, HIV/AIDS, reproductive health, and street children's health. In chapter one, Leshabari and Kaaya discuss the challenges of "Youth and Development" from a health prospective. The authors discuss a variety of developmental problems that youths experience. These include the issue of early, unprotected sex that puts them in danger of HIV infection. One growing problem for many Tanzanian youth is being recruited to traffic in and to use narcotic drugs. As a solution to such problems, the authors emphasize greater parental responsibility in guiding and providing information for young people. They also propose the introduction of new programs in schools that focus on "living or life skills," and they suggest the need for improving communication between youths, communities, and families on issues regarding sexuality and sexual behavior. The authors see communities, families, the education system, and religious organizations as institutions that can play an important role in socializing youths well.

Chapter two by Leshabari *et. al.* examines the issues of youth mobilization and unprotected sex as key factors in the spread of HIV/AIDS. The authors raise two important points. The first is that Tanzanian youths tend to be more vulnerable to HIV/AIDS than the general population. Second, there is a gender difference in the age at which infection with HIV occurs. The authors argue that one of the main factors contributing to this difference is a variance in the age of the sexual partners of male and female youth; male sexual partners of female youth tend to be older than the female sexual partners of male youths. The other key argument advanced by the authors is that poverty is a driving force, particularly for boys, in making them very mobile, moving from one place to the other in search of greener pastures. During this period, the likelihood of boys becoming vulnerable to risky sexual behavior is great. As a result of this, the authors argue that poverty is one of the contributing factors in the rapid spread of HIV/AIDS. While it may not have been the case initially, AIDS now appears to be most severe among the most impoverished segment of the population where the risks of starvation and lack of basic needs are high. Hence, according to the authors, fighting poverty must be one of the major steps towards fighting the rapid spread of HIV/AIDS.

The third chapter, by Kaaya and others, deals with contextual aspects in relation to reproductive health information among school youth in the Rombo District in Tanzania. The authors examine issues relating to sexuality among youth and how the nature of the economy as a whole leads to the increasing commercialization of sex. In brief, the authors argue that the lack of appropriate psychosexual socialization structures during the transition period into young adulthood—that is, the gradual disappearance and/or lack of relevance of traditional "rites of passage"—and the rapid cultural change due to the sweeping winds of globalization and modernization— are creating a new generation of youth—a generation that has not previously been seen in Africa in general or in Tanzania in particular.

The fourth chapter by Lugalla and Mbwambo looks at the fate of street children and the implications of street life on children's health. The authors examine the factors which appear to explain why the government is failing to provide viable solutions to this problem. The authors argue that the government has made no attempt to understand street children in terms of where they come from, their reasons for leaving home, how they survive and meet their daily needs, what problems they experience, and how they resolve them. The authors argue that street children are a product of social and economic factors. They are the neediest persons in the society but the least assisted. Once again, it is noted that that any attempt to address this problem is likely to succeed only if overall societal factors, particularly equity issues and poverty, are addressed.

Part two of the book is composed of chapters six, seven, eight, and nine, which focus on "Reproductive Health and HIV/AIDS." Chapter five, by Mwaikambo, looks at the impact of HIV/AIDS on children. Chapter six, by Kaaya, Mbwambo, and Leshabari, assesses the impact of HIV/AIDS on women and children in the Morogoro Region. Both chapters confirm with concrete data how HIV/AIDS is especially affecting children and women. These two chapters not only call for more government resources to be invested in children and women's health, but also for programs that can empower women and children socially and economically. The chapter by Kaaya, et al. also suggests the importance of having guidelines that can assist primary health care workers in managing opportunistic infections that enhance or are associated with HIV/AIDS. The authors suggest the need to use social support network structures that exist in rural areas in assisting families that have been affected by HIV/AIDS.

In chapter seven, Kapiga presents a comprehensive analysis of the history of HIV/AIDS in Tanzania, its current status, and what has been done to both understand its dynamics as well to control it. He examines a variety of responses that Tanzania has adopted so far in order to confront the epidemic. He also assesses the strengths as well as the weaknesses of these responses and interventions, and he finally suggests what ought to be done in order to win the struggle against HIV/AIDS. Kapiga's chapter also shows that there is a big discrepancy between condom knowledge and condom use. His data show that although condom knowledge is high, condom use is still very low. He therefore suggests that more effort is needed in order not only to impart information, but to identify effective strategies that can be used to promote safer sexual practices and condom use in Tanzania.

Chapter eight, by Kwesigabo *et al.*, examines the current trends of HIV/AIDS in the Kagera region. The chapter, which is a result of a longitudinal study on HIV/AIDS in the Kagera Region, presents positive news. Kwesigabo et al. show that there is a declining trend in the prevalence of HIV/AIDS in Kagera. What is not yet clear is whether this is unique for Kagera or a trend also occurring in other regions of the country. The chapter also looks at associated behavioral factors. Since this was the first region to record AIDS cases in Tanzania (in 1983), the findings presented in this chapter suggest that something positive is happening in the country which may well be a result of the interventions which have been made to prevent the further spread of HIV/AIDS. What is evident from this chapter is that even various epidemics like AIDS can be halted at any point in time if the government, the people, and other stakeholders are willing and committed to act.

Part three of the book is devoted to "Mental Health." Chapter nine by Kaaya and Leshabari examines the status of depressive illness and primary health in sub-Saharan Africa by using Tanzania as a case study. The authors discuss the magnitude of the problem and identify the kind of bottlenecks that hinder the smooth functioning of mental health services in the country. They point to a lack of coordination and of financial resources as major problems in this regard. In order to improve mental health services, the authors suggest that mental health should be defined broadly and, as such, be placed centrally on the country's health agenda. They also suggest that mental health programs derived from the formulation of comprehensive country-based mental health policies would contribute to improved planning and implementation of mental health activities at individual, community, and service provision levels.

Chapter ten by Ndosi discusses the challenges of psychiatry in terms of economic deprivation and social change in Dar es Salaam. He examines the nature of the urbanization process that is taking place in Tanzania and how this process is accompanied by a variety of problems which tend to impact mental health negatively. Ndosi argues that rapid urbanization in Tanzania has led not only to poor housing, overcrowding, poor sanitation, unemployment, and escalating poverty, but that all of these changes contribute to increased stress and to the development of significant mental health problems. While these problems are increasing through rapid urbanization, mental health facilities have become inadequate, leading to a situation whereby many mental health patients remain unattended. Ndosi's chapter reveals how inappropriate policies of regional development can trigger social processes of change that are detrimental to people's health. For example, Ndosi associates poverty and rapid urbanization with delinquent behavior among youth and their involvement in drug abuse and drug peddling. He points to a study of drug abuse related admissions in Dar es Salaam which found that the majority of patients were single, unemployed or underemployed males below the age of 30 years. In order to address these problems, Ndosi suggests the importance of adopting comprehensive national policies that do not isolate health problems from overall development policies. He is of the opinion that policies that aim at promoting rural development can be of great help in limiting rural-urban immigration.

The eleventh chapter by Kilonzo and Simmons is an attempt to reappraise the requirements for the future development of mental health services in Tanzania. They examine the historical development of mental heath services by beginning with the traditional system and moving to the western model of mental health care. After this historical analysis, they present the current burden of mental disorders in Tanzania and examine the efficacy and appropriateness of the Tanzanian National Mental Health Program. The authors also discuss the success of a community mental health care team in Dar es Salaam and the effectiveness of psychiatric agricultural rehabilitation villages in dealing with mental health patients. Their chapter shows how a community-based approach can be effective in dealing with a variety of mental (and other) health problems.

In chapter twelve, Ndosi and Waziri discuss the nature of parasuicide in Dar es Salaam. They present the different types of parasuicides and the methods most commonly used by people to commit suicide. The authors argue that there is a strong determining association between the worsening socio-economic situation in Tanzania and increasing suicide rates. They cite poverty, unemployment, and "difficult conditions of life"—particularly in terms of meeting basic necessities — as creating despair and hopelessness, and thus, factors which form an impetus to commit suicide. The authors also mention that the increasing trend of social conflict in Tanzanian society also contributes to an increase in suicide. These conflicts include misunderstandings between parents and children, husbands and wives, and girlfriends and boyfriends. For example, "freedom" demanded by modern children tends to interfere with the type of firm and strict parental control that is common in a traditional African society. This leads to severe misunderstandings and conflicts between children and their parents or caretakers.

The last part of the book deals with "Poverty and the Political Economy of Health" in Tanzania. The chapters in this section examine the relationship between poverty, growing inequity, and the negative impact on the health of the majority of poor people in vulnerable positions. The chapters argue for the importance of using a political economy approach in understanding prevailing health problems in Tanzania (as well as elsewhere).

Chapter thirteen by Lugalla describes the impact of the well-known World Bank/ International Monetary Fund policies of structural adjustment on women's and children's health. The main argument presented by Lugalla is that structural adjustment policies (SAPs) have had a negative impact on people's health. These policies have not affected all people in the same way, and Lugalla shows with concrete data how these policies have disproportionately affected Tanzania's most vulnerable social groups such as women, children, and the poor.

In chapter fourteen Kopoka performs another examination of the association between poverty and rapid transmission of HIV/AIDS among the young women of Africa. He argues that poverty forces an increasing number of urban and rural young women to engage in high-risk employment opportunities like working as bar/housemaids. The amount of money these women are paid is too small for them to live comfortably. As a result, they are forced to adopt a variety of high-risk survival strategies including survival sex. Kopoka cites the structural changes that are taking place in Africa and on a global scale as the main factors behind the existence of grinding mass poverty in many countries in Africa. The poor become particularly vulnerable to sexually transmitted diseases and HIV/AIDS. Poverty forces many young women to practice survival sex. In order to stop the further spread of HIV/AIDS, Kopoka concludes that the struggle against HIV/AIDS can only succeed if accompanied by efforts aimed at addressing the situation of poverty in both urban and rural areas.

In the last chapter (fifteen), Heggenhougen presents a seminal discussion on structural adjustment, de-facto violence as a result of social inequity, and globalization. He describes how these policies and processes affect people's health and human rights. He argues that the majority of the world's population is now living in a period characterized by increasing globalization. The accelerating process of globalization is expanding global economic opportunities without distributing them equitably. The playing fields of globalization more often than not slope against the interests of poor countries (UNDP 1997) and against the poor in all countries. In order to make his point, Heggenhougen presents some sobering statistics that confirm that globalization is not accompanied by an equitable distribution of economic rewards or social justice. The data show that the difference between rich and poor nations is increasing as is the difference between the rich and the poor within countries. The Human Development Index, developed by UNDP and based on a number of social health and human welfare indicators, had been improving for some countries but have now fallen in as many as 30 countries (UNDP). According to Heggenhougen, a growing under-class is being created, which has severe health implications.

Although Heggenhougen's observations reveal what is going on in the world in general, his observations are also true for and focus on Tanzania. The adoption of structural adjustments and the winds of globalization do not appear to produce smiling Tanzanian faces as far as their health is concerned; instead, these processes of social change are creating crying faces, which reflect misery and conditions of poverty, squalor and ill health. In order to address these issues, Heggenhougen suggests that policies must focus on "an examination of the root causes of inequality and the growing pauperization of the world."

Conclusion

Reviewing the fifteen chapters of this book, it is evident that the processes of social change and development in Tanzania have had positive but also serious negative consequences for people's welfare. Using concrete data, the chapters confirm the differences in health status between most Tanzanians today. They identify not only the main health problems in Tanzania, but also the particular groups of people who are most severely affected by these problems. Each chapter attempts to suggest what ought to be done to address these problems.

It is our belief and expectation that this book will be of interest to policy planners, students, and all those who are concerned with both public health in general, and particularly, with the relationship between development, economic growth, and people's health and welfare in developing countries in general but particularly in Tanzania. The book attempts to highlight, with available data, that unless policies and development strategies listen to the voices of the poor and put poor people first, the health outcomes not only of the poor but of the nation as a whole will be severely curtailed. The authors believe that there was a time in Tanzanian history when policies of development paid a great deal of attention to the equitable provision of health and educational services for all Tanzanians, and based on the current signs of growing health and social welfare disparities, that there is a need to examine contemporary policies and development strategies to see how they can be amended to fulfill the endeavor set in motion at the beginning of Tanzania's independence. We hope the readers of this volume will keep this in mind. The development of Tanzania can neither be imported nor carried out by outsiders. It is the Tanzanians themselves who must (re)direct the wheel of development—of social development—in a positive direction. The purpose of this book is to point to issues which differentially affect groups of Tanzanians and to suggest new approaches which may lead to making Tanzania a nation of people who are healthy, productive, and happy.

PART ONE

YOUTH AND HEALTH

Chapter One

Youth and Development in Tanzania: Challenges from a Health Perspective

Melkizedeck T. Leshabari and Sylvia F. Kaaya

Introduction

Tanzania is an East African country covering 939,000 sq. km and with a population estimated at 30 million. Over the past quarter of a century, the urban population has grown from 5% to 21% of the total population (UN, 1992). While the average annual population growth rate of the country is 3.4%, that of the urban population is 11.3%. The increase in the urban population is related to both a natural increase and rural to urban migration, though the latter is of greater significance (Chacha, 1994; Mongula, 1991). Half of the increase in urban population is reported in the capital city, Dar es Salaam. The contribution of industrial output to the national economy is currently at 25% of the gross national product. With a per capita annual income estimated at $120, Tanzania is amongst the poorest countries in the world (Haub and Yanagishita 1992). Rapid socio-cultural and economic changes characterize the country with attendant implications for the health status of its population—particularly its youth.

The onset of youth is heralded by adolescence, a period of rapid physical and psychological growth during which the adolescent forges an individual identity in the adult world. For the adolescent, despite this period being one of fun, excitement, adventure, risk-taking behavior, and experimentation, society expects them to make important decisions regarding their future and to resolve problems that relate to themselves and the wider society. Psychological coping skills acquired during the socialization process are used to their maximum. Young people in Tanzania today live in a rapidly changing world and are faced with challenges that range from mixed messages and changing views on what is acceptable behavior to the downside of urbanization such as drugs, violence, and poverty. The changing socio-cultural and economic context within which adolescents grow forces them to make choices regarding behavior and lifestyle that they would not have had to make in the past when society and its expectations were well-defined and homogenous.

Writing about youth requires that some attention be paid to the various ways this population sub-group is conceptualized within local contexts. For the majority, particularly rural traditional groups in the country, the measurement of advancing maturity using age as a ratio scale is a new phenomenon. Indeed, in many communities there is more importance placed on the locally constructed concepts regarding maturity and adulthood as internalized during the process of socialization. Hence, a 13-year-old married mother has a very different position and status compared with a pregnant school girl of similar age. The young married mother is conferred the social status and responsibilities of an adult, while the schoolgirl remains a child despite her being at a similar level of psychosexual and biological maturity.

The problem of defining youth as a concept not only occurs at local community levels but also within public institutions such as law enforcement, health, education, and other social services. The issue under consideration in these institutions plays a more important role in defining a young person than where they are on a spectrum of developing maturity or acquisition of development tasks. The acceptable age of enrolment to compulsory primary education ranges between 5 and 13 years due to variations in parental and school teachers' views on an appropriate age at which to send children to school (BEST, 1990). Problems of resources sometimes dictate whether health services consider patients children or adults, and hence, the size of available beds may determine who is admitted to a pediatric ward and who is admitted to an adult medical ward. Pediatric wards with cots limit the age of patients to seven years, while wards with regular beds may admit children aged up to 12 or 15 years. These are just a few examples.

Assumptions made in the local operationalization of the concept of youth sometimes ignore the fact that this population sub-group may have special physical, psychological, and other needs. Institutions dealing with various youth-related issues tend to view youth from a specific perspective and fail to have a comprehensive view of the population sub-group. This may have implications when planning services that target the needs of adolescents and youth. For the purpose of this chapter, youth refers to people aged 10 to 24 years. Adolescence will refer to the age group of 17 years or younger and teenagers will refer to boys and girls aged 13 to 19 years. The concept of "adolescence" is restricted to young people who have specific psychological and physical needs and deserve special attention due to the stage of human development to which they belong. Within this definition of youth, age groups 10-14 years or 15-19 years and 20-24 years can be discussed separately depending on the issue in question. We approach this exploration of Tanzanian youth from a health and social perspective that tries to demonstrate the various vulnerabilities of Tanzanian youth that often result from both a lack of awareness of their needs, and hence, a lack of comprehensive, focused planning for this age group.

In a quest for health for all in Tanzania, one strategy has been to emphasize the health of children below the age of five years. However, this may have been at the expense of other vulnerable groups such as older children. The success of concerted immunization and other preventive health programs has decreased infant mortality from 137/1000 live births in 1975 to 115/1000 live births in 1988 (Bureau of statistics, 1994). A larger proportion of these children now survive to become adults in an environment that, we argue, is ill prepared to deal with the needs of a rapidly growing youth population. In this chapter, demographic trends in the youth population and the context within which health and education services for this population sub-group are provided will be explored. Available evidence on social and health problems will be discussed, as will potential needs in the future in the areas of research, services, and policy.

The Demographic Profile of the Youth Population

The Population Profile of Tanzanian Youth

In the last two national censuses, youths constituted about a third of the population in Tanzania (Bureau of Statistics, 1982 and 1992). In actual numbers, the youth population increased by 230% between 1967 and 1988 and by 45% between 1978 and 1988 (Bureau of Statistics 1971, 1982 and 1992). Interesting patterns emerge when age, sex, and locality desegregate census data is analyzed. While the rural youth population doubled between 1967 and 1988, the urban population increased eight times. The rural female youth population doubled over the twenty-year period, while the urban female youth population multiplied almost nine times. Similarly, rural male youth doubled, while their urban counterparts multiplied seven times during the same period.

Table 1: *The Number of Times the Youth Population Increased Between 1967 and 1988 by Age, Sex and Area of Residence*

Age group (yrs)	*Rural*			*Urban*			*Total*
	Male	*Female*	*Total*	*Male*	*Female*	*Total*	
10-14	2.1	2.3	2.2	9.8	11.4	10.6	2.5
15-19	2.1	1.9	2.0	7.2	8.6	7.9	2.4
20-24	1.9	1.6	1.7	5.7	7.2	6.4	2.1
Total	2.0	2.0	2.0	7.3	8.8	8.0	2.3

Source: *Computed from 1967 Population Census Vol. 3 table 202 p25 and 1988 Population Census: Basic Demographic and Socio-Economic Characteristics Table 1. p.1*

Teenagers account for much of the observed increase in the urban population. Despite a general decrease in the rate of growth of the youth population in the period between 1978 and 1988, the urban increase remained higher than that of rural youth (Bureau of Statistics, 1982 and 1992). Though a natural increase may explain the observed variation in locality-specific rates of increase, it is also likely that large numbers of youth migrate from rural to urban settings in search of better living conditions.

Tanzania has experienced rapid urbanization over the past generation. The family, particularly in urban centers, is changing from extended in nature to a conjugal nuclear and neo-local residence. Until a few years ago, in an effort to strengthen national identity and break tribal boundaries, there was a deliberate move to have people work in localities outside their ancestral villages and tribal groups. Although this policy had a positive effect on nationalism, people were cut off from social interactions with the extended family and the social controls on parenting practices and behavior that such interactions enforced. The current increasingly prohibitive costs of travel make visits to home villages more infrequent, further narrowing the circle of interaction between family members. Traditional child rearing practices, internalized during the psychosocial development process of the current cohort of parents, are applied to children whose realities are far removed from those of their parents.

There are difficulties related to contextual relevance in the transfer of parenting practices to environments in which social structures no longer support some of our traditional values and norms. In emphasizing this, one author notes, "we should avoid attributing motives and measures to the young that were appropriate to their ancestors, but that are not so relevant to them now" (Liljestrom *et al.* 1994). One change that may obviously arise that may impact parenting practices is a loss in the traditional sense of community. While, in the past, adults in communities were actively involved in setting boundaries and providing discipline amongst children regardless of whether they were the biological parents or not, reports from Kyela, a rural district, indicate that this is no longer an acceptable practice (Leshabari *et. al.*, 1996a). There are also indications that parents and adults sense a decreasing "hold" over the thinking, experiences, and decision-making processes of the young (Omari, 1977; Leshabari *et al.*, 1996a). Omari (1977) notes that parents have lost, to a large degree, their role and authority over their children, and the emerging social institutions have only assumed partial responsibility or introduced a different role and meaning altogether from that of traditional institutions. These changes may be a result of cultural diffusion and a lack of homogeneity in norms and values in many Tanzanian communities. The development of a new set governing parenting practices is, hence, not surprising. This is an area of study yet to be explored in Tanzania.

In the existing socio-cultural transitional period, there are bound to be contradictions within and between families and communities regarding parenting and limit-setting for children and youth that may have a negative impact on particularly first and even second generation urban dwellers in Tanzania. One such transitional effect is a lack of awareness on the part of adults and parents of the challenges children and youth in contemporary Tanzania face in their growth to maturity. This lack of awareness may inadvertently prohibit parents and the wider society from equipping young people with the necessary skills and providing enabling environments for adequate growth and development. Omari (1977) predicted that one of the outcomes of these changes would be an increase in divorce rates amongst young couples as cultural structuring of the concept of marriage and its meaning changes and the social and psychological support offered by the extended family in resolving marital conflicts decreases.

The Marital Status of Youth in Tanzania

Evidence indicates a decline in the proportion of married youth in the country that correlates well with the introduction of compulsory primary education in 1967. The summary shown in figure 1 shows a decline in the proportion of married youth in each successive census year, this being more significant for females compared with males. In 1988, almost a third of females aged between 10-24 years were married, compared with under a tenth of male youth of similar age.

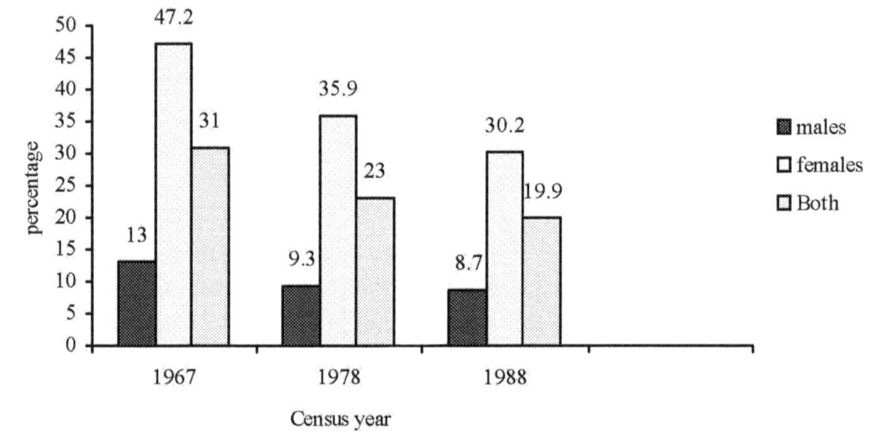

Figure 1: *Percentage of married youth by age and sex extracted from 1967, 1978 and 1988 census data.*

Source: *Computed from 1967 Population Census Vol. 3 table 202 p 25; 1978 Population Census: Basic Demographic and Socio Economic Characteristics table 2 p 12 and 1988 Population Census: Basic Demographic and Socio-Economic Characteristics table 4 p 18.*

Much of the decline in married youth is attributed to a decrease in the proportion of married females in the 15-24 year age groups. The variations in proportions of married female and male youth indicate that females do not marry men within their own age cohort, suggesting they become wives of older men. It is unclear in what contexts courtship between female youth and older men occurs and how societal norms and values moderate such courtship to its conclusion in marriage. As there are less defined social controls on behavior in urban compared to rural areas, sexual relationships between relatively older men and young girls in urban settings may partly reflect traditional age differences in the choice of intimate partners. The phenomenon of older men having loosely-defined sexual relationships with young girls in urban settings in East Africa has been called the "sugar daddy" phenomena and has been reported by other authors in urban areas of East Africa (Schoepf, 1992, Lwihula, 1996). The "sugar daddy" phenomenon connotes exploitation of girls by older men where economic gains on the part of young girls are an important factor that maintains the practice. However, this may be too simplistic an explanation as it portrays adolescent girls as passive and innocent victims; this may be misleading. A study of complicated urban teenage abortions indicated that many of the girls had conceived with much older men, and only a small proportion indicated that their partners were well off financially (Leshabari et al., 1994). This suggests a need for a further exploration of this phenomenon that includes broader socio-cultural and psychological contextual variables such as women's status, self-image, esteem, and self efficacy, as well as factors that define gender power relations and how these relate to wider social and political structures in contemporary Tanzania.

Information that exists on the traditional structuring of sexuality in communities in Tanzania indicates that sexuality shaped the patterns of social, economic, and political lives within many communities (Mbunda, 1991). Concepts of age and maturity could only be understood within the framework of sexual development and the basis this formed for the social allocation of jobs. In many communities, sex was viewed not only as a source of physical pleasure, but as central to reproduction, production, and a host of complex sets of interdependent relationships, roles, duties, and rights. Sex was sanctioned and controlled by ensuring it occurred within the framework of marriage. At this juncture, it is possible to argue that girls traditionally tended to marry men who were older than them, sometimes as second or higher index wives, in a balance of power that favored men. In many traditional societies in the country, marriages are generally arranged by parents and are utilitarian in nature with more value invested in the kinship ties created by marriage than in the individual relationship of the new couple (Wilson, 1951). Haram (1995) noted that dowry – a system where the intended groom's family pays a set amount of goods or cash for a bride – was the only legitimate way of gaining access to a woman's sexuality. Payment of dowry gave men rights over wives and the children they bear. But it is important to note that dowry and marriage was also linked to complex systems of social organization, roles and obligations, and clan and community survival including assurance of paternity (more so in patriarchal societies).

In present day Tanzania, particularly in urban settings, arranged marriages are less prevalent than in the past. The widespread availability of formal education has contributed to a significant reduction in female youth marriages in Tanzania as well as in other parts of sub-Saharan Africa (Bledsoe and Cohen, 1992). The longer period of being "single" that is sometimes referred to as a bio-social gap has implications for sexuality and pre-marital sexual behavior and practices in a changing socio-cultural context. Changes that have occurred in the cultural structuring of sexuality, the development of heterosexual intimacy, courtship, and marriage, in the light of the rapid changes in the cultural and socio-economic contexts, are not very clearly understood. Bledsoe and Cohen (ibid) note that financial constraints often result in marriage becoming a lengthy process, where young people may live together before sufficient funds for a respectable (traditional) union can be acquired. It is unclear to what extent these relationships culminate in legal marriages. Amongst youth that do get married, there is little information on the stability of these unions. The census data on divorce rates among youth is perhaps an early warning of disturbing patterns if divorce is considered an indicator of societal instability.

Table 2: *Percentage of Divorced Youth by Age, Sex and Census Year*

Age (yrs)	*Census year and sex*								
	1967				*1978*			*1988*	
	Male	*Female*	*Total*	*Male*	*Female*	*Total*	*Mak*	*Female*	*Total*
10-14	8.2	3.0	3.8	5.7	3.9	4.2	5.1	3.9	4.2
15-19	3.1	3.6	3.6	3.7	4.3	4.3	2.7	3.2	3.5
20-24	3.7	4.3	4.1	4.0	5.3	5.0	2.5	4.7	4.2
Total	3.6	4.0	3.9	4.0	4.9	4.7	2.6	4.2	3.9

Source: *Computed from 1967 Population Census Vol. 3 table 202 p 25; 1978 Population Census: Basic Demographic and Socio Economic Characteristics table 2 p 12 and 1988 Population Census: Basic Demographic and Socio-Economic Characteristics table 4 p 18.*

In 1978, only 1.43% of all Tanzanians were divorced, but by 1988, this proportion increased to 3.8% (Bureau of Statistics, 1992). Census data computed and summarized in table 2 indicate rates amongst youth were higher than in the general population during both census years, that female youth have higher rates of divorce than their male counterparts, and over time, divorce rates among female youth are increasing. Males who marry at 14 years or younger appear to have higher rates of divorce than older age groups, though their actual numbers are so low that the significance of variation in rates of divorce is questionable. We hypothesize that the higher rates of divorce amongst female youth are transitional effects of socio-cultural change. Assuming greater social stability and consistency in rural compared with urban areas, it would be expected that divorce rates amongst female rural youth would be lower that that of their urban counterparts. This hypothesis can only be tested out with the 1978 census data that was desegregated by urban/rural areas of residence (Table 3). Indeed, the 1978 census data shows divorce rates were higher in married urban than in rural youth, the differences being particularly pronounced in female youth aged 20 - 24 years.

Table 3: *Percentage of Divorced Youth by Age, Sex and Area of Residence in 1978*

Age(years)	*Area of residence and sex*					
	Rural			*Urban*		
	Male	*Female*	*Total*	*Male*	*Female*	*Total*
10-14	6.3	3.9	4.2	2.0	4.4	3.9
15-19	3.6	4.3	4.2	3.5	4.5	4.4
20-24	4.0	4.8	4.6	3.6	7.5	6.5
TOTAL	4.0	4.6	4.5	3.6	6.5	6.0

Source: *Computed from 1978 Population Census: Basic Demographic and Socio-Economic Characteristics table 2 pp. 12.*

The data supports the assumption that urban environments may contribute to lower stability of marital unions that involve youth, with married females aged between 20-24 years in an urban locality being most vulnerable. Unfortunately age, sex, and area of residence was not desegregated in the 1998 census data report making it difficult to validate this observation. The increasing divorce rates amongst young couples is a trend that needs to be followed up, and one hopes that future census data will collect information that will allow this type of analysis. Stability of marriage is important not only for the welfare of couples, but also for their children. Psychosocial skills required in adolescence and youth that allow for development into mature and responsible adults such as trust, self-assertiveness, confidence, and self-determination are often internalized during early childhood. Child rearing in present-day Tanzania will increasingly be solely the responsibility of biological parents, without the safety net that was previously provided by the traditional extended family system.

Youth and Education in Tanzania

Since independence in 1961, the government has done a commendable job with respect to increasing the level of literacy from a rate of less than 10 % in the early 1960's to rates above 90% by 1988 (World Bank, 1992). This success was achieved through an adult education campaign and concerted efforts to transform the existing colonial education system. A previously racially segregated education system was reformed by legislation that aimed at developing a unified national system with no racial or religious distinctions; these attitudinal changes were embodied in the 1967 Policy of Education for Self-reliance introduced in the primary education system. The intention was to develop a type of education that nurtured self-responsibility and collective self-help, integrating technological skills with the values and attitudes of a developing socialist community (Mosha, 1988). Since the majority of the population resided in rural areas, practical agricultural skills were particularly emphasized. Schools developed agricultural projects both for training pupils as well as to raise funds that helped reduce recurrent expenditure funding from the government.

The Education for Self-reliance Policy was, however, not sufficiently articulated by implementers who were unable to communicate its meaning to communities served by the schools. Despite the introduction of agricultural and other vocational activities in primary schools, the assessment of pupils' competence remained academic with a focus on passing examinations and gaining admission to the few places available for secondary education. The criteria for the success in primary education remains the number of pupils who pass school-leaving examinations and proceed to public secondary education. Outcomes in terms of proficiency in agricultural and other vocational activities were not officially or unofficially recognized, and for pupils graduating from primary schools there were few readily available jobs in rural areas (Kamm, 1977). To date, parents continue to perceive self-reliance activities as "stealing" time from the "normal" teaching curricula. In an assessment of parents' attitudes towards education in rural Tanzania, Cooksey et al. (1993) noted the disenchantment of parents who did not feel children benefited from the agricultural activities they performed. Parents felt that the labor of children was being exploited and links were not made between the school's agricultural earnings and benefits in terms of the financing of school activities.

Universal Primary Education, introduced in 1977, required by law school enrolment of all children aged between seven and 13 years. This policy emphasized an approach towards mass education at primary and adult education levels and took place during the villagization program when policy ensured that each village in Tanzania had at least one primary school (Lugalla, 1993 pp. 191). The impact of these policies was encouraging, with an increase in the number of enrolled pupils in primary schools nationwide from 2.2 million children in 1977 to 3.8 million by 1993 (BEST, 1994). Net school enrolment, however, fell from 60% of 7-13 years olds in 1978 to 47% in 1988. A longstanding economic crisis in the country since the early 1980's, compounded by structural adjustment policies, led to a decline in public spending for education with far-reaching implications for the implementation of education policies. Between 1978 and 1988, the proportion of the Gross Domestic Product that was allocated to education dropped from 5.2% to 2.2% (Lugalla, 1993). The school environment is currently characterized by poorly maintained infrastructure that lacks basic furnishings and other facilities. There are shortages of teaching facilities including teachers, and less well trained assistant teachers introduced as part of the Universal Primary Education Policy have gradually taken full responsibility for teaching with adverse repercussions on the quality of education provided. These are evident factors that do not motivate pupils or teachers in their learning and teaching environments.

The extension of gains in primary to secondary levels of education has been much slower than was anticipated. The public secondary school system remains one of the smallest in the world, and in 1980, it was only able to cater for 2.4% of primary school graduates (Kahama, 1986). By 1988, the proportion of primary school graduates accepted into both private and public secondary schools had risen to about 10%, a figure that remains unacceptably low (BEST, 1990). Encouraging measures are in place to increase the numbers of secondary schools through community efforts. The pressure to build more secondary schools, however, to a large extent has ignored the need for important input such as teachers and teaching and learning materials. The problems related to the quality of education provided by primary education are hence reproduced in secondary education settings. Between 1989 and 1993, the number of students sitting their final O-level examinations after completing four years of secondary education increased from 24,068 to 35,025. However the proportion that pass with a distinction (Division one passes) declined progressively from 7.1% in 1989 to 2.3% in 1993. This decline was mirrored by the increase in those who failed the examination from 12.7% in 1989 to 19.8% in 1993 (BEST, 1994).

Lugalla (1995) notes that parental attitudes towards education are influenced by the social, economic, and cultural conditions of their environments. These regional variations in parental attitudes create inequities in access to education for young people. Parents from agrarian areas that have experienced land shortages tend to orient both male and female children towards the urban job market and commercial activities rather than farming. Such parents are willing to invest in the education of their children compared with those from pastoral and agrarian communities who have not experienced land shortages. Some studies indicate that variations in parents' perceptions on the importance of children applying themselves to school work as opposed to helping out in household economic activities may be important factors that explain school absenteeism and drop-outs (Cooksey *et. al.*, 1993, Lugalla, 1995; pp. 59). Children whose parents are professionals or administrators (most of whom are urban dwellers) are also more likely to access educational facilities compared with children of peasant farmers. In 1974, a survey in seven secondary schools revealed that only 38.2% of students came from homes of full-time peasant farmers who comprised 90.2% of the workforce according to the 1967 census. About 12% of students came from homes of professionals or administrators who comprised 1.5% of the workforce (Kahama, 1986). These regional and socio-economic biases have permeated all levels of higher education in Tanzania (Lugalla, 1995). With the current economic crisis that has generated cost-sharing policies in the provision of social services, these inequalities in access to education are bound to increase if measures are not taken to ensure more equity. Despite paying high taxes, parents also pay increasing informal contributions to an education system in gradual transformation from a previously perceived "free" social service to one where direct contributions are made by parents in a Cost-sharing in Education policy. Many parents in a survey of rural schools were of the opinion that urban parents and those with money would be the main beneficiaries of the existing public education system (Cooksey *et. al.*, 1993).

Trade liberalization in the early 1990's in Tanzania brought with it some positive but double-edged changes in the education system the impact of which it may be too early to assess. Private enterprise primary and secondary education was deregulated during this period. In response to dissatisfaction with the quality of the public education system, mushrooming private primary and secondary schools have characterized the past decade. The government has continued to regulate to a certain extent the curricula of these schools through the registration process and regular supervision by the Ministry of Education and Culture through school inspectors. A school textbook trade industry is growing in response to demand, and the country is seeing more bookshops opening, though mainly in urban areas. Both locally published and imported textbooks predominantly for primary and secondary schools are now available for sale. These are all promising developments, but have far reaching political implications for a country that had an emphasis on socialist policies that encouraged access to education for all.

Employment Opportunities for the Youth in Tanzania

The growth of the Tanzanian population has exceeded growth in the service and industrial sectors of the economy with implications on employment opportunities. Each year the primary school system in Tanzania produces over 360,000 graduates that join an unemployment pool to which the youth already constitute the majority (BEST, 1994). Among the few who join secondary education, the increasing numbers that fail their O-level examinations and do not secure an O-level Certificate of Education add to this pool of unemployed youths. The proportion of economically active teenagers and youth is reported to be higher in rural areas—at 62% compared with only 45.4% in urban areas (Bureau of Statistics, 1992).

The migration of youth to urban areas can be linked to both unstable economic conditions in rural areas as well as to an attitudinal mindset that is encouraged by a lack of social and economic incentives that could have made work in a rural setting attractive for primary school graduates (Chacha, 1994). Lugalla (1995) notes, as is the case elsewhere in the world, in Tanzania, there is a direct association between the educational level attained and employment opportunity, income and socio-economic status. This means that given the geographic differentials between rural and urban areas in access to education, youth from rural areas are unlikely to find a job with ease in the urban areas to which they migrate. They consequently risk transforming a state of rural poverty to poverty in an urban setting to which they are unaccustomed and in which they may be more vulnerable than their urban counterparts to the ravages of urban poverty. Many rural migrants to urban areas experience difficulties in securing both employment and accommodation and are forced to live in make-shift houses in squatter settlements that lack basic social service facilities (Lugalla, 1997).

In response to the economic crisis in Tanzania, a significant informal economy has developed in urban areas over the past ten to 15 years. The income-generating activities in the informal economic sector range from selling vegetables and hawking to carpentry and tailoring. These activities have provided a niche for survival for many young urban migrants. An urban sub-culture of the "*mmachinga*" petty trader is evolving. The term *"mmachinga"* is a colloquial street term that was used to describe people from Southern Tanzania from where it was assumed young people who were on the streets in Dar es Salaam came. It is now evident that young people on the streets of Dar es Salaam come from many regions of the country (Lugalla and Mwambo, 1999). The "*machinga*" is often a young male petty trader who hawks his wares at strategic positions on pavements. The government response to this phenomenon, which has not been very effective, has been to institute by-laws to curb such informal sector activities including forceful removal of these young men off the streets. More effective interventions are necessary that focus on the predicament of the young person in Tanzania and facilitate an increase in employment opportunities for both rural and urban youths.

A serious consequence of large numbers of unemployed youth on the streets in urban areas is an increase in youth gangs within which criminal activities often evolve. This has implications for law enforcement agencies as well as public security. Experience in the West indicates that unemployment can directly or indirectly increase the risk of psychological distress in persons without previous psychological vulnerability (Montgomery *et al*., 1999). Psychosocial difficulties amongst adolescents and youth often manifest themselves in maladaptive coping strategies that breed problem behavior. Balmer *et al.* (1997), in a study amongst adolescents in a slum urban area in Kenya, note the difficulties adolescents experience in developing a coherent and consistent set of personal values that would govern their behavior in a setting of cultural diversity. Dysfunctional coping strategies that could be injurious to health that were reported include use of drugs—which ranked first—while alcohol use and sex for favors ranked fourth and fifth respectively, the latter being of particular concern amongst adolescent girls. Although survival may be a major motive that could explain problem behavior amongst urban East African youth, the possibility of psychological problems in unemployed and under-employed youth that is directly or indirectly linked to their employment status needs further exploration. An understanding of youth involvement in crime and violence in urban areas in Tanzania is an area of public health significance that requires a multidisciplinary approach in its exploration and the development of relevant interventions.

The Health Status of Tanzanian Youth

Though Tanzania can boast a decrease in infant mortality, the health status of children aged 6 to 18 years and older youth aged 19-24 years remains a gray area in as far as our understanding and knowledge is concerned. Due to the large youth population in the country, the declining economy, and sporadic droughts and floods, one would expect youth to feature significantly in morbidity and mortality statistics, particularly for prevalent communicable diseases. Unfortunately, retrievable national morbidity and mortality data are rarely desegregated to allow for reflection on their health status partly because this population sub-group has not been a focus for health-related interventions.

Recent evidence from a large morbidity and mortality surveillance system that has been in place since 1992 provides some hope that this situation will be rectified (Ministry of Health and AMMP, 1998). The surveillance system covers representative cohorts from an urban area (Dar es Salaam region), a high socio- economic status rural area (Hai district), and a low socio-economic status rural area (Morogoro rural district). Mortality rates amongst youths in the sentinel surveillance populations are summarized in figure 2. Mortality rates increased with age in the youth sub-groups, particularly for youths in the poor rural district of Morogoro Rural where rates were highest for older female youth at 11.8 per 1,000 population. At 6.4 per 1,000 population, older female youth in the urban study area of Dar es Salaam ranked third in mortality statistics.

The female death rates in the more affluent area of Hai District (compared with Morogoro Rural) were consistently lower than the rates for males in the same area for all the youth age groups. There appear to be factors in the urban and poor rural area that increase the risk of death amongst female youth compared with males, while factors related to affluence in a rural setting are more protective for female than male youth.

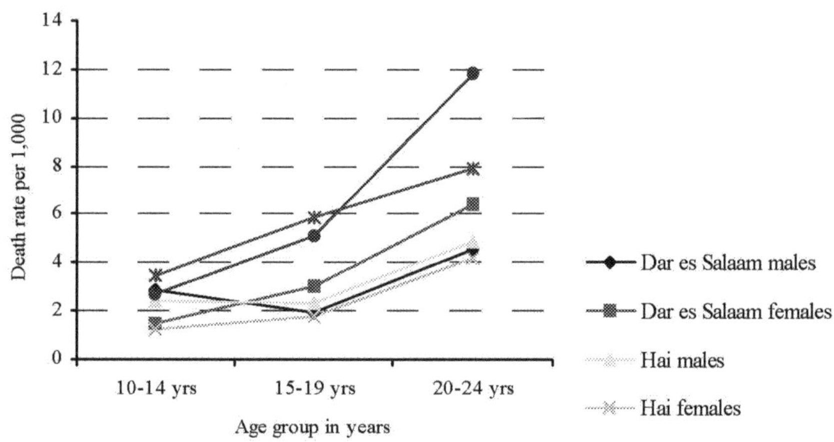

Figure 2: *Mortality rates among youth by sex per 1,000 population in Dar es Salaam, Morogoro and Hai between July 1992 and December 1995*

Source: *Health Statistics Abstract, 1998; Vol. 1 Morbidity and Mortality Data. Ministry of Health, United Republic of Tanzania, Issue no. 6, July 1998*

Broad classifications of causes of death revealed infectious diseases to be the most common, followed by injuries as summarized in Table 4. Infectious disease was the most common broad cause of death in both males and females in the three sites. Youth in the poor rural site were more likely to die of infectious disease than urban female youth. In all the sites, injuries were the second most common cause of death amongst male youth, while maternal causes were the most common among urban female youth and females from the poor rural sites. It was interesting to note that in the more affluent rural area, injuries were the second most common cause of death amongst females, as was the case for males in the same area. It is worth noting that injury control has not been given much emphasis by either public health professionals or communities.

The findings call for more focused qualitative studies to explore the reasons for the gender variations in the causes of death noted above.

Table 4: *Causes of death in AMMP areas: Percentage of Death Attributable to Broad Causes by Age and Sex for Youth 10-24 Years July 1992- December 1995*

Causes of death and age groups in years	*Sentinel surveillance sites, gender and percentage of deaths*					
	Dar es Salaam		*Hai District*		*Morogoro Rural District*	
	Males n=119	*Females n=167*	*Males n=226*	*Females n=183*	*Males n=286*	*Females n=333*
Infectious diseases	47.9	61.7	44.7	47.5	60.1	67.9
Injuries	23.5	5.4	25.7	14.7	20.6	4.2
Non-infectious diseases	22.7	9.0	22.1	21.8	17.1	10.8
Maternal causes	-	16.2	-	10.4	-	14.4
Uncertain	5.9	7.8	7.5	5.5	2.1	2.7

Key: n= all deaths in age group 10-24 years
Source: Robert Mswia (1999)

There is very little information on the health status of youth in schools in the country that would allow some reflection on health status and morbidity in this population. A mailed questionnaire to 50 District Medical Officers indicated no retrievable studies on the health status of primary school children or any health examination of the same population (Malentlema, 1977). Health services provided for schools by the Ministry of Health were minimal and involved mainly advice on sanitation and hygiene and the occasional examination of pubescent girls for pregnancy. Only five District Medical Officers reported they had provided a first-aid box in some primary schools. Though the School Health Programme has been in place since 1921, a recent review noted very minimal implementation of activities due in part to poor coordination across the five government sectors (Ministries) whose collaboration is essential for action at the school level (Leshabari *et. al.*, 1996b).

In many cases, health care for adolescents in the country is integrated within general health services. Under the current public health services, pediatric services cater for children up to the age of 7 years, and children above this age are treated in services that cater for adults, with the exception of children with handicaps or congenital/hereditary disorders. Mental health services have very recently started providing formal outpatient services for children and adolescents, but this is restricted to one consultant hospital in the capital city. In the absence of school health services, an obvious gap exists in health care provision for this population sub-group. Surveys in selected areas indicate a range of health-related behavior patterns with adverse consequences for young people. These range from sexual to drug-use behavior that will be reviewed briefly below.

Youth Sexual Behavior and Related Health Problems

There are several pointers that indicate a decrease in the traditional control over youth sexual behavior in contemporary communities. Data from several school-based surveys and a few community-based studies indicate sexual exposure amongst youth in school is higher than what is assumed to be the case. Current arguments in some sectors of society against exposing youth to reproductive health information and services for fear this might prompt promiscuous behavior are unwarranted given the evidence from existing data that shows a significant proportion of youth engage in unprotected sex. Many do so in an atmosphere of ignorance and misconceptions, thus exposing themselves to the health consequences of unprotected sex. A school-based survey conducted in 1985 revealed the rates of sexual exposure varied from about 18% among young boys aged 12 years or younger to over 85% among young men aged 20 to 24 years. The corresponding rates among girls varied from 5% to over 86% respectively (Mbunda, 1988). A school-based urban study revealed that nearly half of adolescents aged 14 years or younger have had sex at least once, and this proportion increased to nearly 60% among teenagers aged 18 years or older (Leshabari, 1988). More recent urban and rural-based surveys provide very similar rates (Kapiga *et. al*., 1992; Lwihula *et. al*., 1996; Seha *et. al*., 1994; Klepp *et. al*., 1994; Leshabari *et. al*., 1997).

Much of the above data was collected in the context of Knowledge Attitudes Behavior and Practice Surveys. Both Mbunda (1988) and Leshabari (1988) had reported on the presence of myths and misinformation on issues related to human reproduction in this population of youths. Later studies that used knowledge scales in data analysis confirmed the low levels of reproductive health-related knowledge in urban and rural school youth respectively (Lwihula *et. al*., 1996; Leshabari *et. al*., 1997). From these studies, it was evident that peers were the main source of information on basic aspects related to biological maturity, and young people poorly understood this information. An expressed need for such information was noted. Studies in the area of sexual behavior amongst youth have consistently shown a lack of association between knowledge and sexual behavior, and it is difficult to determine whether knowledge is acquired prior to or after the onset of such behavior.

There are a few studies that have moved beyond knowledge and analyzed in greater depth how factors such as attitudes, perceived social norms, and self-efficacy influence sexual behavior in Tanzanian youth. Klepp et al. (1996), in a survey of 2,026 primary school students of mean age 14.0 years in the Arusha and Kilimanjaro regions of Northern Tanzania, explored the decision to have or abstain from sexual intercourse. They used as a theoretical framework a modification of the Theory of Reasoned Action and were able to demonstrate that attitudes, subjective norms, self-efficacy, and reported life-time frequency of sexual intercourse accounted for 26% of the variance in the intention to have sexual intercourse within the next three months. Pupils from rural schools expressed more restrictive attitudes and subjective norms towards having sexual intercourse than urban pupils, though urban pupils were more confident that they could resist pressure to engage in sexual intercourse than rural pupils. In this survey, 63% of boys and 24% of girls were sexually active. The authors note that silence on issues related to sexuality between adults and children in the study areas contributes to unfounded perceptions of norms related to pre-marital sex amongst pupils. They also note the need for reproductive health education programs to begin at an early age in the study populations before sexual activity begins. More studies such as these are important given the diversity of ethnic groups in Tanzania to allow for planning of interventions that focus on core needs in wider school youth populations.

Studies addressing youth sexual behavior have utilized a narrow concept of sexual behavior. While it is quite possible that a variety of different types of sexual behavior are being practiced, available data is limited to heterosexual vaginal sexual practices and offer no information on anal penetrative sex (heterosexual or homosexual) or non-penetrative sexual behavior currently in practice. Although kiswahili words ("*msenge,*" "*basha*") for homosexuality are fairly common, especially in urban areas along the coast, not much is known about the extent to which this behavior is practised. Non-penetrative sexual practices may also occur amongst youth including practices such as masturbation, but they remain largely undocumented. It is important to be familiar with a variety of existing non-penetrative sexual practices in order to have a pool of potential choices for advocating safer sex among youth (Liskin, 1989; AHRTAG, 1993).

A more serious problem concerning the available data on youth sexuality and sexual behavior in Tanzania is lack of information on the contexts that are associated with reported sexual experiences. An understanding of the context within which sexual behavior takes place is important for planning interventions focusing on reproductive health. This is primarily because human behavior is influenced not only by awareness and knowledge of the consequences they produce but also by the antecedent cues or contexts that preceded them (Baldwin and Baldwin, 1986). These situational contexts are more sensitive to effective behavioral change than focusing on the behavior alone.

Consequences of Pre-marital Youth Unprotected Sexual Intercourse

Since a substantial proportion of youth is sexually active, the potential for damaging consequences is high. These range from unwanted pregnancies to sexually-transmitted diseases (STDs) including HIV/AIDS. Worldwide, 15 million teenage girls aged 15-19 years give birth each year and 80% of them come from developing countries (Senderowitz and Paxman, 1995). In Latin America, 50% of all young women give birth by age 20 years, as do 65% in Africa and 54% in Asia (Population Reference Bureau, 1990). Much of the data available on unwanted pregnancy in Tanzania is from the school population. School pregnancy is a major cause of primary school dropout in Tanzania. Statistics from the Ministry of Education provide only a glimpse of the extent of the problem. This is because of the logistical difficulties in compiling data centrally in a country as large as Tanzania. Data from schools in remote villages may rarely reach district education authorities. The following data must at best, therefore, be considered an underestimate. Records from the Ministry of Education for 1992 show that a total of 46,204 pupils dropped out of primary school (approximately 2% of the primary school population). Half of these were girls (49%), and 13% did so due to pregnancy. Mpangile and Mbunda (1993) noted that the majority of 298 urban schoolgirls who dropped out of primary school due to pregnancy over a three-year period were in their fifth or higher year of study.

Although the extent of unwanted pregnancies among youth at a national level is not known, female youth admitted to gynecological wards with complications of induced abortions can serve as a proxy measure. A study of 300 women with early pregnancy loss at an urban tertiary care facility indicated 52% had an unwanted pregnancy, and 61% decided to terminate the pregnancy. The majority of these patients were under 25 years of age (Justesen *et. al.*, 1992). A similar study conducted in public hospitals in Dar es Salaam revealed that out of 965 consecutive admissions with diagnosed abortion complications, 455 had induced an abortion, a third of whom were teenagers (Mpangile *et. al.*, 1993). Further analysis revealed that teenage girls received minimal social support from the time they conceived to when they were admitted to hospital with a complicated abortion. Relatives, particularly mothers, were the major source of support. Despite public opposition to contraceptive services for youth, it appears that, when parents are faced with a pregnant unmarried daughter, it is not unusual to arrange for an illegal abortion as a solution to the crisis (Leshabari *et. al.*, 1994). The problem of induced abortion amongst youth is not restricted to urban areas but is also common in rural areas. Ignorance about modern contraception methods, lack of psycho-sexual counseling and contraceptive services, and the illegality of abortion may contribute to the magnitude of this problem.

Apart from unwanted pregnancy, sexually transmitted diseases (STDs) also comprise a potentially significant problem. The extent of STDs among youth is also generally unknown at a national level, but given the large number of youths who indulge in unprotected sexual intercourse, STDs are among the major problems they may have to cope with. One study involving 1,253 patients with sexually-transmitted diseases drawn from various parts of Tanzania revealed that nearly 75% were below the age of 30 years (Msamanga, 1986). The peak age group among males was between 20-24 years, and it was lower among females at 15 to 19 years. Data from sexually transmitted disease and antenatal clinics in Dar es Salaam also indicate that youth are vulnerable to chronic STDs (Mhalu *et. al.*, 1992; Mwakagile *et. al.*, 1996). Mwakagile *et. al.* (1996) note that STD prevalence amongst women surveyed was 45.3% amongst teenagers compared with 29.2% in adults. Information from the National AIDS Control Programme indicates that youth are a seriously affected population sub-group (NACP, 1994). HIV prevalence rates among teenage male blood donors (15-19 years) increased from 0% in 1987 to 4% in 1992 while that among teenage girls increased from 0 to nearly 14% within a year. This phenomenon has already been observed in Sub-Sahara Africa where women are infected with HIV not only earlier but also more often than men, at a rate of three women to two men (Fleming, 1994). The differences in transmission rates between males and females are difficult to explain. The above findings contradict available sexual behavior survey data where more male than female youth report sexual behavior. This suggests either gender differences in the types of sexual partners of youth or the influence of culture on the responses of youth in surveys—a culture that portrays "good girls" as virgins and as passive in sexual matters and "proper boys" as masculine and active in sexual matters. The fact that female youth are involved in relationships with older men perhaps contributes to their vulnerability to HIV infection. Older men are more likely to be sexually experienced with a wider range of sexual partners, and hence have a higher chance of having contracted the HIV/AIDS virus that they may then transmit to their young sexual partners.

Information surrounding care seeking behavior of youth with STDs or choices regarding treatment facilities are not that well known. Yet background information of this type is important, especially for health education on STDs amongst youth. Some studies have shown that drug stores both prescribe and dispense treatment for STDs. The types of drugs prescribed and dispensed and the dose of drugs provided are more a function of the ability of the patient to pay rather than appropriateness of the drug to the type of STD and the required dosage (Temu and Leshabari, 1992). Observations during fieldwork in a village in the Kyela district revealed that STD treatment was easily available from any one of the five village drug shops, and injections were administered on request. Despite the illegal nature of this practice, due to drug shortages at the public health center, many villagers were happy with services rendered by the shops. Few were probably aware of the dangers of indiscriminate drug use, particularly drugs given in injection form from such sources where the infrastructure required to ensure sterility was often not in place.

Social and Psychological Consequences of Youth Sexual Behavior

An awareness of the extent of youth sexual exposure and its implications appears slow in reaching adults, service providers, and policy makers in the country. This is liable to generate a situation where young people may experience enormous social and psychological problems related to their sexual behavior that are rarely, if at all, brought to the attention of significant adults. It is quite likely that the initial sexual experience for many youths is quite traumatic, especially under existing circumstances where there are little, if any, counseling services for adolescents. Anecdotal accounts and preliminary data from a rural area in North East Tanzania indicate that much of the information youth get on issues related to sex is from listening in on conversations of older brothers and sisters, peers, or from written material (Leshabari *et. al.*, 1997). The trauma of unwanted pregnancy, especially among schoolgirls, is reported to exert enormous psychological and social problems on both the girls and their parents (Puja and Kassimoto, 1994).

Studies in the West have reported links between psychological distress, psychopathology, and sexual behavior, especially amongst adolescent girls. The fact that culture shapes the experience and expression of psychological distress makes methodological issues in the study of such distress inherently complex, and the fact that mental health professionals in the country are few and far between perhaps further explains the lack of any systematic studies. Sexual socialization in various cultural societies varies to some extent, though in many cultural groups, virginity at marriage was and probably is still highly prized (Mbunda, 1991). In many ethnic groups, premarital pregnancy was not tolerated, and girls who conceived or boys who impregnated risked either being ostracized or, in the case of the boy, forced to marry the girl. Children born out of wedlock were in some areas called "bush children" and usually did not get the same social and psychological support enjoyed by legitimate children. The social forces that control sexual behavior appear to be less effective as the traditional structures they supported decline, and there is increasing social tolerance of premarital sex and pregnancy, particularly in urban settings. However, the stigma of a child born out of wedlock remains, and the implications for both the young mother and her child are unclear. These are areas that require exploration in research.

Alcohol, Substance Abuse and Other Risk-taking Behavior

Risk-taking behavior is part of the nature of adolescence, but raises concern when it increases vulnerability to health-related consequences and poor health. The range of risk-taking behavior amongst Tanzanian youth varies from hanging outside moving vehicles to various criminal activities in a setting where mob justice and certain death is common (Kaaya *et. al.*, 1998). Youth are over-represented in persons who abuse and trade in psychoactive substances as well as in those who participate in various criminal activities such as illegal migration, often as stowaways on ships. Of particular concern has been the increased visibility of the abuse of both licit and illicit substances amongst youths.

There are indications that alcohol consumption amongst youth is on the increase. More than half of seventy-one elders in peri-urban and urban communities in the country, when interviewed, felt more youths were taking traditional alcoholic beverages than in the past (Nikander *et. al.*, 1992a). More youth, particularly females, were getting involved in the production process, and the beverages were increasingly brewed for commercial rather than ceremonial purposes. Informants from communities in the Kyela district of Southern Tanzania suggested that excessive alcohol use amongst youth interfered with judgment regarding sexual behavior and may have increased their vulnerability to HIV infection (Leshabari *et. al.*, 1996a). In a study involving 1,913 consecutive injury victims at Muhimbili Consultant Hospital, raised serum alcohol levels were noted and thought to be partly responsible for the injury in one of every five victims. Serum alcohol levels were highest in females aged 15-25 years and males aged 25-30 years (Nikander *et. al.*, 1992b.). There is very little information on the types of risky behavior related to intoxication world wide except in the broadest terms, that is, intoxicated individuals take more chances (WHO, 1993).

Investigations into community attitudes, knowledge, and practices regarding substance abuse which covered four regions in the country indicated that cannabis and khat are the two major illicit substances abused with a lifetime prevalence of 3.8% and 3.7% respectfully (Kilonzo *et. al.* 1992). Though only 0.1% had ever used heroin, there are concerns regarding the use of less traditional drugs with higher addictive, and hence, abuse potential, that the general population is less knowledgeable about. A survey of 1,100 secondary school students in Dar es Salaam with a mean age of 17.6 years revealed that 63% reported non-medical drug use (Kaaya *et. al.*, 1992). Of these, a third reported lifetime use of a white powder they called "*unga*" (literally translated as powder/flour, it is also the street name for heroin), a fifth reported having used stimulants, and only about 5% reported the use of cannabis. The study was conducted about a year after the first reports of heroin availability on the streets, and police records at this time indicated that "*unga*" peddled on the streets in urban areas contained a wide variety of substances ranging from starch and adulterated heroin to pure heroin (Kilonzo, 1992). Though curiosity could account for the large numbers experimenting with "*unga*," it was remarkable that a high proportion (above 80%) were aware of the effects of cannabis, which was used by very few, while only 7% were aware of any health hazards of heroin use.

There have been significant changes in the patterns of availability and use of illicit psychoactive substances in Tanzania. The country has become more established as a transit point in the Southern Corridor traffic of drugs from

Asia to Southern Africa, as well as to the West. A spill-over effect of narcotics, particularly heroin, is increasingly becoming a problem, and a market is gradually growing. Hospital records indicate that 2 - 3 new cases per month of heroin dependence report for help, the majority being below the age of 24 years. There have also been sporadic cases of intravenous drug use amongst both males and females, an indicator that points to a higher degree of abuse of heroin than health services are currently aware of. Judging from the patterns observed in other developing countries where heroin use and dependence is more established, such as Nigeria and India, the drug use problem in Tanzania is bound to escalate.

In addition to the use of drugs, there are increasing numbers of youths being recruited into the drug trade. Mass media and police reports indicate an increasing number of Tanzanian youth who are apprehended in foreign countries in Asia and even Latin America on narcotics trafficking charges. While only 4 Tanzanian nationals were apprehended on narcotics charges abroad in 1981, the figure for 1986 rose to 35 (Kilonzo, 1992). Several have also been apprehended at ports of entry into Tanzania, many risking their lives by swallowing large numbers of plastic pellets containing heroin. From 1980 to 1985, a total of 6,019 persons of Tanzanian nationality were apprehended at border posts and within the country on drug-related charges, of whom 7% were below the age of 16 and 49% were between 16-25 years of age. The arrests on drug charges and seizure records for 1990 alone showed an alarming increase with 2,111 individuals apprehended, 13,279 kg of cannabis, 2.2 kg of heroin, and 1.5 kg of cocaine seized in the country. While these records could partly be attributed to improvements in detection of substances of abuse by law enforcement agencies, they raise concerns regarding the escalation of availability of substances of abuse on the streets in urban settings of the country (ibid.). The returns of the drug trade are high, often amounting to millions of shillings, an aspect that makes many youth feel the risks are worth the bonus to be had from trafficking in drugs. The fact that only a few among the youth who traffic and trade in drugs are actually apprehended reinforces this view. This view of gains outweighing risks is likely to worsen the use, traffic, and trade in narcotics given the current situation of insufficient opportunities for secondary and tertiary education and high unemployment amongst youth. There are very few interventions in place that address substance use amongst adolescents. Health services have several infrastructural barriers to the management of dependence which is currently dealt with by mental health services. Aspects related to substance abuse are currently not a focus for school health in the Ministry of Education and Culture neither is the subject taught in teachers' training colleges. For substance use prevention amongst youth to move beyond rhetoric to action in Tanzania, there needs to develop more working links between the school health programs sections of the Ministries of Health and Education and NGOs working in the field of substance abuse prevention. There is also a need for more active political will demonstrated by more funds being allocated to both ministries to allow for needs assessment; development of curricula for both teachers' training colleges and education institutions; as well as for the development, execution, and evaluation of school-based interventions.

In the last 10 years or so, rural to urban migration has extended to illegal migration outside the country's borders amongst youth. It has become a usual occurrence for the mass media to report long lists of names of young people apprehended and returned from neighboring countries and of late from South Africa. This is a phenomenon mostly observed in male youth who stowaway on foreign ships at local ports. Stowing away has become a fad that is reinforced by the need to appear "in," and many youths take the risk. The small proportion of illegal migrants who manage not to be caught and returned home, or who manage to settle and prosper in their new residences abroad, are further reinforcing factors.

What Needs to be Done?

Many suggestions have been put forward on what needs to be done in order to minimize youth-related problems, especially the consequences of unprotected sex. These include more parental responsibility in providing information to young people and more programs in schools to develop "living skills." Yet little is known of the ability or willingness of parents to take up this role, and suggestions of introducing family planning education and services to school youth have been resented, due to the assumption that, in so doing, the young people will be introduced to promiscuity. One of the probable reasons behind this lethargy may be the cultural barriers that exist regarding communication on issues regarding sexuality and sexual behavior within and between communities and families that have either been insufficiently investigated or ignored by various sectors involved in health care delivery.

There are very few interventions that focus on risk/problem behavior such as substance abuse, unprotected sex, or repeated criminal activities in the youth population. There are a few NGOs and research projects that have carried out interventions in some of these areas. However, many interventions are conducted as projects rather than programs, and problems of sustainability once the project ends prevent work from continuing even when evaluation reveals successful outcomes. In addition, many of these intervention activities are poorly coordinated, running the risk of replication in a setting where resources are scarce. The available evidence suggests that the problems of youth are multidimensional in nature, and hence require coordinated multi-disciplinary approaches that involve parents, social services, health services, education services, religious organizations, and the community at large.

There are aspects of the family's role in socializing children that can be beneficial in building appropriate living and social skills useful in helping young persons deal with problems they encounter in a more positive manner. These include the provision of security and stability, which allows for communication and the development of self-assertive, confidence, and determination skills. The education system provides a setting where children and youth can be accessed with health promotion information and skills. In such settings, there needs to be more focus on the emotional development of children and youth which entails, amongst other things, having pupils at the same level of maturity in class to facilitate the accomplishment of the developmentally appropriate tasks that will enhance psycho-social growth. Identification of children with emotional difficulties and assisting such children is a role that can be performed by teachers. This task can only be feasible if there is less emphasis on quantity and more focus on quality in the education system so that teachers are motivated to focus more holistically on the needs of their students.

Religious organizations can also contribute to the socialization process by not only imparting religious morality, but also accepting the reality of problems that do exist within this population sub-group. The problems in the youth population will not go away so long as key players in the lives of young persons are prepared to bury their heads in the sand and deny the existence of problems. Acknowledging the problems would be a first step towards understanding and planning appropriate services for youth such as assisting in providing recreational activities that are constructive and healthy for their development. In addition, the society itself can contribute towards addressing youth problems by each community working towards developing programs that are culturally acceptable for youths in the area.

Despite the reported poverty in many communities in the country, it is also true that youth and the problems they experience have not been an area of focus in community programs. There is a need to increase awareness of the plight of young people in communities and to harness existing resources by encouraging people to take responsibility for their own children and youth. Community involvement and participation in intervention programs that focus on youth is important for their future sustainability. There also needs to be a move away from the central government as a key implementing body of programs at the community level to the government providing coordination, regulation, and evaluation of community initiatives and using information from such initiatives to inform policy reviews. This represents a major shift that will require a change in the attitudinal mindset of government workers as well as changes in management and administrative style. To a certain extent, this shift will involve relinquishing both power and resources to others to do the job. However, a shift is necessary if the government is to develop policies that will be conduBroad classifications of causes of death revealedcive to various agents of the socialization process being able to contribute constructively to the healthy development and growth of children and youth.

Chapter Two

Youth Mobility and Unprotected Sex as Key Factors in the Spread of the AIDS Virus in Tanzania

Melkizedeck T. Leshabari, Sylvia F. Kaaya, Japhet Z. Killewo and Jessie K. Mbwambo

Introduction

Since the Acquired Immuno-deficiency Syndrome (AIDS) was first reported in Tanzania in 1983, a considerable effort has been made to control the spread of the epidemic in the country. Among the initial steps taken by governmental and non-governmental institutions was the raising of AIDS awareness in the general public using various communication media including the radio, newspapers, drama, and traditional dances. This step was later followed by the procurement and distribution of condoms to population sub-groups which were assumed to be at a high risk of being infected or of spreading the virus to susceptible individuals in various communities. Due to these efforts, available survey data show the level of AIDS awareness in the society as being over 90% (Kessy, 1995; Ngallaba *et. al.* 1993; Swai, 1995). However, despite the reported high level of awareness, the HIV sero-prevalence rates continue to increase, and it is difficult to predict when the existing infection rates will decline.

In Tanzania, the first AIDS patient was reported in the Kagera region of the Northwestern part of the country in 1983. By 1986, all the 20 regions in mainland Tanzania had reported at least one AIDS patient, while within Kagera itself, the number of officially reported AIDS cases increased from three in 1983 to 1,665 by 1987 (NACP, 1991). During the period of 1983 to 1987, Kagera region consistently reported the highest numbers of AIDS cases when compared with other regions. It was not until 1988 that the Dar es Salaam region ranked first (NACP, 1994). Since 1988, Dar es Salaam has consistently reported the highest number of cumulative AIDS cases, and in 1994, Mbeya region, which had not reported an AIDS case until 1986, was ranked second. The Kagera region ranked third, Coast region fifth, and Kilimanjaro region, which reported only 36 AIDS patients in 1986, was now ranking fourth out of the 20 regions in the country (NACP, 1994). At the national level, the cumulative AIDS case-load increased from three in 1983 to 1,525 in 1986, when all regions reported at least one patient, and by 1994, the country had reported over 50,000 AIDS patients (N4CP, 1995). The doubling time of reported AIDS cases in 1992 was 51 months compared with 156 months in 1993, suggesting a slower growth in AIDS cases during the latter period. However, although these data are considered a true reflection of the trend of AIDS cases, it should be noted that due to under-diagnosis, under-reporting, and delays in submitting reports centrally for compilation, the absolute numbers of AIDS cases are assumed to be higher by a factor of 5 (ibid).

During the early years of the HIV/AIDS epidemic, many rural residents encountered diagnosed AIDS in relatives, neighbors, or friends who had been sent to their home villages from urban areas (especially Dar es Salaam) for terminal care. It is probably due to this reason that the local population in rural villages tend to associate the disease with urban lifestyles despite the fact that their own sexual behavior provided a high potential for spreading of the disease. Such associations between AIDS and urban life styles have been reported among informants in the Kilimanjaro, Morogoro, and Mbeya regions (Setel, 1995; Kaaya *et. al.*, 1995; Leshabari and Kaaya, 1996).

The rate of the spread of HIV-1 infection has been observed to vary both across and within regions. These variations can be explained to a large extent by the migration of people both across and within local communities. Studies from the Kagera region revealed a considerable variation in the prevalence of HIV infection by age, sex, and area of residence within the region (Killewo *et. al.*, 1990; Killewo *et. al.*, 1994). Surveys conducted in 1987 revealed that while the overall prevalence of HIV infection in the region was 9.6%, this varied from 24.6% in Bukoba town to less than 1% in some rural villages (Killewo *et. al.*, 1990). An interesting feature which was revealed in this study was the observation that even within rural villages, infection rates varied from 0.6% to 10%. Higher HIV sero-prevalence rates in urban compared with rural areas have also been demonstrated in the Mwanza and Kilimanjaro regions (Borgdorff *et. al.*, 1993; Klepp *et. al.*, 1995). Borgdoff *et. al.* (1993) show that higher sero-prevalence rates in urban than non-urban sentinel and population samples persisted even after the rates were adjusted for age and sex.

Considerable variations in HIV sero-prevalence by age and sex have also been noted, with overall infection rates being higher amongst women than men. In one study, the female: male prevalence ratio in a population survey was 1.7 in urban and 1.3 in non-urban populations. HIV - 1 infection was noted to be most common in women aged 15 to 34 years and in men aged 25 to 44 years (Borgdoff *et. al.*, 1993). Surveys, as well as sero-surveillance data, have persistently documented higher sero-prevalence rates among female youth than any other gender or age group (NACP, 1995; Borgdoff, 1994; Killewo, 1994; Klepp *et. al.*, 1995).

Several reasons may account for the gender differences in age at which infection with HIV occurs. A potential explanation may be differences in the types of sexual partners of male and female youth. Census data show that female youth tend to get married at an earlier age than their male counterparts. In 1988, while 4.1 % of male youth aged between 15 to 19 years were married, this marital status applied to 29.3 % of females within a simi l ar age range, indicating a difference in ages of partners between these two populations (Leshabari and Kaaya, 1994, table 4). This observation is confirmed by the Demographic Health Survey which revealed that in 94 % of the couples in the survey sample, husbands were older than their wives, while in a third, husbands were 10 years or more older than their wives (Ngalaba *et. al.*, 1993).Other studies have also reported similar findings of variations in the age gap between husbands and wives (Killewo *et. al.*, 1994).

The age gap between husband and wife may in part depend on whether the wife is a first or higher index wife in polygamous marriages. Assuming that the same age differences will apply in intimate relationships with the opposite sex that do not culminate in marriage, the observation implies that female youth are more likely to be involved with sexual partners who have a longer and more variable history of coital contacts; they are therefore exposed to a higher risk of acquiring HIV than male youth from their sexual partners. Other factors which increase the ease with which HIV can be acquired among female youth include the physical immaturity of the vaginal mucosa and the presence of raw surfaces in the vaginal wall caused by physical trauma when virginity is lost. Both factors increase the risk for semen-blood contact and transmission of the HIV virus. It is perhaps these factors, that is, the socio-cultural structuring of sexual partnership and biological vulnerability, that may play a much more important role in transmission dynamics among female youth than the "sugar-daddy" phenomena which has been described elsewhere (Schoepf, 1992).

In view of the above observations, this chapter argues that youth mobility and unprotected sex are key factors in the spread of HIV infection in Tanzania.

Increased youth mobility in the country is evidenced by several anecdotal accounts of an increase in this population sub-group in urban areas as a result of rural-urban migration. Census data show that there has been an increase in absolute numbers of the youth population as a result of both natural increase and increased survival following the success of immunization programs in the country in the past three decades (Leshabari and Kaaya, 1994). However, the sevenfold increase in urban youth compared with the doubling of the rural youth population noted between 1967 to 1988 (perhaps partly) supports these anecdotal accounts.

In 1977, the Universal Primary School Education policy increased the accessibility of education opportunities for school-aged children (Ministry of Education, 1989). However, the sudden increase in this population sub-group was not met with concomitant growth in the number of teachers and other educational resources, leading to a lowering of educational quality throughout the country. In the setting of an economic crisis which did not allow expansion of the productive sectors of the country, youth constituted a highly vulnerable population sub-group to the vicissitudes of socio-cultural and economic changes. Informants in a study using in-depth interviews and focus group discussions to collect data noted that adverse socio-economic changes in the Kyela District of Mbeya Region have contributed to both an increase in youth mobility as well as in health- risking sexual behavior in this population sub-group (Leshabari *et. al.*, 1996). Similar accounts are noted from the Kagera and Kilimanjaro regions (Lwihula, 1993; Talle *et. al.*, 1995). In all of these reports, the struggle to earn a living within the youth population has unfortunately also exposed them to increased internal movements as well as health-risking behavior, including excessive use of alcohol and other substances of abuse and unprotected sexual intercourse. It is the combination of increased youth mobility and health-risking behavior, particularly unprotected sexual intercourse, which has so facilitated the spread of HIV infection that its control is likely to curb the spread to a significant level.

In attempting to make sense of the variations in cumulative AIDS case rates across different regions in the country, available data on reported AIDS cases will be used to analyze regional variations within the context of accessibility by road both between and within regions. The cumulative reported AIDS case rates between 1985 and 1991 are used in this analysis. The analysis is restricted to 1991 as there is no explanation for the increase in case rate doubling times in subsequent years, making it difficult to rule out problems related to data quality. Using this analysis as a framework, the discussion will focus on available data from ethnographic studies that have been conducted as well as small-scale surveys in order to describe factors related to transmission dynamics in the various zones and the role of youth mobility particularly in the spread of HIV in Tanzania.

Association Between Accessibility of a Region and Its Cumulative AIDS Case Rate

In this analysis, an arbitrary grouping of regions into four zones was done on the basis of ease of accessibility by road. The Tanzania-Zambia highway is the major tarmac highway from Dar es Salaam to Zambia. The highway traverses five regions: Dar es Salaam, Coast, Morogoro, Iringa, and Mbeya. At the time the cumulative AIDS cases by region were compiled, this highway had the highest volume of vehicles including those going to Zambia, Malawi, and several other Central and Southern African countries. During an ethnographic study which was conducted in 1992 along this highway, it was found that this route was used by truck drivers and their assistants from twelve different countries in East, Central, and Southern Africa (O'Connor *et al.*, 1992). The regions falling along this major truck route were categorized as zone one. The second zone included regions through which the highway from Dar es Salaam to Rwanda, Burundi, and Zaire passes. This route branches from the first route in the main town of the Morogoro Region (Morogoro town), which is about 200 Km from the city of Dar es Salaam. This truck route does not have an all-weather surface throughout its course, and some stretches are not passable during the rainy seasons. Hence, goods destined for Zaire by road are sometimes sent through the first route via Zambia. The route is also used for goods destined for Uganda by road from Dar es Salaam. The regions through which this route passes include Dar es Salaam, Coast, Morogoro, Dodoma, Singida, Tabora, Shinyanga and Kigoma, which were categorized as zone two.

Regions which do not fall along these two major highways were grouped into two further categories on the basis of their road networks and accessibility throughout the year. The first group consists of five northern regions with relatively good all-weather roads. These include the Tanga, Kilimanjaro, Arusha, Mara, and Mwanza regions, and they constitute zone three. Zone four regions were those which are not easily accessible by road for part of the year due to lack of all-weather roads or have poor communication structures within and across them. These include the Lindi, Mtwara, Rukwa, Ruvuma and Kigoma regions. Kagera region was not included in zone four, despite not being easily accessible by road, as there are factors specific to this region which will be discussed below. Using this classification, the cumulative AIDS patients per 100,000 population was computed for each zone, and the results are summarized in table one below.

Table 1: *Cumulative Reported AIDS Cases per 100, WO by Road Accessibility in Tanzania*

Category of Regions	*1985*	*1986*	*1987*	*1988*	*1989*	*1990*	*1991*
Zone one	0.9	8.7	33.1	79.8	127.4	205.3	307.7
Zone two	0.6	5.8	21.3	48.8	83.7	121.4	169.0
Zone three	0.4	1.8	8.1	21.7	32.1	51.3	93.1
Zone four	0.0	0.9	2.7	10.2	18.7	42.2	77.3
*Kagera	24.3	63.9	125.5	161.5	191.8	238.6	291.1

Source: *Computed from National AIDS Control Programme, Report No. 6, May 1992, Table 1*

Data in table 3 generally show that the cumulative number of reported AIDS cases has been increasing over the years since 1985, and the zone falling along the Dar es Salaam to Zambia highway is the most seriously hit. This was followed by the areas along the highway from Dar es Salaam to Rwanda, Burundi, and Zaire. Areas with a poor road communication network have the lowest cumulative AIDS patients per 100,000 population, indicating that the HIV virus was introduced to them much later compared with areas with good inter-regional or inter-district road communication.

Mobility, Migration Patterns and Disease

Although not much is known about contributory factors to this pattern of HIV transmission in the country, migration patterns of people within and across regions, coupled with differences in behavior which facilitate HIV transmission within local communities, to a large extent explain the observed phenomena. Technically, the spread of any infectious disease is worsened by migration of people, especially when this occurs under circumstances where factors which facilitate transmission in susceptible communities are unknown or where there are inadequate facilities to contain the disease (Anarfi, 1993). The major truck routes facilitate movement of people, especially long-distance truck drivers, from various countries to and from Tanzania. In addition to these international movements, the available highways also facilitate internal movement of people from one area to another within the country, while involved in trade activities or for other official or social reasons. These movements expose local inhabitants in various areas to mobile individuals who are usually high-risk individuals. In addition, the traffic density along truck routes encourages the rapid growth of peri-urban foci, which both serve travellers' needs in terms of food and lodging and become foci for trade activities. Such foci are often associated with large groups of people from differing backgrounds living together either as permanent or transient residents. A potential explanation for the rate at which the HIV virus spreads in a particular region, therefore, includes a combination of the prevailing circumstances which determine when the virus is introduced, the amount of the virus introduced, and the presence of local sexual behavior which facilitates further that spread within communities once the virus has been introduced.

The Case of Kagera Region

Despite the fact that the Kagera region is neither traversed by a major truck route nor easily accessible to urban trade influences with other regions in Tanzania, there are factors that make this region special in terms of the mobility of residents in the region. The initial AIDS patients were reported to be youth who were involved in illegal trade across the border with neighboring countries (Lwihula *et. al.,* 1993). Around the time the epidemic was first reported, the Kagera region was experiencing serious shortages of basic commodities, a phenomena which was fairly common in the country at that time. In response to this illegal cross-border trade of essential commodities was a means of earning easy money—particularly for the youth (ibid). Similar behavior has also been reported among youth in the Kilimanjaro region (Setel, 1995). Through these types of trade activities, many youth acquired large sums of money which raised their status in rural villages and perhaps facilitated social interactions in settings where they were vulnerable to excessive alcohol use and promiscuity. Such youth were attractive to many women, particularly because such interactions not only provided a form of entertainment they could otherwise not afford, but also assured them of basic commodities at a time of economic hardship where the key issue was surviving at that time. The role of movement as a result of trade activities in facilitating the spread of HIV has also been reported in Uganda (Barnett and Blaikie, 1992). These circumstances, however, only partly explain the introduction of the virus to the Kagera region.

In addition to the index cases in the Kagera region, available literature shows that prostitution may have played a role in introducing the virus to this area. Prostitution has been implicated as one of the important factors in the transmission of HIV in several African countries (Van De Perre *et. al.*, 1984; Kreiss 1986; Anarfi, 1993). Rates of HIV infection among prostitutes in Tanzania have been reported to be considerably higher than in the general population (Nkya *et. al.*, 1991). Little is known about the movement of these prostitutes from urban to urban areas, urban to rural areas, or from country to country. Some mention has been made about the role of prostitutes in the AIDS epidemic in the Kagera region (Lwihula *et. al.*, 1993). However, available literature which dates back to the time of early colonialism indicates that prostitution and extended sexual networking was a coping strategy used to lessen the culturally-induced oppression and economic hardships among women from this area (Cory, 1949; Swantz, 1985; Kaijage, 1992). Available literature on prostitution in East Africa specifically mentions women from this area in study samples (Southall and Gutkind, 1957; Obbo, 1980; Rutasitara, 1980; Wilson, 1980; White, 1983; White, 1988; Ngugi *et. al.*, 1988; Little,1992). Given that in many cultural groups in East Africa, individuals residing outside their home villages frequently go back to visit relatives, it is quite possible that such women may have been instrumental in introducing the virus, acquired from scattered urban settings in East Africa, to rural communities in their home villages.

The region also had the unfortunate history of accommodating large numbers of soldiers in transit from both Uganda and Tanzania during the Tanzania -Uganda war in the late 1970's. This period coincides with the probable time when HIV infections first occurred in the communities. During this period of upheaval caused by war, unprotected casual sex and reports of rape perpetuated by soldiers were common and may have contributed towards the introduction of the virus in the area. Despite the fact that the region does not fall within areas which are easily accessible by existing road networks, these special features, which are all related to high mobility in and out of as well as within the region, may account for the processes which led to the epidemic in the region.

Once HIV infection is introduced to a susceptible population, the social and cultural activities which facilitate exposure to the virus will determine the extent and intensity to which the virus will spread. In the Kagera region, as in other areas of the country, loosening of cultural controls over sexual activity has been reported by some authors (Lwihula *et. al.*, 1993; Lwihula, 1995;

Kaijage, 1992). Overnight functions such as weddings, local dances/discos, and culturally sanctioned intra-familial sex have been reported to be among activities suspected to have been associated with unprotected sex and an increase in HIV sero-prevalence in the area. However, circumstances which facilitate HIV transmission within many rural communities appear to be fairly common even though very little systematic documentation exists. In the Mbeya region, for example, excessive alcohol use and promiscuity were closely linked and were reported by informants in the villages of the Kyela District to be among factors facilitating the spread of HIV infection in that area (Leshabari *et. al.*, 1996).

Factors Influencing Transmission Dynamics Along the Major Truck Routes (Zone one and two)

Looking at the situation along major truck routes, several factors influencing HIV transmission dynamics have been documented by observational studies. In one study along the Tanzania-Zambia highway, promiscuity was found to be rampant, and more than seven categories of commercial sex workers were identified; truck drivers and mobile young prostitutes constituted important vehicles for spreading the virus along these highways (O'Connor *et. al.*, 1992). The population of commercial sex workers was noted to be highly mobile both within the different truck-stops as well as to and from urban and rural areas. It was noted that bar owners contributed to the mobility by frequently firing "old faces" and hiring "new faces" among the barmaid population in order to keep truck drivers interested in returning to their place of business. The truckers themselves also frequently moved with their female partners from one truck stop to another. The data also show that sexual partners of the truck drivers were unable to negotiate condom use with long-term partners, had multiple partners, and many offered or were forced/coerced into providing both anal and oral sex (O'Connor *et. al.* 1992)

Although many young girls were aware of the implications of their risky behavior, many claimed the risks were nothing compared with the economic hardships they were experiencing before being involved in commercial sex. The spread of the virus from the truck stops to rural villages can be conceptualized in terms of what goes on at the truck stops and movements of people from the stops to more rural communities. The stops along the highways serve as trade centers where young business men and women from rural villages bring farm produce for sale and where they buy essential commodities to sell in rural villages such as clothes, sugar, kerosene, cooking oil and salt. Casual observations reported by O'Connor *et. al*. (1992) revealed that many of the sexual partners of truck drivers may also form intimate sexual relationships with young men involved in different types of trade activities around the truck stops. These young men, on returning to their home villages, have the potential to pass on the virus to wives and girlfriends. The prevailing circumstances as regards partnership exchange within sexual relationships in these rural communities are what will then determine the extent of the spread of HIV once introduced.

Similarly, girls involved in commercial sex at the truck stops sometimes go to their home villages to visit relatives and friends, and while there, casual sexual encounters with men in the village cannot be ruled out. In one study (O'Connor *et. al*., 1992), a truck stop was abandoned by truck drivers after they had heard that four girls had died of AIDS in that area, depriving commercial sex workers of clients. Interestingly, local resident males, who previously could not afford the fees charged by the girls when they were competing with truck drivers, were able to participate in the commercial sex activities due to the reduced rates caused by the lack of business. Many bars and lodging houses also closed, and bar girls resorted to selling local brews in "pombe" clubs whose clientele were men from the surrounding community. It is through such movements and interactions with various people that the virus spreads from the road-side to rural communities both across and within regions in the country.

Factors Influencing Transmission Dynamics in Zone Four

Although regions in zone four have fairly low reported cases of AIDS, it should be pointed out that, with time, they are likely to experience the problem in epidemic proportions unless steps are taken to introduce preventive measures against the behavior which facilitates transmission of HIV infection. The current situation is most likely the result of poor communication networks. For example, the natural barrier created by the River Rufiji, as well as the lack of all-weather bridges and roads, has limited the movement of large numbers of people in and out of the southern regions at a time when the virus was spreading rapidly in other more accessible regions. However, anecdotal accounts indicate that the lack of social controls over sexual behavior is also a feature in many of the zone four regions, and what was probably lacking was a sufficient number of sero-positive individuals to produce an epidemic.

However, the fact that communication difficulties may also influence the availability of adequate HIV testing kits at surveillance sites, cause difficulties in the supervision of such sites, and a lack of prompt reporting in such areas, cannot be ruled out.

Why the Youth?

The youth are the focus of the following discussion, taking into consideration the fact that they constitute more than a third of the population of the country and are very mobile, particularly with regards to rural-urban migration (Leshabari and Kaaya, 1994). In addition, there is growing awareness and concern among researchers working on teenage sexuality in Tanzania that the sexual and reproductive health of youth in the country is characterized by high rates of unprotected sexual intercourse which consequently has led to high rates of unwanted pregnancies, unsafe abortions, and STDs/HIV infection (MOE; Mpangile, Leshabari and Kihwele, 1993; NACP, 1992; Fuglesang, 1995). Available survey data on rates of coital exposure among urban youth who are in school show that a substantial number of them is sexually active, and many of them are ignorant of the consequences of unprotected sexual activities (Leshabari, 1988, Mbunda 1988, Kapiga *et. al*., 1993). Apart from these observations, information and services for reproductive health targeting youth are extremely rare. Although, of late, there are plans to introduce family life education (including AIDS education) in schools, implementation of such programs has been hampered by controversies surrounding how much to cover and the methods which will be used to impart such knowledge. Meanwhile, increasing numbers of young persons continue to suffer from the consequences of their unprotected sexual behavior, including death from AIDS.

Contrary to the belief that unprotected coital exposure is primarily an urban problem among youth, a recent study involving rural youth indicated an alarming prevalence of HIV and sexually-transmitted infections (STIs). Kessy (1995), in a community-based sample, noted HIV sero-prevalence rates higher than 7% among youth in the Moshi Rural District and prevalence for various STIs ranging between 0.8 % to 19.1%. Trichomoniasis was the most common STI identified among both males and females, while genital ulcer disease was the least common.

Youth Mobility and the Spread of HIV - The Case of Kilimanjaro and Mbeya

The deteriorating economy in Tanzania has created quite an alarming potential for the spread of HIV. Youth in particular are coping with the economic hardships in ways which not only facilitated migration, but also exposed them to risky behavior including excessive alcohol use and unprotected sexual intercourse. As pointed out earlier, the truck stops along the major highways in the country provided easy avenues for youth income-generating activities, including selling of fruit, food, barbecued goat meat, as well as car and truck washing and the providing security for vehicles. This was in addition to employment in bars and lodgings which were important components of the truck stop environment. Many of the female youth in such settings were employed as bar tenders and lodging attendants, which technically made them easily available sexual partners for the truck drivers, their assistants, and others who could pay for their services either in cash or in kind. Youth also featured among the mobile female prostitutes who moved with their partners along the truck routes as well as across countries. Accounts from this ethnographic study indicated that such "business" was so lucrative that mobile prostitutes saw no need to look for paid employment and made the fear of death from contracting AIDS a small risk which they could think about later after attending to the more pressing survival needs of themselves or their families (O'Connor *et. al.*, 1992).

Male youth who were involved in business transactions at truck stops were also at risk of both acquiring and spreading the virus as a result of the partnership exchange dynamics in these settings. In settings outside truck stops, youth also appear to be a very vulnerable population. The findings of high STI prevalence among youth in Moshi rural district (Kessy, 1995) are not surprising given the high mobility of youth in the Kilimanjaro region in general. Apart from the economic crisis which affects all youth in the country, historically, in Kilimanjaro region, a complex interaction has occurred between population growth, landpressure, and cultural change which, according to Setel (1995), has resulted in radical changes in the ritual, educational, and daily-life activities of early adulthood. Since the early 1940's, an increasing number of young men have left the mountains in search of alternative livelihoods to coffee, cattle, and the "*kihamba*" (Setel, 1995 pp 53). Despite the out-migration, the population has continued to grow, and it is of note that young men from the region are scattered all over the country looking for means of survival. Many of these young men have migrated totally or are transient residents in urban areas in East Africa in search of employment or involved in small-scale business. Setel (1995) notes that such businessmen, who view themselves as individuals struggling to survive, are often perceived to have loose morals and a lack of civilized demeanor by elders. This perhaps reflects the inherent difficulties of maintaining cultural mores and integrity given the new lifestyles adopted by many of these young people. Such young men often leave their wives in their rural villages of origin and visit once or twice a year. High youth mobility as a result of various trade activities has also been reported in the Mbeya and Kagera regions (Leshabari *et. al.*, 1996; Lwihula *et. al.*, 1993). These movements to and from rural villages in search of employment or "business" opportunities, coupled with prevalent sexual behavior in this population sub-group, may partly explain HIV transmission dynamics within rural communities.

There are few studies which address the contexts surrounding coital exposure among youth. Although data revealed high unprotected sexual exposure among youth in Moshi Rural district, Kessy (1995) reported that only 18% of her subjects had ever used condoms. This was despite the fact that 36% reported at least two different life-time sexual partners. Unfortunately, an ethnographic study conducted in the area indicates that many youth believe HIV infections come from outside their own communities through prostitutes, businessmen, and female bar-workers. For many youth in the area, sex is part of being adult and living independently, whether or not one is married. Their socially constructed meaning of "sex" is totally unrelated to the meaning assumed during AIDS education based on the biological model of disease causation (Setel, 1995).

High youth mobility has also been shown to occur in the Mbeya region which, like Kilimanjaro, is a border region (Leshabari *et. al.*, 1996). Movements to and from Malawi and other neighboring counties, coupled with youth migration to gold mines in neighboring districts (Makongorosi), were all noted to have contributed to increased exposure to unprotected sexual encounters in the Mbeya region. Village elders noted that drinking and sexual liaisons among both youth and adults are part and parcel of many trade activities (ibid). Due to the deteriorating standards of living and the hardships families were experiencing due to declining economic conditions, some informants reported that parents no longer questioned their daughters on the source of funds used for buying essential items they brought home. A similar situation has been reported from a study which was conducted among the men in Arusha region (Haram, 1995). In the Arusha study, it was observed that for many female youth, sexual relationships were the only means of easy access to items like soap, body lotion, shoes, and nice dresses. In some cases, the home environment can no longer provide guidance to youth in order to minimize the risks they were taking including unprotected pre-marital sex. Risk taking in sexual behavior in these communities appears to be fairly common, and unless drastic steps are taken to address the problem, the epidemic is going to have devastating demographic effects.

There is little documentation on what factors have influenced the emergence of the current pattern of sexual behavior in the youth population. However, decrease in social controls over sexual behavior in general over the past generation or so has been reported in the Kagera, Kilimanjaro, and Mbeya regions (Lwihula *et. al*., 1993; Setel, 1995; Leshabari *et. al*., 1996). Several complex factors have been noted to be at play, including but not limited to rapid socio-cultural and economic changes which have resulted in the disintegration of traditional socialization institutions at such a rapid pace that new institutions to replace them are either inadequate or non-existent (Ornari, 1991; Leshabari *et. al*., 1996). Key informants in a study in Mbeya noted the inappropriateness of the school curricula to the realities of the lives of children. They also noted the effects of exposure to foreign influences such as unsupervised discos and video shows with explicit sexual scenes which perhaps has facilitated inappropriate behavior among youth in the villages (Leshabari *et. al*., 1996). Other behavioral pathologies among youth such as substance abuse have been hypothesized to be on the increase as a result of the rapidity of socio-cultural changes in the country (Kilonzo and Kaaya, 1994). The family as an institution has been noted by several authors to exert less control over its members than in the past, and lack of parental guidance has been reported to be among the factors contributing to health-risk behavior as youth attempt to satisfy sexual curiosity (Omari, 1991; Kilonzo and Kaaya, 1994; Leshabari *et. al*., 1996).

During fieldwork in the Mbeya Region, informants complained of irresponsible youth behavior which was partly blamed on changes in child-rearing practices (Leshabari *et. al*., 1996). This appeared to be the consequence of an interaction of complex factors including but not limited to social cultural changes in gender roles. Traditionally, roles of men and women with respect to what was expected of them in the household were clearly spelled out (Siegrist, 1993). Due to a variety of factors including changes in the ability to provide for the family through their traditional family roles, the position of men as breadwinners in families has weakened. Women are increasingly supplementing household income with new income-generating roles, while men have not changed their behavior relating to their traditional roles at the household level. This contradiction has proved to be fertile ground for marital conflict (Leshabari *et. al.*, 1996). Frequent quarrels between parents were reported to provide an environment where they could not serve as appropriate role models for the behavior of their children. These changes appear to have evolved over the past decade or two, and current observations of youth problem behavior perhaps reflect the impact of such changes on socialization.

Conclusion

AIDS is emerging as a disease of poverty both within and across nations (Johnson and De Cock 1994). The problem appears to be most severe among impoverished segments in poor countries where the risks of starvation and lack of other basic needs are high. Available evidence shows awareness of AIDS and related problems to be high. However, despite considerable efforts made by the National AIDS Control Programme, non-governmental organizations (NGOs), and individuals, rates of HIV infection, particularly among youth, continue to increase, and changes in risky behavior appear to be negligible given the extent of the HIV/AIDS epidemic. Despite evidence of the devastating effects of AIDS in the Kagera Region, aggressive control measures within other regions, especially in rural communities, are not encouraging, perhaps due to a lack of foresight, a reluctance to learn from the experience of others on the grounds that factors which led to the epidemic are different, as well as lack of funds for procuring basic preventive packages including HIV screening tests, gloves, and effective educational and communication materials.

Differences in rates of HIV infection across different regions are due to a variety of factors including ease of physical communication to and from a particular area. The behavior which facilitates transmission of the virus appears to be common in all regions, even though the existence of such behavior has probably not been coherently conceptualized when thinking about the potential health and economic problems of regions which have low case-loads of AIDS patients. The youth appear to be at considerable risk, particularly given that risk taking is among the behavioral norms of this age group, and risks associated with sexual pleasure may be ranked quite low among the array of risks taken by this population sub-group. Many studies which have been carried out in Tanzania do not provide the contexts and the consequences to young people of their risky behavior in unprotected sex, injuries, and alcohol as well as drug abuse. Lack of contextually rich information has created a situation where, due to the relatively higher HIV-sero-prevalence among youth, their risk of acquiring HIV infection has been considered in isolation from more immediate life-threatening risks taken by the youth while coping with the harsh reality of social economic problems. Improvement in the road communication networks to and from various regions provided good avenues for facilitating various income-generating activities among youth. Unfortunately, available data on HIV patterns in the country also show that where migration of people is high due to good all-weather roads, HIV rates are also high. In other words, the blessing brought about by improving road communication infrastructures has also facilitated the spread of the AIDS virus.

Finally, in all regions in Tanzania, it must be realized that HIV infection is now an inescapable fact of life. Unless realistic and effective measures are taken to control the behavior which facilitates transmission across and within communities, it will just be a matter of time before each region is leading in terms of AIDS case-loads. By the time all regions have taken their turn being first in terms of the number of cumulative AIDS patients for every 100,000 people, the loss to this society will be insurmountable psychologically, socio-demographically, and economically.

Chapter Three

Contextual Aspects in Relation to Reproductive Health Information Among School Youth in Rombo District, Tanzania

Sylvia F. Kaaya, Melkizedeck T.Leshabari, G.I. Van den Bergh, K.Klepp

Background

Premarital unprotected sex and its related consequences appear to be fairly common amongst Tanzanian youths. Although data on this problem at a national level is rather limited, available information from selected areas in the country shows unprotected sex among youth varies considerably. In a study involving 1,862 rural and urban youth, nearly 15% of boys and over 5% of girls reported a sexual debut by the age of 12 years, increasing to 85% and 91% amongst boys and girls respectively by the age of 24 years (Mound, 1988). Leshabari (1988), in a school-based urban survey of 657 youth, demonstrated that nearly 61% of boys and over 35% of girls were sexually active by the age of 14 years.

Sexually active youth often suffer the social and health-related consequences of unprotected sexual intercourse. Between 1987 and 1993, at a national level, pregnancy accounted for 10.5% of reported school dropouts amongst girls (Sawaya, 1995). When pregnancy risks compromise a school-girl's future, illegal abortion is often a choice made. Urban-based studies in Tanzania indicate that adolescents and teenagers are over-represented in the population of women admitted to hospitals with illegally induced abortion complications (Justesen, *et. al.*, 1992; Mpangile *et. al.* 1993). In addition to unwanted pregnancy and its health and social ramifications, there is evidence that the prevalence of sexually transmitted diseases (STDs), including infection with the Human Immunodeficiency Virus (HIV-1), may be high in the youth population. Kessy (1996) noted a point prevalence range of 5%-14% for various sexually transmitted diseases in a rural community-based sample of 1,104 youth (10-24 years). Data from the National AIDS Control Project demonstrates a cumulative AIDS case rate of 281 per 100,000 amongst females aged 20-24 years and 140 per 100,000 amongst males of a similar age, suggesting that infection with HIV occurred during adolescence (NACP, 1994).

In order to explore factors which affect sexuality and reproductive health amongst youth in the current Tanzanian context, Van den Berg (1996) noted the impact of macro-level trends on national policies, cultural, religious, political, and economic relations as well as on infrastructures at regional, ethnic, and local community levels. In particular, the effect of economic policies on labor-migration were of relevance to areas such as the Kilimanjaro region, where the reported study is based. The pace of change during the 37 years following the colonial era in Tanzania has created a situation where increased survival due to effective immunization programs is not matched by societal structures to meet the needs of a growing youth population. These needs include education, recreation, as well as job creation, affecting both rural and urban areas of the country (Leshabari and Kaaya, 1994). Due in part to these deficiencies, in recent times there has been an increase in migration of youth from rural to urban areas. Computed census reports indicate a seven-fold increase in the urban male and a nine-fold increase in the urban female youth populations (age 10-24 years) between 1967 to 1988, compared with a two-fold increase in the rural male and female youth population (Leshabari and Kaaya, 1994). Though a natural increase could explain this discrepancy, a large proportion of the dramatic increase in urban youth is a result of rural-to-urban migration. Youth predominate as internal transient migrants working in the informal economic sector as petty traders.

A Historical Analysis of Youth Sexuality in Kilimanjaro Region

Evidence from literature suggests that various members of the extended family in many traditional societies in Tanzania played a significant role as reproductive health educators in the transition from childhood to adulthood (Ntukula, 1994). Amongst the Chagga who reside in the Kilimanjaro region of Northern Tanzania, a cultural analysis of the reproductive lives of young people by Setel (1995) notes the decrease in the historical forms by which values regarding sexuality and adulthood were transmitted. Rituals such as those surrounding male group initiation and circumcision and female circumcision (clitoridectomy) were traditionally combined with puberty training by extended family members—particularly paternal aunts and uncles. The sexuality of young people was strictly guarded and linked to a system of inheritance where stern morality guarded the integrity of paternity. Inherited land, under Chagga custom, was predominantly passed on to the eldest and youngest sons. The latter would take over the homestead and assume primary responsibility for the care of his elderly parents. Hence, control of youth sexuality and associated morality played a role in clan stability and the clarity of inheritance rights over land.

Bride wealth – a marriage system whereby rights to women were acquired through transfer of goods from the groom's to the bride's kin – used to be the only legal way of gaining access to female sexuality and fertility. Caldwell (1989) also places a lot of significance on such transactional aspects of sexuality in studies on sexuality and sexual networking in sub-Saharan Africa. Haram (1995) notes in one area of Northern Tanzania that though, traditionally, a woman's sexuality, reproduction, and labor could be exchanged for its equivalent—bride wealth—the limitations on what goods could be exchanged have become blurred over time. There are indications that economic crises may foster a variety of non-traditional sexual partner strategies (Bujra, 1975). The free-flowing nature of current female sexuality has created a situation where a woman may barter her sexuality in exchange for a job opportunity, money, education, or school fees.

The Economy and Sexuality in Kilimanjaro

Between 1921 and 1948, the population density on the slopes of the Kilimanjaro mountain grew from 26 per Km^2 to 50 per Km^2 (Maro, 1975). Such changes in and of themselves resulted in radical changes in the ritual, educational, and daily-life activities of early adulthood. Setel (1995), in his analysis, noted the impact of land shortages in the Kilimanjaro Mountain slope homelands of the Chagga on aspects related to sexuality and sexual relations. Inherited plots of land grew too small to sustain families and increasing numbers of particularly young men left the mountain slopes in search of alternative livelihoods from the 1940's onwards. Provided that wives who remained behind maintained the land, clerical and teaching jobs for men became status occupations. Many young men were forced to live away from the mountain, coming back yearly for the now famous "Christmas pilgrimage" to visit families left on their land (Setel, 1995; pp. 53). The colonial employment policy, where men working in towns were not permitted to move to such areas with their families, also encouraged the seasonal migration of men from rural to urban settings where non-agricultural jobs were available. Despite this out-migration, between 1948 and 1975, the population in the region grew from 267,700 to 660,000. Setel (ibid.) noted that by the 1960s and the 1970s, clan patriarchs no longer articulated the language of legitimacy in sexual affairs to groups of young men. Young men tended to learn about sexuality through day-to-day experience in school, town, or the market-place. Young women, on the other hand, learned through a combination of personal experience and an apprenticeship system where the instructor, often an older female schoolmate, emphasized sexual technique rather than, as their aunts once did, marital responsibility

In rural areas of the Kilimanjaro region, a shift from working the land to trade activities amongst youth is alluded to by Setel (1995). As either part of the increasing commercialization of sex or a number of other inter-related contextual factors, youth have a higher tendency towards pre-marital and extra-marital unprotected sexual experiences with more than one partner (Setel, 1995; Leshabari *et. al.*, 1996a; Lwihula *et. al.*, 1996). Some of these contextual factors include the settings within which trade activities occur, alcohol use, and a decrease in purchasing power at household level. In addition, changes in the roles of men and women at the household level have influenced parenting styles and the degree to which parents and other significant adults are able to supervise and counsel children and youth. Given the realities of the daily lives of Tanzanian youth, it would be important to explore the extent to which they are equipped to deal with their developing sexuality and choices regarding sexual behavior.

Reproductive Health Knowledge and Sexual Behavior

Any study of adolescent sexuality and sexual behavior inevitably confronts the topic of reproductive health knowledge and its impact on sexual behavior. Throughout the world, formal education per se for women is the single most consistent correlate of their low fertility (Bledsoe and Cohen, 1993). How, precisely, education impacts on reproductive behavior is less clear. One simple argument may be through raising the age for first marriage for women (ibid.). However, this would not necessarily protect adolescents and youth from sexual activity prior to marriage. Several authors have noted that formal education may influence values surrounding sexual behavior in the sub-Saharan setting. Formal education has been reported to erode deeply ingrained cultural and familial constraints on pre-marital sexual relations (Cherlin and Riley, 1986; Worthman and Whiting, 1987; Adeokun, 1990). The greater sexual autonomy provided for women by formal education, as well as Western ideals of "romantic love" with one partner, may both lead to earlier ages of sexual debut and more frequent sexual encounters. As it is not possible to reverse these influences of formal education, a third potential impact of education on sexual behavior amongst youth is through the imparting of knowledge and social skills that would induce avoidance of pre-marital unprotected sexual experiences and their consequences. It is on this potential influence of education on youth sexual behavior that the authors base their arguments.

Few studies have reported in a comprehensive manner the level of reproductive health knowledge in the youth population of Tanzania. However, there are indications from data reported by Leshabari (1988) and Fundikira (1985) that the level of such knowledge amongst school children may be low. In a more recent study conducted by Lwihula et al. (1996), involving 681 urban school youth with a mean age of 14.8 years, of those who had heard of menstruation and wet dreams, only 13% and 7% perceived them respectively as an indication of sexual maturity. In addition, only 26% of boys and 20% of girls were found to have correct perceptions regarding sexually transmitted diseases (STDs). A large proportion of youth in this sample reported peers as their primary sources of information. There is less information from rural areas regarding the extent of reproductive health knowledge. One would assume that the greater intactness of traditional institutions, which formally provided reproductive health information during rites of passage in rural areas, would confer greater reproductive health knowledge on rural youth. This study intended to shed some light on the extent of such knowledge in the Rombo district, which is categorized as rural.

To date, there has been considerable resistance to teaching issues related to reproductive health in the school system in sub-Saharan Africa (Bledsoe and Cohen, 1993). Although there is increasing awareness amongst teachers and parents in Tanzania of the need to impart such knowledge, there is still a lack of clarity regarding who should teach, what should be taught, and when such knowledge should be imparted. Although Tanzania has introduced reproductive health lessons within the framework of family life education in primary and secondary schools, the course is not yet offered in teacher training colleges. It is questionable, given the problems related to clarity and cultural sensitivity, whether teachers would feel confident and competent enough to teach the related topics in the absence of formal training in teacher training colleges (Sawaya, 1995). There is minimal information from youths regarding whom they would prefer to provide reproductive health information. It is hoped that data presented here will fill some of these gaps. The findings reported in this article are extracted from a wider study which aimed at exploring factors which were associated with rural school youth reproductive knowledge and the extent to which other health-risk behavior such as smoking, alcohol consumption, and pre-marital sex is practised.

METHODOLOGY

A cross-sectional descriptive study was conducted which involved a random sample of 658 school youth that were in the final two years of primary school or the first two years of secondary school. Data was generated using both quantitative and qualitative methods concurrently.

Sample Selection

The Rombo district in the Kilimanjaro region was selected as a study site due to its rural character and the fact that it borders the neighboring country of Kenya, and hence would be subject to socio-cultural and economic changes, in part, as a result of border trade activities. A two-stage random sampling approach was used. Twelve primary schools were randomly selected from a sampling frame consisting of 123 primary schools in Rombo Rural District of Kilimanjaro Region, while all twelve secondary schools in the district were selected. From each selected primary school, one class was randomly selected from a list of all six or seven classrooms. A similar procedure was used to select from one or two classes in the secondary schools. All the selected students were administered a self-report questionnaire. Participants for focus group discussions were selected from the same target population, but from classes that were not involved in fillingout the survey questionnaire. This procedure was used in order to minimize contamination of the focus group discussions (FGD's) by issues raised in the questionnaires. Two major methods were used to generate data: structured, self-administered questionnaires and focus group discussions.

The Structured Self-administered Questionnaire

A 112 item self-administered questionnaire that consisted of six major sections was used. These included: demographic characteristics of the respondent and parents/guardians; youths' primary and preferred sources of reproductive health information; leisure-time activities; conformity to peer expectations; reproductive health knowledge; and history of sexually related and other risky behavior.

Focus Group Discussions (FGD's)

These were conducted to explore the contexts surrounding the acquisition of reproductive health information, the extent to which unprotected sex was perceived to be a problem, and the processes that surrounding unprotected sex among school youth. The FGD's were exploratory in nature, with between 8 and 10 participants. Gender was an important selection criterion due to the sensitivity of the themes that were to be explored and the assumptions of differences that would exist in male and female perspectives on issues related to sexuality and reproductive health. Three gender categories were agreed upon: female, male, and mixed males and females. The number of groups to be conducted per category was established in the field when no new information was noted to be emerging after conducting a series of group discussions in any one category. Focus group discussion participants were suggested by class teachers on the basis of their ability to discuss and debate on various issues and were recruited by the research team on the basis of their willingness to participate in a discussion after the purpose of the study was explained to them. The results obtained from both instruments related to reproductive health knowledge are presented and discussed in this article.

Data Analysis

Data were entered and cleaned using SPSS. Proportions were used to compare sex differences in demographic characteristics, and chi-square tests were used to gauge the significance of differences. The reproductive health knowledge items were divided into three knowledge sub-scales: a 25-item scale measuring knowledge on biological maturity and fertility control, a 16-item scale measuring STD knowledge, and a 22 item scale measuring HIV/AIDS knowledge. Each correct response was scored as one point, and the scales had good internal consistency with reliability coefficients of 0.79, 0.82, and 0.8 respectively. Mean scores were determined for the various knowledge scales, and ANOVA tests were used to gauge the significance of differences by gender and age. Short field and process notes collected during each FGD were transcribed on the same day, and discussions were held within the research team regarding the emerging core categories which were summarized and used to provide more in-depth insights into the reported quantitative data.

Results

Background Demographic Information

The study sample consisted of 658 school youth with a mean age of 14.9 years (+/- 1.8 SD) of whom 54.7% were females. The majority of the respondents were adolescents aged 15 - 17 years, and girls were generally younger than the boys were. Nearly 21% of the girls were 14 years or younger, compared to 16% of the boys. Almost 60% of the respondents were in primary school. The majority had grown up in a predominantly rural environment, and only 10% were raised in urban areas.

Table 1: *Distribution of Demographic Characteristics of School Youth by Sex*

Characteristic	Males %	Females %	Total (%)
Age (Years)[a]			
12-14	16.4	20.6	118(18.7)
15-17	58.4	64.3	389(61.6)
18+	25.2	15.1	124(19.7)
TOTAL	286	345	631
Grade in School[b]			
Primary 6	22.5	25.4	157 (24.0)
Primary 7	38.1	32.9	231 (35.4)
Secondary 1	26.1	9.2	112 (17.2)
Secondary 2	13.4	32.4	153 (23.4)
TOTAL	304	346	653
Religious Affiliation			
Catholic	90.1	91.5	586 (90.9)
Protestant	6.3	6.7	42 (6.5)
Moslem	2.6	I. 1.2	12 (1.9)
Others	1.0	0.6	5 (0.8)
TOTAL	303	342	645
Upbringing Predominantly			
Urban	9.9	10.5	65 (10.2)
Urban + rural	18.4	17.7	458 (18.0)
Rural	71.8	71.8	115 (71.8)
TOTAL	294	344	638
Lives with (during term time):			
Both parents	43.8	39.7	265 (41.6)
Other relatives	26.8	18.1	142 (22.1)
Peers in dormitories	11.0	24.2	116 (18.1)
Other adults	5.0	4.5	61 (9.5)
Single Parent	7.7	9.7	56 (8.7)
TOTAL	299	343	642

[a] Chi-sq = 10.46, p =0.0054 [b] Chi-sq= 53.72, p = 0.0000 [c] Chi-sq= 23, p = 0.00034

Source: *Research Findings*

Just over two-fifths of the students lived with both parents, and over a quarter lived with relatives other than their parents. While the proportion of boys living with other relatives was slightly higher than that of girls, female students were more likely to report being boarded at school compared with the males. Less than a tenth of the students lived with a single parent. The inhabitants of the study area were largely Catholics, reflected in the 91% of pupils who were Catholics. Other Christian denominations constituted less than 7% of the total sample. (See Table 1).

Focus Group Discussions

There was relative ease in initiating and maintaining group dynamics within the FGD's. Three were conducted per week, each by a team of one facilitator (MTL or SFK) and a trained recorder. A total of 18 FGD were conducted out of which five consisted of boys only, five were girls only, and the rest involved both boys and girls. The introduction of soft drinks as well as the setting of the discussions— often while seated on the grass in a secluded area of the school compound—went a long way towards encouraging openness in the FGD's. The mixed FGD's provided more diverse core categories than the single gender groups, and hence it was not until eight had been conducted that it was felt that no new information was emerging. This point was reached after conducting five FGD's with the single gender groups. The "boys only" FGD's had an average of 8 participants, ranging in age from 14 to 19 years, while the average number of participants for the "girls only" groups was 8.2 with and age range of 12-17 years. There was an average of 8.6 participants in the mixed gender FGD's; 36 were girls and 34 were boys with an age range of 14-19 years. Three of the "boys only" FGD's involved secondary school students compared with only one of the "girls only" groups. Three of the mixed gender FGD's involved secondary school students. Primary school students were involved in the remaining FGD's.

Awareness of Reproductive Health Issues

About 52% (343) of the sample had fully attained pubescence measured by onset of menarche or breaking of the voice amongst boys (social pubescence). Of the 276 who could recall and document the age at which they attained pubescence, the mean age at social pubescence was 14.9 years (+/- 1.2 at 2SD). About 70.0% (N=343) reported they had talked to an adult about pubescence when they had attained this state, though when the total sample

Table 2: *Percentage of Rombo School youth Who Were Aware of Menstruation, Wet Dreams, Sexual Intercourse, STDs and AIDS by Age and Sex*

Characteristic	Percentage of Youth who were aware of [% /N=denominator[a]]											
	Menstruation			*Wet dreams*			*Sexual intercourse*			*STDs*		
	Male	*Female*	*Total*	*Male*	*Female*	*Total*	*Male*	*Female*	*Total*	*Male*	*Female*	*Total*
Age (years)	12.8	26.8	21.2	17.0	4.2	9.3	36.4	29.6	32.2	19.1	18.3	18.6
< 14	47	71	118	47	71	118	44	71	115	47	71	118
15-17	14.4	48.2	33.7	28.7	14.4	20.6	54.8	48.2	51.0	27.5	31.1	29.6
	167	222	389	167	222	389	166	218	384	167	222	389
> 18	41.7	71.1	54.0	48.6	25.0	38.7	76.8	76.5	76.7	44.4	40.4	42.7
	72	52	124	72	52	124	69	5	12	72	52	124
TOTAL (N)	21.0	47.2	35.3	31.8	13.9	22.0	57.3	48.5	52.5	52.5	29.9	30.1
	286	345	631	286	345	631	279	340	619	286	345	631
Level of education												
Primary school	8.1	21.3	14.9	18.3	8.4	13.1	42.8	27.3	34.1	18.3	16.8	17.5
	186	202	388	186	202	388	186	198	384	186	202	388
Secondary school	40.5	83.3	63.8	55.4	22.2	37.3	82.4	78.3	80.1	52.9	47.9	50.2
	121	144	265	121	144	265	119	143	262	121	144	265
TOTAL (N)	20.8	47.1	34.8	39.9	14.2	23.0	58.5	48.7	53.3	31.9	29.8	30.8
	307	346	653	307	346	653	305	341	646	307	346	653

[a]*The numbers below each proportion, represent the denominator on which the percentage is based*

Source: *Research Findings*

was taken into consideration, only 32.1% (N=658) had ever talked to a parent regarding their sexual development.

Given the stage of psychosexual development of the respondents, exposure to issues related to biological and psychological changes associated with menarche and spermache in human growth and development was anticipated. Surprisingly, while more than half of the students had heard of sexual intercourse, only 22% had heard of wet dreams, 30.1% had been exposed to information on STDs, and 35.3% on menstruation. Exposure to information on these items increased with age, and higher proportions of secondary school students reported such exposure compared with primary school students. The higher exposure to information on sexual intercourse, compared with exposure to basic issues related to biological maturity and STDs, increased with age and gender, as well as in secondary and primary school students (See Table 2).

As a result of the advent of the HIV epidemic, there have been intensive AIDS control campaigns in the country, so attention was paid to how many Rombo school youth had heard of the disease. Generally, awareness of HIV/AIDS was relatively high compared with other reproductive health issues. Over 90% of the respondents reported to have heard about AIDS. The discrepancy in responses to exposure to information on HIV/AIDS and STDs suggests that HIV/AIDS may not be conceptualized in the same way as other STDs in this population.

Although the extent of exposure to reproductive health issues increased with age, there was considerable variation by sex. Girls, as opposed to boys, were more likely to be exposed to information on menstruation. Boys, on the other hand, were more likely to have heard of wet dreams than girls were. Common local terms for these phenomena were used in the questionnaire, making it unlikely that these were novel terms to the students.

Sources of Information on Reproductive Health Issues

The primary sources of information for students who reported they had heard of the explored issues relating to reproductive health were explored and the responses obtained are summarized in Table 3. Peers were the major primary source of information on menstruation and wet dreams and were second to the mass media for information on sexual intercourse. Peers, however, featured less prominently as sources of information on the consequences of unprotected sexual intercourse such as STDs, AIDS, and prevention of STDs and pregnancy. This observation was supported by FGD's data where personal experiences regarding biological maturity and sexual relationships with the opposite sex were the main categories emerging regarding the content of discussions on sex among young people.

Table 3: *Percentage Distribution of Primary Sources of Information on Biological Maturity and Consequences of*

Information Source	*Frequency of primary sources of information on (%)*											
	Menstruation		*Wet dreams*		*Sexual Intercourse*		*STDs*		*AIDS*		*Prevention of STDS*	
	Male (N=60)	*Female* (N=163)	*Male* (N=112)	*Female* (N=57)	*Male* (N=184)	*Female* (N=171)	*Male* (N=104)	*Female* (N=111)	*Male* (N=275)	*Female* (N=318)	*Male* (N=310)	*Female* (N=657)
Peers	16.7	35.6	35.7	14.0	22.8	25.1	6.7	11.7	3.6	4.7	0.6	1.4
Teachers	33.3	20.2	15.2	12.3	10.3	12.3	18.3	24.3	2.5	5.7	3.9	4.6
Other relatives	11.7	12.3	16.1	19.3	9.8	9.3	3.8	3.6	4.0	4.0	2.6	1.4
Mass media	18.3	5.5	17.8	29.8	39.1	39.2	37.5	30.6	67.6	63.8	17.7	13.2
Father	10.0	24.5	4.5	19.3	3.8	5.8	3.8	8.1	6.9	2.8	3.2	1.7
Mother	3.3	0.6	1.8	-	1.6	-	-	-	2.9	1.8	1.9	1.4
Health worker	-	0.6	5.3	3.5	8.7	4.7	23.1	15.3	9.4	7.9	65.8	73.2
Religious leader	3.3	-	2.7	-	3.8	3.5	4.8	5.4	2.9	8.2	4.2	1.7
No response	3.3	0.6	0.9	1.7	-	-	1.9	0.9	-	0.9	-	1.1

Source: *Research Findings*

The mass media featured highly as a primary source of information for all the items explored—except for menstruation. Though health workers featured low as a primary source of information on biological maturity and sexual intercourse, they were more likely to provide information on the consequences of unprotected sexual experiences. It was of interest to note that amongst youth who had ever heard of wet dreams and menstruation, a larger proportion reported fathers as primary sources of information than mothers. This was particularly so for girls, though the type of information provided by fathers was not explored nor mentioned spontaneously in the FGD's.

The proportion of school youth who identified teachers as a primary source of information on the health consequences of sexual activity was low, although there have been attempts to integrate aspects relating to human reproductive health into the school domestic science (Primary schools) and biology (Secondary schools) curricula. However, this could probably be due to what students described as the "difficulties" teachers had in communicating with them on issues related to sexuality and human reproductive health, as will be reporting in the FGD findings below.

The data indicated that students would prefer to be informed on various reproductive health issues from sources that differed from their primary sources. Generally, students would prefer to hear about the various reproductive health items explored from, in order of most preferred source, teachers, health workers and parents (See Table 4). The preferred sources were also reflected in all the focus group discussions.

There were no significant differences in terms of gender in the proportions of students who preferred the various sources of information. The findings suggest that the most frequently reported primary sources of reproductive health information derived from these data (peers and the mass media) were used as a result of lack of access to information from other socially recognized and sanctioned sources rather than by personal preference.

FGD Findings on Contexts Surrounding Acquisition of Reproductive Health Information

The students generally agreed that information about menarche (*kuvunja ungo*) and spermache (*wakati wa kubalehe*) was scarce. In support of the quantitative data, in almost all the FGD's, there was agreement that both boys and girls experienced overt manifestations of puberty without any prior

Table 4: *Percentage Distribution of Preferred Sources of Information on Different Reproductive Health Issues by Sex*

Information	**Frequency of Preferred Sources of Information on (%)**									
Sources	*Menstruation*		*Wet dreams*		*Sexual Intercourse*		*Prevention of STDS*		*Prevention of Pregnancy*	
	Male- (*N=154*)	*Female* (*N=193*)	*Male* (*N=149*)	*Female* (*N=165*)	*Male* (*N=175*)	*Female* (*N=209*)	*Male* (*N=292*)	*Female* (*N=320*)	*Male* (*N=279*)	*Female* (*N=325*)
Health Worker	40.9	30.6	38.2	35.1	45.1	37.8	22.9	37.1	20.4	18.1
Teachers	31.2	39.4	37.6	40.0	32.6	33.5	44.9	54.7	45.2	40.3
Parents	19.5	24.3	15.4	17.6	12.0	19.1	6.8	6.6	6.4	9.2
Mass media	2.6	1.0	4.0	1.2	3.4	2.9	10.6	8.7	10.0	18.5
Religious leaders	1.9	2.1	4.0	1.8	4.6	2.9	9.2	5.9	10.0	3.7
Peers	2.6	1.0	0.0	2.4	1.1	0.9	2.4	2.8	6.4	7.0
Others	1.3	1.6	0.7	1.8	1.1	2.9	3.1	0.9	1.4	3.1

Source: *Research Findings*

preparation for the events. Parents did not appear to discuss such issues with their children, as was illustrated in a mixed-gender FGD amongst secondary school students in their second year of study where it was reported that "... Parents do not teach these kinds of things..." with reference to issues surrounding puberty. In both boys and girls only FGD's amongst primary and secondary school students, a common statement regarding the experience of menarche and spermache was, "…everyone just gets taken by surprise by the changes they experience in their bodies."

Information regarding puberty appeared to be acquired after girls achieved menarche and boys' voices started to break. Boys appeared, from this data set, to be as disadvantaged as girls were in terms of adult sources of information regarding pubescence. In a male primary class 7 group, there was consensus on the statement, ".... when you reach sexual maturity, you explain and talk about what happens to your friend." This method of acquiring information from a peer's experience of puberty was a recurring theme in all the boys only focus groups. It was also noted that some boys can talk to their grandfather (babu), but it was difficult to talk to fathers or other relatives such as mjomba (maternal uncle). While the boys felt that maybe mothers talked to their daughters about menarche, evidence from the girls' FGD's indicated that this was not the case. A female secondary school group put it in the following way:

> "Many youth do not know anything about menarche and spermache, and this is because the parents do no tell the truth about these matters. It would be fine if, when young people realize their bodies are changing, they could say so to their parents and be taught by them."

FGDs with girls in their final year of primary school revealed that mothers would talk to their oldest daughter about menarche and expect that she would communicate such information to younger female siblings when they achieved menarche.

Teachers were a source of reproductive health information reported in some of the FGD's. However, it was also generally accepted that there was a selective process involved in access to such information, as is illustrated by the following statement made in an FGD with girls in the first year of secondary school: "however, information on matters related to sex is given to only a few of us, as teachers would choose those children who seemed to be older and the younger ones were not told anything at all." In would appear that when girls were selected for such information-providing sessions, these did not form part of the normal structured teaching activities in the school curriculum.

The primary school curriculum provides for some reproductive health information in the domestic science course. In many of the FGDs, it was noted that teachers would ask students to read the relevant chapter in their textbooks and promise to teach the topic at a later date, but the promises would rarely be fulfilled. Many of the students felt this was because teachers felt too shy or embarrassed to teach the relevant topic. In one FGD it was noted that "teachers feel ashamed to talk about such topics as the genitals," which were referred to in Swahili as sehemu za siri (literal translation - secret parts). In all the FGDs there was expressed need for information regarding biological maturity. Indeed, despite the reluctance of teachers to teach the subject in a didactic manner, some students did get information from textbooks. In a primary class FGD of six boys, it was noted that information on biological maturity is available in science and sayansi kimu (domestic science) textbooks. However, questions asked by students after the FGDs confirmed the lack of adequate understanding of this information amongst the students. These included questions like "what does spermache/menarche mean?;" "when can a boy make a girl pregnant?;" "at what age can a girl become pregnant?"

Extent of Reproductive Health Knowledge

Despite the level of exposure of students to terms relating to reproductive health, there was evidence of a lack of a deep understanding of the issues from their low performance on the 63 items of the composite reproductive health knowledge scale (CRH) where the mean score was 12.75. Within the sub-scales, the mean scores for knowledge on biological maturity and fertility control (BMFC scale; 6.08 for 22 items) and sexually transmitted diseases (STDs scale; 4.4 for 16 items) were lower than those for HIV/AIDS (9.2 of 25 items).

Analysis of variance (ANOVA) of mean scores by gender and age revealed that female students scored significantly lower mean scores than males on all the knowledge sub-scales and that older youth were better informed then their younger counterparts. Lower mean scores were particularly noted in all the age groups on the STDs and the biological maturity and fertility control knowledge scales (see Table 5).

It was of interest to determine the extent to which variations in mean scores by gender were influenced by differences in age distribution of male and female youth in the study sample. Analysis revealed that the significance of variations in scores disappeared in the two-way interaction between age and gender, (BMFC, p=0.131; STDs, p=0.424; HIV/AIDS, p=0.113) suggesting an age effect in all the three knowledge scales by gender.

Table 5: *Knowledge mean scores on the biological maturity and fertility control (BMFC), sexually transmitted diseases (STDs), HIV/AIDS and the composite reproductive health (CRH) knowledge scales by gender and age*

Knowledge Scales and Age in Years	*Males (N)*	*Females (N)*	*Total[a] (N)*	*p-values*
BMFC				
12-14	5.91 (47)	3.96 (71)	4.74 (118)	0.011[b]
15-17	6.35 (167)	5.61 (222)	5.93 (389)	0.000[c]
18 and above	7.78 (72)	7.87 (52)	7.81 (124)	
STDs				
12-14	4.21 (47)	2.65 (71)	3.27 (118)	0.000[b]
15-17	4.84 (167)	3.93 (222)	4.32 (389)	0.000[c]
18 and above	5.88 (72)	5.42 (52)	5.69 (124)	
HIV/AIDS				
12-14	9.53 (47)	7.2 (71)	8.13 (118)	0.005[b]
15-17	9.46 (167)	8.62 (222)	8.98 (389)	0.000[c]
18 and above	10.85 (72)	10.79 (52)	10.82 (124)	
CRHS				
12-14	12.17 (47)	9.17 (71)	10.36 (118)	0.008[b]
15-17	13.46 (167)	11.91 (222)	12.58 (389)	0.000[c]
18 and above	15.39 (72)	15.77 (52)	55 (124)	

Key: [a] *Information not available for 26 students with incomplete response on the scales;* [b] *p = significance of variations within gender groups;* [c] *p= significance of variations within age groups*

Source: *Research Findings*

Discussion

Some limitations need to be taken into consideration when interpreting the findings. The authors were aware that there was very little information or study on what youth need to know regarding reproductive health given the current socio-cultural environment in which young people grow. However, data indicating low age at sexual debut in both rural and urban youth populations suggests the need for adequate information to allow young people to make informed decisions regarding issues relating to their reproductive health. Despite the lack of information on acceptable norms regarding the extent of reproductive health information amongst youth, the developed scales were noted to have good internal consistency. During focus group discussions, it was clear that young people had some awareness of items on the scales measuring concepts such as biological maturity, fertility, contraception, and STDs including AIDS.

In selecting the sample, authors were aware that secondary school students represent a selected group of students who score exceptionally well in primary school and are selected to join the few positions available for secondary education. Currently, the secondary school facilities in Tanzania can only cater for 10% of the 300,000 yearly graduates from primary schools in the country (BEST, 1994). Despite the limitations, the data provides some hitherto undocumented information regarding issues relating to reproductive health knowledge amongst school youth in the study area from which general conclusions can be drawn.

Many people who are opposed to adolescents' and youths' rights to reproductive health information and services assume this population sub-group is socially insulated from such information. There is also a belief that exposing them to such information and services might not only increase understanding and influence more socially acceptable and healthy sexual behavior, but also tempt them to practise what they have learned. Other studies have shown that access to counseling and contraceptives, let alone reproductive health information, does not encourage earlier or increased sexual activity amongst youth (Grunseit and Kippax, 1993). The reported lack of having heard of biological aspects relating to sexual maturation was an issue of particular concern as the majority of primary school youth in the sample, upon graduation, would not be exposed to a formal learning environment where such information could be acquired. To date, there are negligible formal reproductive health services which target the youth population in Tanzanian communities. Little is known about how youth that are not in school acquire necessary reproductive health information before they become adults. Evidence from the reported data indicates that little remains of the emotional and spiritual guidance or the knowledge-providing functions that initiation ritual and other traditional socialization practices once had. The traditional informal sources of reproductive health information, which include adult extended family members, were no longer in operation in this rural community as only 2.0-17% of students reported this group as a primary source of information on the various reproductive health issues explored.

Parents did not feature as highly as traditional or current primary sources of reproductive health information. Although the study did not explore parents' own reproductive health knowledge or their ability/willingness to pass on such information to their children, there are studies from Uganda which report that, culturally, parents cannot talk to their children about issues related to sexuality (Huygens *et. al.*, 1996). This observation may be applicable in many traditional societies in East Africa, including the study area. Where traditional systems of imparting social skills to youth as they relate to gender roles and relationships with the opposite sex exist, little is known about the coverage of various components of reproductive health. While it is important for males and females to be exposed to information on the biological changes associated with both menarche and spermache, it appears relatively fewer male than female youth knew about menstruation and the opposite was the case with respect to awareness of wet dreams. Generally, these findings suggest a cultural, gender-selective process in the type of reproductive health information the youth were exposed to and/or desired. This bias needs to be explored and reduced in interventions aimed at increasing reproductive health knowledge in this population.

Exposure to information on sexual intercourse appeared to exceed exposure to basic reproductive health knowledge on menarche, spermache, and the consequences of unprotected sexual intercourse. This trend persisted irrespective of age, sex, or grade level of the school youth. The relative lack of having heard of sexually transmitted diseases was of particular concern, as one would assume that giving or searching for information on sexual intercourse would be closely linked to some exposure to information on its consequences.

There may be several reasons for this trend that can be implied from the data. First, the exploratory nature of young people at this stage of psychosexual development may result in youth actively seeking information on sexual intercourse or focusing more on such information than on more basic information on biological maturity. This may be particularly so given the observed lack of formal sources for such information. Perhaps a second reason may relate to the nature of the primary sources for such information. The major sources of information on sexual intercourse were peers and the mass media. Evidence indicates that peers may not be sufficiently informed to provide adequate reproductive health information while the mass media does not allow for didactic interaction where the consequences of sexual intercourse and related concerns can be discussed and provide meaning for young people. The variations in responses to having been exposed to information on STDs and HIV/AIDS suggest HIV/AIDS information transmitted by current mass media campaigns find an audience in the youth population. A high awareness of HIV/AIDS amongst urban school children in Tanzania has also been noted by Lwihula et al. (1996). A lack of a deeper understanding of HIV/AIDS necessary for risk-reduction measures is, however, prevalent in this population. This interpretation is supported by the relatively low scores on the HIV/AIDS knowledge scale suggesting that the messages received from the mass media may not be sensitive enough to allow in-depth analysis and personalized meanings of the messages for the youth population. This indicates a need for more youth-focused mass media messages on HIV/AIDS.

It appeared from the reported primary sources of information that few responsible adults were involved in providing reproductive health information to young people. The assumption that traditional institutions which provided such information in the past are in existence may be erroneous and increase the vulnerability of young people to potential reproductive health consequences as a result of ignorance, misinformation, and pressure to indulge in unprotected sexual intercourse. Community perceptions on acceptable reproductive health information and who should impart such information to young people would be an important prerequisite for any potential intervention to provide information and services for the youth population.

Though the formal education system is a major institution for the socialization of young people in Tanzania, the proportion of school youth that identified school as a primary source of human reproductive health information was low. There have been attempts to integrate aspects related to human reproductive health into the school domestic science (Primary schools) and biology (Secondary schools) curricula in Tanzania. However, the focus group data revealed a consensus on teachers' avoidance of topics that focused on human reproduction. This raises concerns regarding the adequacy of the domestic science and biology syllabus in providing reproductive health information. Although reasons for the reluctance of teachers to provide didactic sessions for issues related to human reproductive health were not explored, communication with Ministry of Education and Culture officials indicated that reproductive health education does not form part of the curriculum in teachers training colleges. This may suggest that what was interpreted by students as teachers' unwillingness to provide a didactic session in human reproduction may be a reflection of the lack of teaching skills in this subject. A recent school health situation analysis raises other concerns about the school environment and the reproductive health particularly of female students. Many schools were noted to lack facilities that would afford the necessary privacy and maintenance of personal hygiene for menstruating girls (Leshabari *et. al.*, 1996b). This suggests perhaps a general lack of a systematic and a coordinated focus on the reproductive health-related needs of young people in these learning environments.

The reproductive health knowledge scores demonstrated by this data were generally lower than the impression created by other surveys where the concept of reproductive health knowledge was measured and interpreted on a single item basis (TDHS, 1993; TKAPS, 1995). The use of single test items has the disadvantage of being unable to differentiate between simple recall of basic facts and in-depth understanding of issues. Yet, if knowledge is to be translated into practice, the level of understanding has to go beyond simple recall of a fact or basic comprehension of fundamental components to a personalized analysis of what was learned. Provision of reproductive health information needs to address what Levitt *et. al.*, (1991) have termed personal meanings given by youth to different types of sexual risky behavior. Such personal meanings are conceptualized as the primary filter through which specific new skills, experiences, and information relating to risk-taking behavior pass. Failure to address the personal significance youth give to risk information does not allow for analysis and synthesis beyond an understanding of conceptual meanings to the ability to anticipate the personalized impact of consequences of sexual activity in a real-life situation.

Unprotected sexual intercourse can be viewed as one of the types of risky behavior to which young people are and will increasingly be exposed to in Tanzania given the pace of socio-cultural changes in the country. Levitt et al. (1991) note that psycho-educational programs may not in themselves bring about anticipated behavioral changes amongst youth if the powerful influences of the temperamental predisposition to engage in risk-taking-behavior and the socio-cultural environment of young people are not taken into consideration. While little is known of the former in the Tanzanian context, the high-risk nature as regards sexual behavior in several communities in Tanzania—given rapid socio-cultural change—has to be acknowledged. In order for information to reduce sexually related health risks among youth, research needs to focus on intervention programs which not only provide information to youth regarding such risks but also develop social management skills including provision of accessible and acceptable services for youth.

In conclusion, these findings imply a need for more focus on the psychosexual socialization of youths in Tanzania. Such socialization needs to be a process that includes the roles of a variety of people such as parents, teachers, health-care workers, and the community in general. The data available suggests a lack of appropriate psychosexual socialization structures during the transition period into young adulthood. The gradual disappearance and/or lack of relevance of traditional "rites of passage," as a result of increased ethnic heterogeneity and rapid socio-economic and cultural change, has created a reproductive health information and living skills development vacuum amongst youth in many rural and urban communities. There is a need for the innovative use of existing structures to ensure a smooth and safe transition to adulthood. This includes increased awareness on the importance of appropriate parenting practices and improvement within the formal school system of both the provision of information and the development of the specific social skills adolescents require in order to make informed and healthy choices regarding sexual behavior.

Chapter Four

Street Children and Street Life in Urban Tanzania: The Culture of Surviving and Its Implications for Children's Health

Joe L.P. Lugalla and *Jessie K. Mbwambo*

Introduction

During the past ten years, Tanzanian cities have undergone rapid changes that have transformed the urban environment as well as the lives of millions of people who live in this setting. The impact of these changes is affecting almost everybody, particularly the urban poor. One of the growing social problems associated with these changes is the tremendous increase in unsupervised children either living alone or working on urban streets. The number of urban street children - *watoto wa mitaani* (Swahili name for street children)—has increased rapidly during the last decade in Tanzania. This problem is especially acute in big cities like Dar es Salaam, Arusha, Morogoro, Moshi, Tanga, Mbeya, and Mwanza where the rates of urban population growth have been exploding amidst an intensifying and severe social and economic crisis. The rapid population growth has been associated with an increase in the number of children living alone on urban streets or spending most of their day on the streets in the quest for survival. Most of these children have, for various reasons, either abandoned or have been abandoned by their families and have migrated to urban areas in order to earn a living. Their rapid increase in number at a time when Tanzania is experiencing great financial constraints raises concerns and calls for immediate attention.

Currently, urban street children are seen as a problem which further compounds the nature of the urban crisis. Politicians, policy-makers, and urban planners seem to be helpless in their efforts to either resolve the problem or to assist street children and have so far failed to prescribe plausible solutions which are realistic, down-to-earth, and concrete. In fact, the official government attitude towards street children has been very negative. Street children are considered to be hooligans, vagabonds, and prone to commit crimes. As a result, they have been a target of harassment by law enforcement organizations; there are many cases of street children being beaten by police, detained, and sometimes repatriated to their rural homes. Nevertheless, these draconian measures have not provided long-term solutions to this social problem. The number of urban street children has continued to escalate every year.

Why is this so? One reason the government has failed to provide viable solutions to this problem stems from the fact that the government is ignorant about urban street children in Tanzania. It has made no attempt to understand who these children are and where they come from, their reasons for leaving home, how they survive and meet their daily needs, what problems they experience, and how they surmount these problems. A lack of this crucial information has led to the adoption of policy solutions that deal with the symptoms of this problem rather than the causes.

In order to address this information gap, the authors, who are Tanzanians, conducted an in-depth study of street children which was carried out in Dar es Salaam in 1994-95. The main objectives were: first, to identify structures and processes that generate and perpetuate the increasing number of street children; second, to understand the historical background of these children, the socio-economic characteristics of their families, how they meet their basic daily needs, the problems they confront, and how they surmount them; and third, to examine the implications of this culture of street life upon children's health.

Methodology and Study Area

The study was conducted in the city of Dar es Salaam between October 1994 and August 1995. This city was chosen because Dar es Salaam, with an approximate population of 3-4 million, is the largest city in Tanzania; since colonization, it has taken the lead in terms of urban population growth and has accommodated over one-third of all urban dwellers in the country for the last three decades (Lugalla, 1995). Recent information from UNICEF (Dar es Salaam office) shows that there are about 5000 street children in Tanzania, 40% of whom reside in Dar es Salaam.

Dar es Salaam city is divided into three administrative districts - Kinondoni, Ilala, and Temeke. While Kinondoni and Temeke are predominantly residential areas, the Ilala district contains most of the commercial and government administration activities. It is the business district of the city that accommodates more street children than the other two districts. It is for this reason that we chose the Ilala district for our in-depth study.

The study was carried out in two phases: the pilot phase and the in-depth study. During the pilot phase, we visited all three districts in order to get an overview of the magnitude of the problem. This phase helped us to identify different types of street children. UNICEF and other agencies tend to define street children on the basis of the frequency with which they sleep on the street and the degree of contact they maintain with their families (Knaul, 1995[a]). Consequently, there are two main classifications: "children *of* the street" and "children on the street." Children *of* the street include those who live and sleep alone on the streets and have almost no family contact; children on the street are those who spend most of the day on the streets, but have homes, maintain family ties, and normally return to their homes in the evening to sleep. Some operate in marginal jobs, and others have flooded the informal sector.

The pilot study identified these two categories of street children in Dar es Salaam and observed that the "children of the street" were more vulnerable and at higher risk than "children on the street." We therefore decided to focus our in-depth study on the more vulnerable group. We began by identifying five street children (three boys and two girls) and establishing an informal, close, and friendly relationship with them so that they became familiar with us. The children were informed of the purpose of the study and were asked to participate in it. Thereafter, these children introduced us to their friends, who in turn, introduced us to other friends.

Information was gathered by means of informal and unstructured interviews with individual children and with ten focus groups. We also designed a questionnaire that included questions about their general demographics, their historical background, and the socio-economic characteristics of their parents. Although it was in our interest to make sure that there was an equal representation of both boys and girls, we encountered a variety of difficulties in attaining this parity. First, cultural sanctions for girls are stronger, and thus they are subject to more controlled supervision or monitoring by their families. The chances of their being able to run away from home are slim. As a result, there are fewer girls living on the streets in Tanzania. Second, even if girls do manage to run away from home, most of them end up living with a family for whom they begin work as domestic servants. As they grow up and become independent, they often join the entertainment industry as barmaids, hotel attendants, or prostitutes. Third, even if they do not work as domestic servants, those who are close to puberty are picked up by pimps or police. There is ample evidence in Tanzania that street girls are harassed and even detained by the police more than street boys. Fourth, street girls are always vulnerable to physical and sexual assault, making street life less attractive to girls than to boys.

All these factors contribute to the existence of a smaller number of girls living and surviving on the streets than boys, which is reflected by the number of girls we interviewed. However, one should not think that girls who work in marginal jobs as domestic servants, in the entertainment industry, or as commercial sex workers are faring well. Evidence from India and South America of the magnitude of exploitation, oppression, and child sexual abuse experienced by these girls is overwhelming (Patel, 1990; Knaul, 1995[a]).

Our research process included a participation dimension, the aim of which was to give the children a chance to have their own voices heard, or, as Blanc-Szanton (1994) has argued, to allow children to be participating subjects in, rather than the objects of, research. They participated in all levels of the research by assisting in identifying areas where most children spend their day and night time. Some assisted in redesigning our questionnaire, and those who could read and write administered some of the questionnaires under the supervision of our research assistants, most of whom were social science students from the University of Dar es Salaam. The children themselves mobilized other children, identified meeting locations, and suggested meeting times.

The approach of involving street children in our research effort made our fieldwork easier and led to valuable and immediate results. Through their assistance, we managed to establish three main meeting areas. One area was near a famous car parking lot situated between Sokoine Drive and Samora Avenue and between Avalon Cinema, the United Nations Building, and the City Council of Dar es Salaam. Most street children prefer this area because some work there informally as "parking boys," car washers, or car security guards. The second area was the Mnazi Mmoja grounds where the up-country bus terminal is located. Street children like visiting this area because of the kind of activities which link Dar es Salaam and its countryside. Some earn their living here by working as on-and-off baggage loaders. The third area was near Uhuru Co-education Primary School playground. This area is quite close to the Kariakoo area, which accommodates the biggest market and low and middle-income shopping areas in Dar es Salaam. It is also close to the city transport bus terminal. Street children flood this area during the day because of the economies of scale or comparative advantages offered by this area in so far as their survival strategies are concerned.

WHO ARE THE CHILDREN OF THE STREET?

Knowing who the "children of the street" are in terms of their age, gender, place of origin, and social and economic characteristics is the first and most important step in designing policies which would have a positive impact on these children. Knowing about their historical backgrounds and the socio-economic characteristics of their families is crucial in that this information helps us to understand why these children are living on the streets. "Children of the streets" are distinctly different from "children on the street" or "children living in poor residential slum areas" of Dar es Salaam.

One main characteristic of the "children of the street" is that they live alone on the streets without proper or reliable shelter; they have lost contact with their parents and, as such, they do not enjoy parental protection, love, and care. All 200 children involved in our study were of the street in these ways. The fact that these children are totally alone means that they are fully responsible for their own lives. They plan different survival strategies on their own. They develop themselves materially, culturally, and morally. Also, as a majority of these children (80%) migrated to Dar es Salaam when they were between eight and ten years old, they became uprooted from the traditional forms of cultural socialization, and hence are completely divorced from their families' ways of life. Only 36 children (18%) stated that they knew their home language and could still communicate in it fluently. In general, these children are not only "homeless" or "roofless," but they are also culturally "rootless." This characteristic not only describes their state or situation but distinguishes them from other children of the urban poor who also flood the streets of Dar es Salaam, but who return home to their families at the end of the day. The fact that these children are unique in these respects demands that they require special attention which is necessarily different from that given to "children on the street."

The ages of the 200 children we interviewed ranged from eight to sixteen years old. Only 4 of the children were aged eight, and 12 were aged sixteen. The remaining 184 children (92%) were between the ages of ten and thirteen. All children said they had migrated to Dar es Salaam from up-country regions. Eighty-seven children (43.5%) stated that they had migrated from the Dodoma region, followed by Tabora and Lindi, both at 11%; 19 (9.5%) came from

Mwanza, and 14 (7%) came from Shinyanga. This means that 82% of the children came from these areas (see Table 1).

The vast majority - 188 - of the children (94%) had migrated from rural areas, while only 12 (6%) had come from other urban areas. A total of 105 children (52.5%) stated that they had been living on the streets for more than five years and only 30 (15%) had been living in Dar es Salaam for less than a year. As many as 190 (95%) said that they had never been to school and did not know how to read and write while only 10 (5%) said that they had attended primary education. However, in-depth information revealed that only 4 of these children managed to complete the seven years of primary education. The remaining 6 dropped out of school when they were in the fourth grade. Of those who attained school, none of them were girls, an indication of how difficult it is for girls to get an education in rural Tanzania.

There are ecological and historical reasons why the majority of these children came from the rural areas of the regions shown in Table 1. Of the 21 regions of Tanzania, these regions experience severe drought. They have arid and very infertile lands, and agricultural production survives by sheer luck. Dodoma is more or less a semi-desert due to severe drought, and overgrazing has had disastrous environmental impacts in the Mwanza, Shinyanga, Mara, and Tabora regions. Lindi, Mtwara, and Ruvuma are regions which have been forgotten by official policy planners as far as development is concerned. They were considered labor reserves by the colonial government, and it is doubtful that the post-colonial state has tried to reverse this situation. In general, these regions experience severe underdevelopment and chronic poverty seems to be the norm rather than a temporary phenomenon. Information derived from the Planning Commission of Tanzania shows that these regions account for a great number of migrants who become beggars in urban Tanzania.

In order to get a picture of the children's family household profiles and the social and economic background of their parents or families, we began by asking them to describe the dominant economic activities of their parents. Since all of them (including those from urban areas) indicated agriculture was the dominant economic activity, we asked them to estimate the size of land their parents or families owned. After describing to them what an acre looked like, only 18 children (9%) reported that their parents used to own land which exceeded two acres. The parents of the remaining 91% of the children owned less than two acres. All of the children reported production for subsistence as the main occupation of their parents. They also complained about poor productivity on these small pieces of land due to drought, poor soil, and poor and archaic methods of social organization of production. This study data also confirms data in the UNICEF study which observed that 80% of households in Tanzania derived their economic livelihood from small-scale food crop production based on rain-fed land and hoe technology. The median size of holding was 0.7 hectares (UNICEF, 1990).

Table 1: *Place of Origin and Educational Status of Our Sample of Street Children, Dar es Salaam*

Origin				*%*	*Education*		
Region	*No. of children*	*From Urban*	*From Rural*		*None*	*Primary*	*Secondary*
Dodoma	87	81	6	**43.5**	79	8	-
Tabora	22	22	-	**11.0**	22	-	-
Shinyanga	14	14	-	**7.0**	14	-	-
Mwanza	19	18	1	**9.5**	17	2	-
Lindi	22	22	-	**11.0**	22	-	-
Mtwara	12	12	-	**6.0**	12	-	-
Mara	10	10	-	**5.0**	10	-	-
Morogoro	5	3	2	**2.5**	5	-	-
Ruvuma	9	6	3	**4.5**	9	-	-
Total	200	188	12		190	10	-
%	**94**	**6**			**95**	**5**	**0**

Source: *Research Findings*

We also asked them about the size of their families and whether they had lived with both parents prior to being on the streets. While 29 children (14.5%) reported coming from monogamous marriages, 84 (42%) originated from polygamous marriages. Sixty-six children (33%) came from single (formerly married or unmarried) parents. Of these, 66, 47 (71.2%) had been living with either their biological or stepmothers only. Twenty-five out of the 30 girls belonged to this category. The main reason for this trend is that, in most cultures in Tanzania, girls prefer living with their mothers rather than with their fathers in the event of divorce or separation. Twenty-one children (10.5%) indicated they had been living with relatives or other guardians. Their response to the question of family size shows that more than two-thirds (78%) came from large families that had between six and fifteen children. All children stated that their mothers had never attended school and did not know how to read and write. Only 31 children (15.5%) reported that their fathers had attained primary education.

It is very interesting, however, to note that although the fathers seemed to have access to education, 133 children (66.5%) identified their mothers or female guardians as the main economic providers. These findings point to an inversion of roles in the families of these children. The dominant patriarchal tradition of Tanzania requires that fathers be the head of the household and the main economic provider at the same time. Among the objective difficulties are workloads borne by the mother and how this, in turn, affects her relationship with her children. Rizzini rightly argues that a long and stressful working day has a negative effect not only on the mother's relationship with her children, but also upon her ability to control them (Rizzini *et. al.*, 1994). A more subjective consequence is the transmission of a weak image of the father, who has difficulty in performing the role that society expects of him. In a male-dominated society like Tanzania, this image undoubtedly produces a lot of frustration, increases the father's level of stress, and leads to negative relationships within the family which contribute extensively to family instability. A recent study in Kenya has observed that street children in Nairobi tend to come from female-headed households in slum or squatter areas (Mutuku and Mutiso, 1994). As Rizzini has argued for Brazil, challenging such deeply rooted cultural attitudes causes both objective and subjective difficulties in the dynamics of the family (Rizzini *et. al.*, 1994).

Having collected some information about children's family household profiles, we became interested in knowing their reasons for leaving their families and migrating to Dar es Salaam. We asked each child to state as many reasons as possible. Table 2 presents a summary of these reasons by rank. It is clear that family poverty and poor economics are the main motives for leaving home. Confronted with rural poverty and hunger, the third most common reason for leaving home is the need to look for means of earning money outside the home village. Since our findings show that these children do not retain links with their families (that is, they do not even have their home addresses and have never revisited their homes), it is very unlikely that they migrate to urban areas in order to assist their families back home. Rather, they move to tend to their own personal needs for survival.

Table 2: *Reasons for Leaving Home by Percentage and Rank of Our Sample of Street Children, Dar es Salaam (Population size = 200 Children)*

Rank	*Reason*	*%*
1.	General situation of poverty	100.0
2.	No food at home	90.0
3.	Need to look for a job and earn money	85.0
4.	Parent/matrimonial problems (parent death or separation)	69.0
5.	Bad relationship with family (fights, abuse by parents or stepparents)	62.0
6.	'Bright-light' theory (Children attracted by city life)	12.5
7.	No parents, therefore have no home	8.0

Source: *Research Findings*

The other common reason which forces them to migrate is the nature of social life and social relationships in the family. Sixty-nine percent of the children stated a variety of matrimonial problems including parental separation due to either death or divorce. Sixty-two percent of the children mentioned fights between parents, the cruelty of some stepparents, and abuse as conditions which forced them to run away from their homes.

Only 12.5% of the children mentioned the allure of city life or the need to see the city as an important factor in their decision to leave their homes, and only 8% stated that they had decided to leave their homes because they had lost both parents and no-one in the village was willing to take care of them.

How Street Children Meet Their Basic Needs

Knowing how "children of the street" meet their basic needs is critical. First, it helps us to understand how these children survive and, second, it enables us to map out the already existing urban resources which are being used by these children. This knowledge has considerable implications for policy planning: it can assist us in planning for future intervention policies and strategies. In order to know how these children manage their day-to-day basic needs, we asked them how they got their food, where they slept, where they bathed, what toilet facilities they used, and how they protected themselves.

None of the children had fixed or permanent accommodation. More than half (60%) slept in the streets or on the pavement quite close to shops or other commercial buildings such as cinema halls, discotheques, and theaters. Fourteen percent spent their nights at bus and railway terminals (Gerezani and Mnazi Mmoja areas), and 11% slept in corridors near religious institutions. Ten girls spent their nights as partners of night security guards, while the remaining 20 spent their nights near hotels.

Most of these children (88.7%) reported that they worked informally during the day as car-parking boys, vehicle security guards, car washers, or baggage loaders and used the money they got from these jobs to buy cheap food in shanty hotels commonly known in Dar es Salaam as *'Magenge'* or *'Mama Nitilie.'* Others (10.5%) got their daily food by begging in various restaurants, and 6.5% indicated that they survived by eating leftovers collected from hotels (see Table 3). Information collected from focus group discussants confirmed that some older girls sell sex in order to survive.

Bathing or taking a shower is not considered to be very important. None of the children bathed more than twice a week. The majority (72.5%) used the waters of the Indian Ocean for bathing. Some (18.4%) used public bathrooms located at the central railway station. A few used water from leaking pipes and public kiosks (5% and 4.1%, respectively). They complained, however, about being harassed by both city residents and law enforcement officials when they used these water sources. More than two-thirds of these children used public toilet facilities available in the city, but they complained that most of them were not functioning. Some (14.6%) used hotel toilets, and less than 10% used parks, pavements, roads, and the seaside for their toilet needs. From these findings, the belief that street children primarily defecate or urinate in open streets must be seriously doubted.

In terms of security, four-fifths reported that they depend on their peer groups. The majority of them know each other and prefer living in smaller groups of between three and five children. This not only provides them with companionship, but also comfort and a framework for socialization. This grouping also serves as support and protection from certain kinds of violence. Street girls also have their own security groups. Theirs are often different from those that the street boys use. For instance, some of the older girls associate with older boys who provide them with security in exchange for sexual relationships. Other girls have managed to establish strong contacts with night security guards who are employed in the formal sector. Some of these guards provide the girls with security and shelter in return for sexual favors.

Street Life as a Social Phenomenon Affecting Children's Health

There is no doubt that the unhealthy urban environment in which these children live is a major cause of health problems among them. In order to know their health status and how they seek health care, we asked them to mention the kinds of illnesses they had suffered while living on the streets. All mentioned malaria (fever), diarrhea and stomach-related illnesses, coughing and other respiratory diseases; 43 (21.5%) mentioned scabies and other skin-related diseases; 24 (12%) mentioned headaches; and 7 (3.5%) suffered from eye infections. Infectious diseases seem to be common among street children. Certainly, this is a result of a variety of predisposing factors which include unsafe and unhygienic sleeping areas, the shortage or lack of safe drinking water, unsafe food leftovers, and food collected from garbage bins. Street children also experience the physical problems associated with homelessness such as the lack of latrines. Some studies on urban crisis in Tanzania have noted recently that none of the public toilets in Dar es Salaam city is functional (Lugalla, 1995).

How, then, do they solve their health problems? What is their health-seeking behavior? More than half claimed to get treatment from public hospitals located in Mnazi, Mmoja, and Ilala. Others said they had received medicinal assistance from friends, and others bought medicine from drug stores in town or from traditional herbalists in the city. Others, due to severe poverty, waited for their bodies to recover naturally. Information from focus groups revealed that these children have some degree of knowledge about medicines which cure their common diseases.

Those who work as parking boys also provide security services and often wash the cars they are guarding as well.

Table 3: *How Street Children Cope with Urban Life: Where They Work, Sleep, Eat, Bathe and Use Toilet Facilities*

Work	%	*Sleep*	%
Parking boys	74.5	Street pavement	60.0
Vehicle security guards	74.5	Railway/bus station	14.0
Car washers	74.5	Religious buildings	11.0
Baggage loaders	14.2	Near hotels	10.0
Beggars	11.3	With security guards	5.0
	100		100.0

Eat	%	*Bathe*	%
Hotels (buying)	82.0	In the ocean	72.5
Hotels (begging)	10.5	Railway station	18.4
Hotel leftovers	6.5	Leaking water pipes	5.0
Miscellaneous	1.0	Public water kiosks	4.1
Seaside	2.8		
	100		100.0

Toilet	%
Public toilets	54.5
Railway station	23.7
Hotels	14.6
Parks/roadside	4.4
	100.0

Sources: *Research Findings*

It is clear from the above findings that there are gross inadequacies in providing for the basic needs of street children. They have difficulty accessing sufficient fresh and nutritious food, clean water, reliable shelter, bathing and toilet facilities, and health care. These children do not have contact with their families or relatives. With no family or formal structure for moral, emotional, and psychological support and protection, they truly exist on their own. There is no doubt that such a situation has a serious impact on their psychological health and is not without consequences.

It was beyond the scope of this study to look at the psychological suffering that the "children of the street" are subject to. Street life is associated with psycho-social distress, as studies done elsewhere have confirmed. Especially instructive to the authors is the study done by Cohen *et al.* (1991) using the

Home, Education, Activities, Drug use and abuse, Sexual Behavior, Suicidality, and Depression (HEADSS) psycho-social profile data. The authors of this study found that more than 50% of homeless children in Los Angeles experience depression, over 30% had attempted suicide, and 5% had had suicidal thoughts in the preceding month. Also they report that only 18% of homeless children claimed not to use drugs or any substance. The findings that homeless children have mental health problems are not unique to Los Angeles' homeless children, as is evidenced by a previous study carried out by Bassuk and Rubin (1987) who report depression, anxiety, and behavioral problems as common among homeless children in Massachusetts. Wagner and Menek (1990) found 50% of homeless children in New York needed mental health intervention. Furthermore, homeless female youth who had been sexually abused and are susceptible to binge drinking have been found to be more prone to suicide. As the problem of children of the street worsens and more girls end up on the streets of Dar es Salaam, it will be important for early interventions for this group in particular to prevent fatal outcomes.

Street Life and Sexual Vulnerability

Living independently at this very tender age makes children more vulnerable to both physical and sexual abuse. Cases of girls being raped and boys being sodomized by force are not hard to find. Although our study collected little information about street children's sexuality and the consequent health implications, discussions in focus groups confirmed that street children in Dar es Salaam also lead active sex lives. Both anal and vaginal penetrative sex seem to be common among sexual relations involving both genders, but penetrative anal sex is more common among boys.

None of those who reported having sex had used a condom, and none of the sexually active children had only one sexual partner. This means that these children tend to practise risky sexual behavior. Since sex is offered as a transaction for money or emotional rewards like security, these children, particularly the girls, are forced to accept sexual behavior that is harmful to their health. Since they are already vulnerable, negotiating condom usage or practising safer sex becomes a virtual impossibility. Even if they are interested in using condoms, these are hardly available in Tanzania, and if they were to become available, it is very unlikely that street children would be able to afford them.

Although our informants did not report having suffered from sexually transmitted diseases, studies elsewhere in Tanzania confirm the rampant spread of such diseases among street children. In their study of the sexual experience of the street children of Mwanza in Tanzania, Rajani and Kudrati (1996) confirm that street children are particularly at risk from infection with HIV and other sexually transmitted diseases (STDs) for several reasons: the need to perform 'survival sex' or prostitution; greater freedom to experiment with sex; and lack of adult protection and socialization (Sibthorpe *et. al.,* 1995). This study noted that sex plays a much larger and more central role in the lives of street girls than of boys, especially after puberty. Rajani and Kudrati also noted that the incidence and recurrence of STDs were also proportionately much higher in girls compared with similarly physically mature boys. Eighty percent of the girls had STDs at least once, while 30% of boys were estimated to have experienced STDs during the same period (Rajani and Kudrati, 1996). Street girls are prone to prostitution because they have a much narrower range of options for earning a living (Rajani and Kudrati, 1996). Narratives from street girls themselves reflect a situation of hopelessness and helplessness:

> If I was a school girl, I could say, 'Don't bother me, I want my education.' If I had a business, I could say I was a businesswoman. If I lived in a home, then they would not think of me [sexually] because they would know I had parents (Rajani and Kudrati, 1996).

Under these circumstances, the girls lack assistance and alternative ways of life and are forced to adopt survival behavior which is a risk to their health and reduces their self-esteem. In addition, they risk being beaten and may experience rough sex, while others end up going unpaid for sexual services they have rendered. In general, their suffering is both physical and psychological. There is no doubt that in an era of rampant HIV/AIDS transmission, commercial sex as a survival strategy becomes a death strategy or a death ticket.

Street Life as an Urban Subculture of Survival and Suffering

Street children do not operate haphazardly in the urban environment. Different groups have different zones/areas in which they operate, and any interference by another group can cause serious trouble between the groups. This informal way of zoning areas of operation within the city limits competition for resources among the children and assures their survival. This means that street children are highly organized.

These children tend to follow the normal rhythms of urban life. They usually wake up in the morning and flood the streets in pursuit of their means of survival. Learning from the children's experience, it is certain that their urban movements are highly strategic. They frequently visit religious buildings during worship hours. They know where the churches, mosques, and other religious buildings are located and are familiar with the worshipping days and hours. They are well aware of important religious ceremonies like Easter, Christmas, Idd-el-Fitri, Maulid, and the Islamic holy month of fasting (Ramadhan). According to them, these ceremonies are associated with great prosperity. One boy explained the fortunes associated with these days in the following way:

We get a lot of clothes as presents, also money and food during these religious ceremonies. Most people become very generous and sympathetic with our situation and give a lot. We really enjoy these days. I wish there were more of them. This shows that street children's thinking is well organized, rational, and calculating.

Another example of street children's strategic movements whilst on the streets is their involvement with the police and other authorities. Most of the street children know the names of people from the police force and the city council. When asked how they knew the names of these people, the response from most of them was, "We deal with these people every day. They keep on chasing, harassing, beating and detaining us." One girl responded by saying: "We know them, and they know us too. They are both our friends and enemies! Sometimes they help us, but sometimes they harass and coerce us. You have to know how to live with them." Since 62% of the children stated that they had been involved in confrontations with the police more than twice, there is clear evidence that harassment by the police and civic authorities occurs.

Street children also know other areas which are important for their survival. Most of them consider streets which attract many tourists and areas near religious institutions as prosperous places. Some even know NGO offices that deal with street children. They are aware of the street children rehabilitation centers located in Dar es Salaam, but they consider these centers to be a kind of prison with tough and inhuman regulations. They stated emphatically that they would rather live on the streets than in such centers.

Street children are well aware of the risks and threats presented by the urban environment. Their perceptions of danger vary by age and gender. Some urban areas pose more danger to some social groups than others. Girls and young boys fear frequenting or spending their nights in areas where drunks are common. Most children also tend to avoid spending much time in areas that are frequently patrolled by police. The plight of street children is hard to imagine. Since most of these children hover on the periphery of other people's lives, most people regard them as inconsequential. The urban authorities view them as a menace to the city. They are invariably seen as people who commit crime, thereby inflaming desires to see them eliminated from the urban environment. They are branded with names like '*wadokozi*' or '*wachomoaji*' (pickpockets) or '*wahuni*' (hooligans) (Lugalla, 1995). According to section 176 of the Penal Code of Tanzania, street children are considered to be "Idle and Disorderly Persons" and are therefore subject to criminalization (Lugalla, 1995).

However, in-depth studies on street children reveal a different picture. The study by Rajani and Kudrati (1996) and our own study show that street children are more down-to-earth in terms of their survival strategies and are capable of evaluating themselves. They normally describe themselves as '*watemi, magangwe*' or '*watoto wa maskani,*' meaning tough, very strong, carefree people who hang out. Others call themselves 'Born-Town' or 'Born-Here-Here,' indicating that they are a product of the social system itself and are therefore familiar with and used to this "horrible" life.

The children's accounts reveal how they earn their living, their relations with each other, with police, with city or non-governmental organization officials, and with passers-by. They also reveal the dangers they face, the problems they experience, and what hopes they hold for their future. As with Rizzini et al.'s (1994) observation in Brazil, the Tanzanian children's stories show how mistaken some segments of society are in regarding the lives of these children as worthless. Street children try their best to earn an income in socially acceptable ways. They work as car washers, car guards, or as parking boys. Others have flooded the informal sector where they work as petty traders of a variety of items. Some work as shoe shiners, while others repair the pot-holes in the road in the hope of being rewarded by passing drivers. Those who fall victim to criminal adults become socialized to participate in activities which lack the approval of society like peddling drugs, petty thievery, prostitution, and other illicit ways of earning a living. In such cases, exploitation of child labor is clearly evident. It is very unfortunate that most research studies have difficulties obtaining in-depth information from these children.

Street children have their own ways of maintaining their identity and establishing their peer groups. They normally undergo intensive socialization and initiation processes in order to conform and adhere to specific forms of behavior and practices. Rajani and Kudrati (1996) have shown that *'kunyenga'* (a slang word meaning non-mutual anal penetrative sex) is practised by the street children of Mwanza as a form of initiation rite (a transitional stage in identity formation) which allows one to become a member of a group and gives one access to 'group secrets.' Their study shows how power, authority, law, and order is exercised and adhered to through these initiation rites. However strange this rite may appear, it nevertheless shows us how organized these children are and how they struggle in order to create their own identity and maintain social cohesion. Through this, they share not only information and survival strategies but also emotions. Their groups do not simply provide them with social cohesion, but act as forms of social networks through which information filters from one group of children to the other. These groups replace the family and provide the necessary social assistance which would otherwise have been provided by social networks within the family.

Street children use their groups in order to maintain love, affection, and protection among themselves. Elsewhere, studies have found that because of the conditions of violence and insecurity the children face in their families, they tend to look out mainly for themselves as individuals (Rajani and Kudrati, 1996). These studies have also underscored the support and training functions of street groups, particularly during initiation into street life. Our study has noted that street children in Dar es Salaam live and work in groups. This form of social organization makes life on the streets viable and manageable. Rajani and Kudrati (1996) have demonstrated how highly organized the street children of Mwanza town are. Their organization is modeled upon an idealized view of a family.

The groups of street children have leaders, and it seems that there are informal rules and regulations which require the members of a group to adhere to group leadership and ethics. Leaders are obeyed and highly respected. They play an essential role in protecting and guiding the group. It is the leaders who decide who should be recruited as a new member and who should not. They also perform the role of socializing new members. Via the influence of these leaders, newcomers undergo a variety of processes of social reorientation through which new norms and values which fit urban street life are inculcated and the former rural-oriented family values are disdained. Rajani and Kudrati's study and our own study show that age, physical strength, and length of time spent on the streets (briefly summarized as 'experience') tend to be the main determining factors of who becomes a leader. Street children seem to believe strongly in experience as a bank of wisdom.

Where Does Tanzania Go From Here?

Findings from this study show that many of the pressures forcing children to leave their families are due to economic conditions and family dynamics. This study and many others from all over the world confirm that street children come from desperate, chaotic, and poor families. The long-term strategy of solving this problem requires addressing the root-causes of poverty. But it is very unlikely that poverty alleviation will take place soon enough in Tanzania due to the ongoing severe social and economic crisis there. Abuse, domestic violence, and family disintegration are also among the most commonly cited factors that push children onto the streets. Thus, any intervention must look for possibilities of maintaining harmony and stability within the family by encouraging processes which foster dialogue, love, and affection rather than fights, conflicts, separation and divorce.

While reducing the increasing number of street children may be a long-term priority, in the meantime strategies which help to meet the immediate needs and priorities of street children are necessary. The urgent basic needs for these children include proper and reliable accommodation (shelter), assurance of good food, security (protection), and provision of medical and healthcare—both physical and mental. All focus group discussions reveal that these needs are important and urgent.

The children also know that lack of education and specific productive skills puts them in a more hopeless situation. Most of the children we interviewed demanded education and training in productive skills. The statement below is typical of most street children:

> Look here, my parents are very poor and that is why they did not send me to school. I am sure that if I was educated and had certain skills, I would not be living in this way. I am also sure that if I get some training now, I will be able to manage my own life more easily.

Such assertions confirm that street children know the means through which their life can be improved, but they lack the ability to achieve those means. It is important to understand that street children are not criminals, though some may participate in criminal acts as the only alternative for survival. They are the neediest persons in urban areas but the least assisted. In this case, policies which criminalize them as "idle and disorderly" are coercive policies which stem from the belief that street children are responsible for their situation. We need to be aware that children's remand homes are not a solution in that they do not rehabilitate the street children but simply deal with symptoms of the problem rather than the essential relations.

One way of establishing policies which would have a positive impact on the street children would be to involve the children themselves in developing the policies and strategies which are aimed at assisting them. Characterizing these children as passive actors is inaccurate. Communication between policy-makers, development and health planners, non-governmental and other grass-roots organizations, and the street children themselves is not only important but necessary, if we want to make sure that policies are realistic, down-to-earth, and can bring positive results to both the children and the urban environment as a whole.

As Rajani and Kudrati (1996: 315) have suggested, "We must learn how to avoid paternalism, cultivate real dialogue and listen to the children with respect." Respecting children means allowing them to participate in decision-making processes in matters which concern them and affect their daily lives on the streets. These are indeed difficult processes, taking into consideration the top-down approach in development planning which seems to be the norm in Tanzania. We need to be aware that street children, like other human beings, have experience and are knowledgeable. They know their needs and the problems they experience. They are also capable of planning their own strategies in order to surmount these problems. Official policies and other efforts interested in assisting these children must begin by acknowledging the power and usefulness of this experience and knowledge.

Research experience gathered at 'Kuleana [raising each other] Center' in Mwanza, Tanzania, confirms that recognizing street children's sexual desires as normal and healthy is an essential starting point for effective HIV and STD prevention among street children (Rajani and Kudrati, 1996). This means that we must begin by accepting and acknowledging the problems which street children experience and what they do in order to solve these problems. In designing policies aimed at assisting these children, we must understand that street children's decisions to leave their homes and migrate to cities are probably based on rational economic calculations of the advantages and disadvantages of remaining within the family networks in their rural areas or migrating. The need to improve their lives, experience alternative ways of living, and to escape from hostile family situations appear to be the predominant factors.

What seems to us to be the real challenge for policy planners is to work with these children in order to make their wishes a reality. They should be able to live well and in an urban environment which affirms their dignity, health, and security. It must be clear among policy planners that if street children are helped to a clearer understanding of the potential risks of street life and are trained to protect themselves, they can be empowered to improve their own well-being. We also need to recognize that although these children live alone and do not have contact with their parents or relatives, possibilities of reunion are not out of the question. Policies which simply focus on gathering street children into rehabilitation centers encourage the separation of these children from their homes and from their communities. Intervention strategies should aim at reuniting the children with their families. This means that policies or programs must include their families. These policies must be broad enough so that they also address the situation of rural poverty which the majority of these children have run away from.

It is necessary to differentiate between street children as a 'problem' and the 'problems' of street children. As far as Tanzania is concerned, it is clear that it is the socio-economic and political environment which is the problem. The phenomenon of street children is a result of this social system. It is the chronic poverty facing their rural areas in general, and families in particular, which produces a state of permanent tension in the lives of these children. A culture of consumerism, to which both the children and their parents, relatives, and friends have been exposed, compounds these socio-economic problems. This culture of consumerism contrasts greatly with conditions of abject poverty and squalor, and it motivates some of the children to seek alternative ways of life.

When the family home environment is full of conflict, deprivation, and loneliness, the companionship of peers or street gangs may indeed offer advantages—not the least of which is freedom from family demands and the wid effects of colonial history or social colonization. The picture that emerges from this is that family dynamics play an important role in expelling children from their homes. Studies from Brazil show that families with strained relationships which no longer operate as a collaborative unit, families with a low degree of social cohesion, and those which frequently resort to corporal punishment have a much higher tendency to produce street children (Rajani and Kudrati, 1996).

Long-term policies must therefore aim at fixing the system rather than fixing the children. As Knaul (1995[a]) has argued, normative categorizations of street children are useful in so far as they stress the need to develop tailored programs for particular groups of children at high risk. This study has noted the existence of many children on the streets of urban Tanzania. More work of this nature would provide better insights into the different kinds of street children in terms of where they come from, how they differ, the problems they experience and how they surmount them, and their survival strategies. Policies must distinguish between demeaning sources of income which jeopardize children's development like pick-pocketing, peddling drugs, begging, or prostitution, and those sources that are socially acceptable, like vending, hawking, scavenging, and cleaning or minding cars. Long-term programs must be community based. Community-based approaches are bound to provide better alternatives to the present strategy of institutionalizing children in rehabilitation centers where they are given food, shelter, and education. If community-based approaches incorporate the richness of the traditional African extended family, they can be of great help to children and their families because they can assist street children in getting access to basic subsistence and social services in their places of origin. There is a need for communities to become facilitators in the provision of children's priorities and needs. This is possible if the civil society is mobilized well. These approaches can also address the disadvantages parents and communities experience in a wider socio-economic framework.

Conclusion

Our study shows that the strategies used by street children are still inadequate in so far as meeting their basic needs are concerned. When one looks at their living conditions, they remain "horrible," and the government has been unable to address this situation. Street children use the existing public infrastructure in order to survive; they use street pavements for sleeping, for instance. But an on-the-spot observation of these pavements reveals how unclean they are. Garbage and all types of litter is found on them. If the city authorities could make sure that these pavements stay clean, they would indirectly be assisting these children a great deal. The same applies to public toilets and bathrooms. The public toilet system in Dar es Salaam has not functioned for the last ten years. Street children depend on these facilities in order to relieve themselves. Improving them would not only lead to a cleaner and more healthy urban environment, but in enabling the majority of the urban population to dispose of their human waste hygienically, it would decrease health expenditure related to illnesses from poor waste disposal. The same should be done to improve the availability of clean and reliable drinking and washing water in urban public kiosks. Urban development policy planners must make sure that they understand this survival subculture and must aim at planning for people rather than things like public parks and other recreation centers which can only remain clean if facilities for sanitation and the disposal of garbage and other solid waste are placed in them. A city management which does not believe in this form of planning ideology should not accuse the urban population of being unclean.

As in other developing countries, it is indisputable that poor children in urban Tanzania confront complex problems, but street children confront far more problems. Chronic poverty within families tends to create a vicious circle of poverty. Children of poor families drop out of school or do not go to school at all, like their parents. These children then run away from home and start working in the streets in demeaning jobs at a tender age, putting them at risk both physically and emotionally. As the socio-economic crisis continues, there is an urgent need to address the broad social and economic issues more aggressively. Thorough studies of street children in Tanzania are just beginning. These studies are very important as far as policy formulation and intervention strategies are concerned. They help to identify children in distress, where they come from, how they survive, and their sources of strength—all of which can assist social and economic planners to devise better support systems. More serious work is still needed. Future studies of Tanzania also need to look at gender differences among street children. Such studies are important and urgent. Children of all kinds constitute the nation of the future, and neglecting them amounts to abandoning the health and welfare of generations to come.
Aug. 1997).

N.B.: This chapter was originally published by the *International Journal of Urban and Regional Research,* Vol. 23, No. 2, 1999.

Chapter Five

The Impact of HIV/AIDS on Women and Children: A Case Study of Morogoro Region, Tanzania

Sylvia F. Kaaya, Jessie K. Mbwambo, Sebalda Leshabari

Introduction

A total of 53,247 cumulative cases were reported in Tanzania by the end of 1994. Of these cases, 2,572 were from the Morogoro Region, placing it in the ninth position in terms of regions reporting cases of AIDS in the country in 1994. There has been a gradual increase in the cumulative case rate in the region; the urban areas have been most affected, but rural areas are also increasingly reporting AIDS cases, particularly in areas with high levels of interaction and mobility between and within indigenous populations and migrant workers. This chapter reports on an exploratory rapid assessment of the impact of HIV/AIDS at the family level with a focus on women and children. It will also suggest potential areas of intervention, taking into consideration available resources. This chapter will describe the HIV/AIDS epidemic in Tanzania and place the epidemic in Morogoro Region within this wider context. The study area and methods used to collect information will be described prior to a report on the perceptions of informants on the extent of the epidemic and its impact on lives. This report will be conducted at an experiential level using illustrative family case studies. The implications arising from the information are discussed.

Epidemiology of HIV/AIDS in Tanzania with a Focus on Morogoro Region

Since the first AIDS cases were clinically diagnosed in three patients in 1983 in the Kagera Region, there has been a steady increase in reported AIDS cases in the country (NACP, 1995). By 1995, the cumulative number of AIDS cases reported stood at 81,498. The Morogoro region, with a cumulative number of AIDS cases of 4,605, ranked seventh in the country. These figures should be interpreted with caution as only one in four to six

AIDS cases are actually reported due to lack of diagnostic facilities and other logistical problems in health-care delivery (NACP, 1995).

The National AIDS Control Programme expects to receive data from 24 HIV/AIDS sentinel surveillance sites distributed in 11 regions of the country. In 1995, however, such data was forthcoming from 11 sites distributed in 3 regions and revealed sero-prevalence rates amongst antenatal clinic attendees that ranged from 5.1% to 27.2%. Though the Morogoro region does not have an established sentinel surveillance site for HIV/AIDS, the anonymous screening of antenatal attendees does occur at one rural based missionary hospital. Hospital records indicated an increase in sero-prevalence from 4% in 1991 to 14% by 1994 (Turiani Missionary Hospital Records, 1995). Sero-prevalence amongst blood donors, though misleading, can assist in giving some idea of the HIV sero-prevalence rates in other areas of the Morogoro region. Data were available from the office of the Morogoro Regional AIDS Control Coordinator that revealed a regional average sero-prevalence amongst blood donors of 4.4% in 1994. The highest rates were in donors from the Ulanga district (7.9%), and the lowest rates were amongst those from the Kilosa district (0.8%). Orphans resulting from the death of one or both parents from AIDS constitute a significant social problem in terms of their sheer numbers. The most recent estimate of children under the age of 18 years who have lost one or both parents stands at 200,000 (NACP, 1995). The Morogoro region was placed third with regards to the number of AIDS orphans in the 20 regions of the country.

The spread of AIDS in Tanzania, as in other countries in Sub-Saharan Africa, is predominantly heterosexual, accounting for 90% of disease transmission (Heydmann and Edstrom, 1991; Mhalu, F., 1993). The increasing prevalence of HIV infection is reflected in the increase in vertical transmission to infants. Assuming a 30% HIV transmission rate, the percentage of newborn babies that will be infected is up to 9.8% in various antenatal clinic surveillance sites. Blood transfusion and injections may have been an important mode of transmission, but this is now under reasonable control as blood screening facilities become widely available (Dolmans *et. al.*, 1992). Cultural practices and remedies associated with the use of communal cutting instruments amongst traditional healers (in tribal skin marking, tattooing, incisions for introducing medication, and circumcision) are frequent, and it remains unclear as to what extent this potential blood-blood contact contributes to HIV transmission.

Several studies in various parts of the country indicate that the transmission of HIV infection is highest in urban and peri-urban settings, particularly when these settings are situated along main truck routes (Lwihula *et. al.*, 1993; Killewo *et. al.*, 1994). Furthermore, it appears phases of increasing HIV sero-prevalence exist in rural areas as peri-urban centers develop and migrants in these centers integrate with rural communities. Though there has been little work done on the determinants of the AIDS epidemic in the Morogoro region, studies have been conducted elsewhere in the country, and identified determinants will be reviewed. Lwihula, *et. al.* (1993), note that in rural communities, cultural and socio-economic factors, together with sexual behavior and practice factors are intertwined in complex interactions that would allow for HIV transmission should the virus be introduced. These include, amongst others, increased mobility related to trade activities, sexual networking, and the struggle for female economic autonomy in male-dominated societies that is often associated with sex for money activities (Mnyika *et. al.*, 1994; Culdwick, 1938; Larsson, 1991). In settings where marriage is understood in the context of social structures and clan continuity, childbearing has special significance, and infertility is indirectly linked to HIV transmission. Infertile women are often divorced, and the subsequent struggle for survival is often associated with complex patterns of sexual networking that often include unsafe sexual practices with implications for HIV transmission (Larsson, 1991).

There are studies indicating that prevailing local explanations for HIV/AIDS may in fact be prohibit people taking preventive action towards reducing transmission of the virus. Although there are indications that knowledge of the cause and transmission of HIV/AIDS is high, this theoretical knowledge is not often translated into experiential realities. What exactly occurs during the sexual act that leads to transmission, that is, the mechanisms of transmission, remain a mystery to many. There is also a lack of distinction between being infected by the HIV virus and suffering from AIDS. Hence, a person who has multiple sexual partners and appears healthy may raise questions regarding the validity of the reported threat caused by HIV infection. Reported lay explanations by Lwihula *et. al.* (1993), which include a perception that AIDS only affects selected susceptible people while others are immune to the disease regardless of their sexual contacts, are understandable given the level at which HIV/AIDS knowledge currently exists in communities. In many parts of the country, AIDS has been thought to be caused by bewitchment, breaching of cultural taboos, imported clothes, and the failure of America to control its biological warfare experiments (Lwihula *et. al.*, 1993; Killewo *et. al.*, 1994; Leshabari *et. al.*, 1995).

There is very little documented information on the impact at the family level of the HIV epidemic in Tanzania. In this country, as in many African societies, when a family member falls ill, close relatives— particularly females—are involved in advising on home remedies, initially, and later, as the case may be, on over-the-counter drugs. When such remedies fail and resources outside the home are required, males and elders within the family and clan are involved in the decision to seek help from traditional healers or allopathic health services. For chronic illnesses such as AIDS, females within the immediate and extended family remain the main care providers for ill members (Leshabari *et. al.*, 1995). This may have several implications as women are also relied on for activities involving economic production at household level and within society as well as childbearing. It is unclear to what extent the expected roles and responsibilities of females within families are affected when, in addition to their normal activities, women are required to provide care for chronically ill persons. Other groups within communities that may also be involved in providing assistance to families with a chronically ill member include religious institutions and women's groups—the latter often providing practical and emotional support for bereaved families. Village governments in some areas of the country have adopted these traditional women's support groups during the process of mourning the loss of a village member (Leshabari *et. al.*, 1996).

Several authors have reported on the potential impact of H1V/AIDS on productivity in sub-Saharan Africa (Carswell, 1988; Hunter, 1990). Every death from AIDS of an adult within the productive age group results in the loss of 20 man or 40 woman years of work; the figure is higher for women who tend to leave the work force at an older age (Carswell, 1988). Cultural practices in many societies require a period of mourning ranging from three days to a week, depending on how closely related one is to the deceased. When mortality is high in an area, the required period of mourning in which the community participates further increases the loss in productive man-hours. In an area with high HIV sero-prevalence, it was reported that, in recent years, the number of people requesting leave from employment to attend the funerals of close relatives was on the increase (Leshabari *et. al.*, 1995). These losses may be particularly catastrophic in the agricultural sector as they are not so obvious as the loss of productive man-hours in the industrial and service sectors despite having an immediate impact on affected families and societies in many agriculturally based subsistence economies. Informants in studies in rural areas of the Mbeya and Kagera regions, where the HIV/AIDS epidemic has caused high mortality, note decreased production of both food and cash crops (Lwihula *et. al.*, 1993; Leshabari *et. al.*, 1995). They attributed this primarily to diminishing performance as a result of frequent bouts of illness or death which creates gaps in the available labor force.

Although there have been changes in many of the traditions governing inheritance, widow inheritance, in which the brother of the deceased has conjugal rights over the widow and the responsibility to provide care for her and her children, is practised in some areas of the country. The emphasis is primarily placed on property remaining within the clan of the deceased, even when such property may have been acquired with the assistance of the wife when the deceased was alive. The fact that the deceased may have died of AIDS does not appear to be an issue in such situations, and this may have implications in HIV/AIDS transmission dynamics. High mortality has magnified problems that existed in traditional inheritance practices and their implications for women and children in these times of cultural change. In general, few people in Tanzania prepare a testament prior to death to ensure the security of their immediate family as this was a traditional responsibility of the extended family. This is the case even when death is anticipated. Women deprived of their legal rights after the death of a spouse are reported to be hesitant to use legal measures that would ensure their economic security. This is due to a combination of a lack of resources to follow through the intricate legal issues and fear of reprisal of a supernatural nature (such as angering the shades/ancestors) arising from breaching culturally constructed rules and systems of inheritance (Leshabari *et. al.*, 1995).

The Study Area

The Morogoro Region occupies 73,039 sq. kilometers in central Tanzania and is approximately 8.2% of the total land surface of mainland Tanzania. Morogoro town, the regional headquarters, is a three hour drive from the city of Dar es Salaam, situated on the main road to countries in the South and to Burundi and Rwanda in the North West. Administratively, the Region has five districts (Morogoro Municipality, Morogoro Rural, Kilosa, Kilombero, and Ulanga), 30 divisions, 137 wards, and 457 villages. The region has a total population of 1,222,737 of whom 50.5% are women.

Ninety per cent of the economy of the region depends on agricultural and animal husbandry activities involving 94% of the population. A small proportion (6%) of the population is employed in the public or private sector or may be self-employed in trade activities. The main food crops are maize, rice, yams, and millet, while cash crops produced in the region are cotton, coconuts, cashew nuts, sugar cane, and various types of vegetables. Other economic activities in the region include industries, fisheries, and mining. Gemstones are mined in the Ulanga district, while the Kilombero district has several sugarcane plantations and sugar processing factories. Large numbers of transient migrants who work on plantations or seek fortunes in the mines characterize both of these two districts. The indigenous population sets up "mini-settlements" to provide services such as accommodation and food, as well as the recreational activities of migrant workers. The region's gross domestic product in 1994 was 3,516 million shillings (equivalent to USD 5,409.00 at an exchange rate of 650 TSh. to one USD). The main economic problems identified by regional planning officers are limited regional food stores due to low agricultural productivity and declining performance and the closure of major industries resulting in increased unemployment.

Children under five years of age account for 20.3% of the total regional population. Infant mortality is above the national average of 115/1000, and between 3.5 and 5.8% of children under five are severely malnourished (UNICEF, 1990). The rate of malnutrition amongst under-fives in the region has declined since the onset of UNICEF sponsored Child Survival Protection and Development (CSPD) program interventions in the early 1990's. With the advent of the HIV/AIDS epidemic in the region, it is anticipated that these program achievements will decline as deficiencies in diagnostic facilities will not allow for distinctions to be made between pediatric AIDS and severe forms of malnutrition. An anticipated increased rate of childhood morbidity/mortality resulting from loss of caring adults and the rechanneling of available household resources to the care of AIDS affected family members is also an area of concern. The authors conducted a rapid assessment with the aim of describing the impact of HIV/AIDS at the family level, particularly as it relates to women and children. The study was also intended to collect information on community perceptions of treatment and care options and choices, as well as perceived difficulties in the care of those with HIV/AIDS in families.

Methodology

Case study areas were selected in rural and urban areas in the region. Following communication with the Regional AIDS Control Coordinator and taking into consideration logistical issues related to travel, both an urban

(Mafiga Chini ward, Morogoro Municipality) and a rural (Mlali ward, Morogoro Rural District) site were selected for the case study.

The Case Study Sites

Urban Site

Mafiga Chini ward has a population of 3,850, 1,994 being women and children. The ward has 1,000 households with about 3.7 occupants per household. The ward is ethnically heterogeneous as a result of recent immigrants into a newly developing urban area. The immigrants are both homeowners and tenants. Urban agricultural activities in the ward include the cultivation of green vegetables and maize, though the plots farmed are small as the Morogoro Municipality has subdivided the area into residential plots. Other sources of income amongst residents include employment in the civil service, parastatal and private organizations in the town, as well as involvement in petty trade activities such as shopkeeping, brewing and selling traditional alcoholic beverages, buying and selling charcoal, as well as selling cooked foods. Many of the employed workers also cultivate small plots of land within the ward or on its outskirts in order to augment their income.

The predominant health problems in the ward identified by ward leaders include malaria, diarrheal diseases, HIV/AIDS, and dermatological conditions amongst children. The ward is well served by social amenities such as electricity and piped water supply in the majority of households. Most of the houses are built of burnt brick or concrete block walls with corrugated iron sheet roofing. The road infrastructure is poor, with no all-weather road surfaces. Two primary schools, one nursery school, and a public dispensary serve the ward in addition to a dispensary run by the Tanzania Parents Association (TPA) and a hospital run by Chinese doctors. There were ten bars, three hotels, and several guesthouses in the area. Generally, people living in Mafiga Chini, despite coming from different ethnic backgrounds, lived as a community, interrelating well and helping each other at times of crisis such as illness and death.

The Rural Site

Mlali ward is located in Morogoro Rural District, a 30-minute drive from the center of Morogoro town. The ward population is 2,764, with 1,260 females and 56.5% children under the age of fifteen. Mlali has a total of 532 households with an average of 5.2 members per household. The Waluguru were the predominant ethnic group, and 25% were from other ethnic groups in the country.

Agricultural activities in the area include cultivation of millet, maize, rice, cassava, and sweet potatoes. Large-scale farming of tomatoes, one of the newer major cash crops, has developed in response to difficulties experienced by villagers in negotiating terms with cooperative unions on the growing and marketing of the more traditional cotton crop. Two large-scale farms provide employment for a few of the villagers. The top five medical conditions in the village were malaria, anemia, intestinal worms, skin conditions like scabies, and more recently, AIDS. The village is well served with social amenities, though very few villagers could afford electricity in their homes. The village had six primary schools, a dispensary, a court, and a number of shops and guesthouses.

Data Collection Methods

The Regional AIDS Control Coordinator (RACC) was our point of entry into the region. At the regional and district level, during formative interviews with the RACC, key sectors dealing with AIDS control activities were identified and formative interviews conducted with representatives from these sectors. HIV/AIDS community-based counselors were involved in AIDS control activities at the community level. They visited affected households, suggested participants for focus group discussions, and were assisted by community leaders in the selected case study areas.

Formative Interviews

Formative interviews were held with 13 informants at the regional and district levels. At the regional level, interviews were conducted with the Regional AIDS Coordinator (RACC), the Regional Maternal and Child Health Coordinator (RMCHC), the Regional Social Welfare Officer (RSWO), and the Regional Cultural Officer (RCO). Due to the links between poverty and HIV/AIDS, interviews were also conducted with the Regional Community Development Officer (RCDO) and two Planning Officers associated with the Child Survival, Protection and Development program (CSPD).

At district level, informants included the District Medical Officer (DMO) for Morogoro Rural, the District AIDS Control Coordinators (DACC) for Morogoro Rural and Urban Districts, the District Cultural Officer (DCO) for Morogoro Urban District, and two HIV/AIDS community counselors working in Morogoro Urban District and Turiani ward. Information collected was on available data and perceptions regarding the extent of the epidemic and its impact on women and children.

Focus Group Discussions

Focus group discussions (FGD) were held in the Mlali and Mafiga wards. Age was considered an important variable in the selection of group participants. Youth (15-24 years) and adult (30-49 years) group discussions were conducted separately. Due to the exploratory nature of the study, two groups were thought to be sufficient per age group, hence 4 groups were held in each area. The size of the groups was set at 8-12 participants. Participants were recruited in each of the study areas by the researchers while conducting household visits in selected hamlets, assisted by community-based HIV/AIDS counselors and the chairpersons of hamlets. The purpose of the study was explained, and participants were recruited only after they had understood and agreed to be involved in the study. The following criteria were used in selecting participants:

i) Participants in each group should be, as much as possible, strangers to each other;
ii) Participants should give informed consent (verbal) to participate;
iii) Age range 15 - 24 for 2 groups and 30 - 49 for the remaining 2 groups;
iv) Participants should be in a marital relationship (legal or informal). This was in order to allow group members to discuss freely issues related to sexual behavior.

Household visits were terminated after 32 males and 32 females had been recruited, aged within the two above-mentioned age categories. From the list of volunteers provided, in each of the two case study sites, 16 people (8 females and 8 males) aged between 15-24 and a similar number aged between 30-49 were grouped into four groups. Dates, venue, and time were agreed upon with each group for the discussions. The Mafiga Chini focus groups were held at the municipal dispensary, while the Miali focus groups were conducted at a communal meeting hall. Information collected in the focus group discussions covered 3 themes: local explanatory models for HIV/AIDS, perceptions of the impact of HIV/AIDS at the household level amongst women and children, and perceived needs in households affected by HIV/AIDS.

Household and In-depth Individual Interviews

Community HIV/AIDS counselors were approached to introduce the study team to potential clients from whom study households could be selected. Due to the sensitive nature of being affected by HIV/AIDS, the only criteria for the inclusion of a household was informed consent from the head of household or his/her representative. Two urban households in the Chamwino area of the Morogoro Municipality and 2 rural households in the Mlali and Turiani wards were selected for the household and in-depth individual interviews. In-depth individual interviews were conducted with the main care provider in each of the selected households. The main care provider was defined as the person who provided actual physical care for the ill family member. Information on changes in roles and responsibilities as a result of being affected by HIV/AIDS, as well as changes in household income and the perceived burden of care within such families, was collected from the households. The main care provider was also interviewed alone to assess perceived needs.

Changes in Instruments

As a result of information collected during the formative interviews, minor changes were made to the focus group discussion guide. These included being more specific in the exploration of changes in inheritance traditions over time, particularly as these traditions related to the support of widows and orphans. This was because it was observed that traditional patterns of inheritance had changed, perhaps due to the influence of religion and cultural diffusion.

RESULTS

Composition of the FGDs

Focus groups were composed of 12 participants each. The mean age of adult participants was 35 years while that of youths was 23 years. The majority of the urban participants were employed or engaged in petty trade activities (16 of 24), while 20 of the 24 rural participants were subsistence farmers, the remaining were either teachers or village government workers. Despite the gender mix in the group discussions, group dynamics developed rapidly, and lively discussions occurred in all the groups, though women sometimes had to be prompted to participate.

Perceptions on the Extent of HIV/AIDS in Morogoro Region

All the informants during the formative interviews expressed concern regarding the rapid spread of HIV/AIDS in the region. HIV/AIDS sero-prevalence statistics from the routine anonymous screening of antenatal attendees at missionary hospitals were noted to be more reliable as HIV screening kits became more consistently available. Informants also noted that more people were suffering from tuberculosis and that there had been an increase in adult mortality compared with previous years. A HIV/AIDS community counselor from a missionary hospital reported that 62 children had lost one or both parents from HIV-related mortality between 1992-1994. Most of the informants anticipated an increase in vertical transmission as HIV sero-prevalence increased amongst women of childbearing age.

HIV infection appeared to be more prevalent in urban settings and trade foci (gemstone mining areas, sugar-cane plantations, areas surrounding large factories as in Mtibwa, and at Kilombero). However, most of the informants were aware that the disease was also affecting rural inhabitants. Although the three main tribal groups in the region are the Wakaguru, Waluguru, and Wapogoro, informants noted that extensive immigration into the region since independence has resulted in a lot of cultural heterogeneity. Migrant workers employed on the sugar plantations as well as immigrants in the rapidly developing trade foci enter the region. A major highway traverses a large part of the region with trade developing around truck stops, further increasing the interaction of indigenous populations with people from outside the region.

The reported interaction and mobility is perceived as a "double-edged sword." While opportunities for employment and income-generating activities are enhanced by the mushrooming of trade, the nature and context of sexual partnership which develops in these settings is perceived as setting the stage for behavior which increases the risk of HIV transmission such as excessive alcohol use, promiscuity, and commercial sex networking.

Local Explanatory Models for HIV/AIDS

Participants in all the focus group discussions (FGD) agreed that there was an awareness in communities of HIV/AIDS as a sexually transmitted disease. Discussions revealed that adults (30+ years) in both urban and rural areas perceived HIV/AIDS to be a big problem in their areas, while the youth noted it was a problem in the region, but not necessarily where they resided. Many of these youths agreed the disease was a threat that interfered in their relationships with the opposite sex by generating fear of possible infection.

Adults in both rural and urban areas agreed that one contracted AIDS through sexual contact with an infected partner. Discussion of HIV transmission in the youth groups was often associated with themes related to morality. Hence transmission risks were associated with extramarital sexual encounters, irrespective of the number of partners, and "amoral" sexual behavior described by the Kiswahili terms "*zinaa*" (indiscriminate sexual intercourse) and "*umalaya*" (promiscuity). In both adult and youth FGDs, participants were unclear exactly how the sexual act could transmit HIV infection, suggesting either an inadequacy in health messages being provided or a lack of synthesis. Participants in all the youth discussions did not feel a person was at risk if they had a steady partner who appeared healthy. Health educative discussions at the end of the discussions indicated that it was possible for people to understand the mechanisms of HIV transmission.

Myths relating to HIV/AIDS causality, transmission, and prevention were reported in the youth group discussions. There was consensus in one such group that transmission of HIV infection could occur through eating uncooked foods bought from street vendors such as salads. Transmission was explained by ingestion of foods contaminated by a street vendor who was HIV positive. One's own urine, drunk early in the morning, was reported to be a preventive measure against HIV/AIDS infection in another young adult group discussion. These misconceptions regarding transmission and prevention of HIV did not arise in any of the adult group discussions.

In all the FGDs, participants agreed that it was difficult to determine whether a person with a chronic illness was suffering from AIDS. It was further noted that persons who knew they were HIV sero-positive rarely disclosed such information to others for fear of being shunned and neglected. Peripheral health facilities such as health centers and dispensaries do not have facilities for screening, and even when AIDS is suspected, health workers are reluctant to reveal their suspicions to patients. There was consensus that when AIDS is suspected by health workers, patients are told vague causes for their symptoms or that the tests have revealed no disease. Suspicions of the possibility of HIV/AIDS infection are often created by several factors amongst relatives. These include a diagnoses of Tuberculosis, "TB ya mifupa"(Tuberculosis of the bones), or "malaria sugu"(chronic malaria), as well as a prescription for a mild analgesic when a patient appears very ill. Despite these suspicions, relatives rarely act on them. Informants from the adult discussion groups in both the rural and urban groups were in agreement that this lack of action is because few people are prepared to accept that a relative has AIDS. Lack of certainty on the diagnosis from health care providers feeds into this attitude of silence. In all but two of the group discussions, there was agreement that chronic ill health and lack of a definitive diagnosis results in seeking traditional systems of care where a more acceptable supernatural causality with greater potential for intervention can be provided. This, however, was not specific for

HIV/AIDS, but a common response to chronic illness in the area.

Despite the reported silence or difficulty in acknowledging HIV positive sero-status in family members, it was clear from all the groups that an awareness of how AIDS presents existed in the community. There was agreement that a vague diagnosis from a health facility, coupled with one or more of the following symptoms: chronic ill health, recurrent fever, weight loss, general body weakness, abscesses, and skin ulceration, often results in rumors that the ill person has AIDS. This was reported with a lot of sadness in the adult FGD while the youth tended to be more humorous and jocular in their accounts, suggesting either the confidence youths have in their own invincibility or a coping strategy to counteract fear of HIV/AIDS.

Stigma and HIV/AIDS in Morogoro

There were particular patterns that emerged regarding attitudes towards HIV/AIDS and the impact of the disease as perceived by participants in the focus group discussions. In all the groups, there was agreement that attitudes towards HIV/AIDS were largely negative. The disease is considered to be shameful and related to promiscuity and amoral behavior. Several issues arose relating to themes of stigma and its impact at the household level amongst those affected by HIV/AIDS. Despite an awareness that heterosexual transmission is the main mode by which the disease is spread, there is still a fear of transmission from touching or even breathing the same air a sick person. As a result, there is a lot of anxiety amongst caregivers and neighbors, often manifest by an avoidance of any close contact with ill persons. Participants in five group discussions noted that, at times, emotional support may not be welcomed in affected families as neighbors and friends may visit out of curiosity rather than concern for the ill health of a fellow human being.

Emerging categories relating to stigma and HIV/AIDS were also evident in the formative interviews. A counselor gave examples of households whose members were avoided by villagers because of fear that the whole family was infected following an AIDS related death. Such attitudes, he noted, increase the burden of care in affected households. In the household case studies, though a sense of being rejected/ostracized by the community was alluded to, it was not clear whether the reasons were a perceived economic burden or an aversion to household members caring for an AIDS victim. This is demonstrated in one of the urban household interviews summarized below as case study 1.

Case Study 1: (Urban)*

MS is a 38 year-old grandmother and a widow who lives in the Chamwino area of Morogoro Municipality. She lives in her own mud and wattle 4-roomed house with two of her four children. Saidi is 19 and Amina is 21, and three grandchildren. MS has not been feeling well for about a year, and attributes her ill health to an attack of typhoid and loss of her oldest daughter from AIDS, four months prior to the interview. She has no source of income, and depends on financial assistance from her two independent older daughters who live away from home and are relatively consistent in the money they send each month. When her husband died, MS refused to be inherited by her brother-in-law who had a large family who depended entirely on his financial support. Amongst her grandchildren is Asia who was orphaned after her mother's death from AIDS, and is two and a half years and fortunately healthy. MS worries, however, about Shanifu, Amina's son, who is malnourished and more recently her son, Saidi, had herpes zooster infection. Although Saidi and Amina are both employed, MS has no control over what they contribute towards food in the household. She has had a difficult year caring for her daughter and is depressed and looks older than her age. She receives moral as well as material support from her brother-in-law but minimal assistance from neighbors or friends. Many of her friends are no longer visiting her but she is not sure why. MS has heard rumors that her daughter had AIDS, and her symptoms prior to her death (episodic fevers, frequent bouts of diarrhea and severe weight loss) are suggestive. Amina, however, strongly believes that her sister had cancer. MS feels they should have sought help from traditional healers, and feels guilty that she was unable to access such care despite acknowledging her financial limitations. She has limited contact with her own biological family, and constantly worries about her ability to continue taking care of her orphaned granddaughter. She wonders "what will happen if my daughter in Dar es Salaam can no longer send money?"

The above case study highlights issues relating to loss and mourning, uncertainty regarding cause of illness and death, and diminished support from neighbors and friends. The emotional toll from caring for an ill daughter until her untimely death is evident. MS's anxieties over her ability to take care of her orphaned granddaughter mask the unspoken fear "is my grand daughter also infected?" This was implied in her insistence that the child was "luckily" healthy and was never explicitly stated during the interview. Female family

Note: The names in case studies are not the real ones.

members who take on caring roles for ill relatives were reported by the community-based counselors interviewed to be often depressed, exhausted by frequent anxieties including trying to meet the ill person's needs and fear for their own HIV sero-status. They also noted that, should a partner of a person with AIDS want to be tested for HIV, often the lack of sufficient HIV screening kits would prohibit it.

More possible evidence for stigma is demonstrated by a case study of a 43 year-old person living with AIDS who had difficulty disclosing his HIV status to his wife and family. The summary of this case study is outlined in case study 2 below:

Case Study 2 (Urban)

WM is a 43 year-old male who resides in Chamwino ward with his wife and seven of their nine children, four of whom are below the age fifteen. WM had a serious chest infection in 1992, when he was screened and tested positive for HIV. He left home after being informed of his sero-status, and only returned 2 years later after his health deteriorated and he could no longer work. He has been unable to disclose his sero-status to his wife, and claims to be abstinent. A six-month old child in the family suggests that during his absence his wife had another child. He retired from his job in June of 1994, having worked for twenty-three years. The family lives in an uncompleted six-roomed house constructed with cement blocks that they own. His retirement benefits were used to begin the construction, but he has since sold many of his assets to pay for drugs he has required over the past two years. A pit latrine that collapsed during the rainy season has not been repaired, as there is no money to buy the logs to lay on the latrine floor. WM's health is currently poor. His wife looks relatively healthy, has no physical complaints but looks depressed and frequently avoids eye contact. All the children except for Selemani who is four years of age, appear healthy. Selemani shows signs malnutrition. He is very thin, has hair changes and a protruding abdomen.

WM's wife has stopped working as she has a young child and the patient to care for. She has not been able to attend to her farm work this year. Increasingly the three older children, whose ages range between 12 and 18 years, are taking on more house work and money generating activities like selling groundnut to help their mother. Dua, who is nine years old, has not yet started school, as there is no money for his enrolment and fees. WM's family visited regularly during the initial stages of his illness, but they stopped coming once they suspected he might have AIDS.

WM returned home in the terminal stages of his illness. Though still unable to disclose his HIV sero-status to his wife, we were informed by the counselor visiting the family that rumors that he suffers from AIDS had already circulated, and his relatives had immediately stopped visiting and offering support. His wife, the main care provider, was unable to explain the abandonment by her husband's relatives, though this was keenly felt. She did, however, note that his relatives had in the past relied on her husband for financial support.

In both of the two case studies, the immediate economic impact of HIV/AIDS at the household level is demonstrated. Decrease in household income results both from the lower productivity of able-bodied adults due to increased caring roles as well as diversion of available resources for the purchase of drugs. The case studies demonstrate concerns that were raised in formative interviews regarding economic impacts at the household level when affected by HIV/AIDS. In most of the formative interviews, it was noted that the limited resources available to households are used in a search for reasons why a family member has been infected or for a possible cure from numerous traditional healers. Often, this entails the cost of traveling long distances to make contact with a recommended healer and the cost of the upkeep of the ill person and an escorting family member in addition to treatment costs. Informants also noted that those affected are in the prime of their lives, and the family depend on their income. Loss of a job as well as loss of productive man-hours through illness means that a major source of family income is eroded.

The Psychological Toll on Women and Children Affected by HIV/AIDS

In the above examples, the potential stress on women who are caring for loved ones suffering from AIDS can take many forms. In addition to the fears generated by the progressive deterioration of the loved one's physical health and the arduous tasks of providing care, underlying fears regarding transmission as well as dealing with financial demands in a setting of decreasing support from family, neighbors, and friends creates additional stress. The psychological impact on children when either of the parents became ill from AIDS was an emerging theme in the household interviews. Children have been noted to be tense, anxious, and fearful, and in some cases, school performance drops. This impact on children is demonstrated by case study three reported below. However, no data exists on the extent of emotional reactions or the rate of school dropouts amongst children in HIV/AIDS affected households. In the four households studied, despite all the households having school-aged children, only two had children going to school. In the rural household, there were older independent children who were taking care of the educational needs of the youngest child in the family. One of the urban households had failed to enroll a child in school due to financial constraints attributed to the expense of providing care. Also evident in the two urban case studies and case study four is the presence of malnutrition in the younger members of the family.

The distress of the female care providers was evident in this case study, as were the emotional effects on the younger children. However, due to perceived obligations, many are willing to provide care. In this particular situation, there were five relatives residing in the home in addition to her four children. The degree of support offered by the presence of extended family members in the home needs, however, to be balanced against available resources.

Case Study 3 (Rural)

SS is a 44 year-old widow, head of household with six children, two of whom are below the age of 15 years. She has been bedridden and mute for the last four weeks, lying in the back room of her four-roomed burnt brick house in Miali village. She is surrounded by her mother and four female cousins from an adjacent village who have been living in her home and taking care of her for the past three weeks. Her brother arrived from Morogoro a week ago with her older children who are independent and live in Dar-es-Salaam and Morogoro.

One of her female cousins and her brother have been informed by the Rural Medical Aid (RMA) who works in the village dispensary that she probably suffers from AIDS, and does not have access to HIV screening kits. Care is currently home-based, and three days prior to our visit she had been hydrated with intravenous fluids, after having yet another bout of diarrhea. SS's female cousins take turns to turn her regularly to avoid bedsores. The RMA had visited with the RACC a day before our visit to provide gloves and a plastic sheet to keep the bedding dry. One of the cousins asks, "what do the gloves mean, could we also get this disease?" Her female relatives lament about their "*shambas*" (farms) which they have been unable to tend for the past three weeks. Some of them have husbands who will take care of the crop but one has no husband. They ask each other, "What of our children and grandchildren at home? Are they well?" One of them gets up from the interview to check on the food they are cooking for the two younger ones who are about to come back from school. One of the cousins notes, "it is hard for us to come and care for her but it is an obligation, she is our younger sister."

Another notes that every time Saida (10 years old) comes back from school, she creeps quietly into the house and stands by the door to her mother's room where she cries silently. She has to be coerced to go in and say hello to her mother. After the interview, the cousin who has been informed of the diagnosis pulls one of the members of the research team aside and asks, "do you also think it is AIDS? If it is, please help me to tell her children as they feel that we do not provide enough care and that we should send her to another traditional healer." SS passed away two days later.

During the formative interviews, counselors noted that visiting extended family members who come to assist in the care of the ill family member may be many, and they increase the demand for food and drink in affected households already desperately short of financial and material resources. This was evident in this case study where several of MS's relatives had moved from their own homes to come and assist in her care.

Case Study 4 (Rural)

MI is 64 years of age and is the head of a household situated in Madizini village in Mtibwa. She is providing care for her widowed stepdaughter MM who is 27 years old and has AIDS. The family lives in a compound with five other houses that belong to other members of the clan. The houses are made of mud walls and are thatched with grass. Around the houses are orange, coconut and mango trees from which fruit is harvested and sold to other villagers during relevant seasons. They also have a few groves of sugar cane. The whole family appears healthy except for MM and her two-year-old son, Edgar. Edgar has moderate to severe malnutrition and is currently receiving treatment and food supplements from a missionary hospital.

MM married her late husband ten years ago at the age of 17 and is mother to two daughters who are seven and five, and a son who is two. MM has had recurrent anemia for the last four years at times necessitating blood transfusion. During the same period her late husband developed recurring illnesses and was retired from his place of work on medical grounds. MM and her husband left for his home village after his retirement but within a week of arriving there, her husband committed suicide. After the loss of her husband, MM had another bout of severe anemia that required blood transfusion. On discharge from hospital, her neighbors helped sell all her personal effects to raise money for her bus fare back to her home village in Mtibwa. She returned home in a very poor physical state about three months prior to the interview. Her family is aware of MM's positive HIV sero-status and that she has AIDS. They are very supportive and accepting of her state though they wish a cure could be found to ensure that their beloved one does not die.

Though they know that the illness is incurable, they still send her to traditional healers to find the "genie" that sucks her blood away. The family members do not segregate her in any way. Their neighbours and her friends do not visit on a regular basis because she has a longstanding illness. They call her a "Bwagala person" meaning she is frequently admitted to Bwagala Hospital (the local name for Turiani Hospital). The main care provider is her stepmother who sleeps in the hospital with her, and also cares for her children. Due to MM's illness the family has been unable to farm and, coupled with two very dry seasons in the area, this means there will be no harvest this season. The family has however subsidized their income by working as laborers on other farms to get money to assist in both paying for medical services and buying food for the family. Although they are sorrowful about the patient's suffering they are accepting the eventuality. They pray that a cure for AIDS can be found. The interview was in an environment where the family was at peace with itself and with the patient in accepting her illness. The illness is openly discussed in the household but terms such as "the new illness" or the "untreatable illnesses" are used.

Despite the observations of extreme distress in the first three case studies reported, the strength of the extended family in providing support for care providers in the home is demonstrated by the last case study. The household reported in case study 4 was rural and had the advantage over other households of having several extended family members residing in the same homestead.

The household was located close to a missionary hospital that had facilities for screening for HIV, and hence the counselors were much more confident and experienced in disclosing HIV positive results to patients. Themes relating to stigma did not arise in either the household interview or the individual interview with the care provider. It was also of interest to observe the relative ease with which AIDS was discussed in this household. As the patient is very ill and will most likely die in the not-so-distant future, the burden of the care of her children will fall on the patient's parents. This was raised as a matter of concern during the household interview by one of the female members of the extended family. She felt that family members were not well equipped to take care of the children, and their paternal relatives were viewed to be negligent as they had not have taken the initiative to come and see the children and preferably take them to their home for care.

Social Support in HIV/AIDS-Affected Households

In all the group discussions, participants noted that in families affected by HIV/AIDS or any other illness, initial support from the neighbors and friends was high. This support is mainly in the form of financial and food contributions, assistance in water and firewood collection, and working on the family's farm. Urban informants reported less support from neighbors and friends during the illness of a family member than rural informants. However, in all the groups, it was noted that support decreased over time when illnesses were chronic. It was felt that people get tired of helping, especially when the sick person continues to deteriorate. During such times, due to the decrease in support, the burden of care on women and on other members of the household caring for a person with AIDS becomes particularly heavy, as reported in two of the case studies reported above.

Information from the formative interviews revealed that traditional institutions that protected the interests of widows and bereaved children, such as the council of elders who ensured trustees took adequate care of widows and children, are no longer an effective control. Furthermore, traditional morality that viewed negligent trustees as causing shame to a clan has also disappeared. These changes had occurred long before the advent of HIV/AIDS. When mortality was not as high as it is currently, communities did not feel as acutely the loss of these institutions. With increasing adult mortality, informants reported frequent conflicts surrounding issues relating to inheritance and care, particularly of widows and bereaved children.

Traditionally, in many of the ethnic groups in the study area, lineage was matriarchal, and maternal uncles on both the father's and mother's side of the family had a lot of power in decisions surrounding who inherited what when the head of a household died. They also took over the care of bereaved children and, in some circumstances, also the older or younger brother of the deceased as well. There were close links between paternal and maternal families that allowed for a sharing in the responsibility of caring for a widow and her children. During the focus group discussions, most of the groups agreed that traditional laws governing inheritance had changed long before the advent of HIV/AIDS. Widow inheritance was noted to have declined over the past 15 - 20 years, and, with its decline, there was also a loss in relevance of many other roles and responsibilities that were linked to the practice.

The decline in widow inheritance was attributed largely to religion—particularly Christianity, which discouraged the practice. Changes in practices governing inheritance were also perceived to be due to increased ethnic mixing and subsequent acculturation as well as socio-economic changes that have decreased the purchasing power of families. It was noted in the rural FGD that the decrease in the purchasing power of households over the years has created a situation where trustees use resources from the estate of the deceased to meet needs in their immediate families. During the in-depth interviews, a female care provider noted "in the past, food was not a problem and the welfare particularly of children was not neglected. Now maternal uncles favor the needs of their children over those of the children of his deceased brother-in-law, resulting in a decrease in the credibility of the maternal uncle as a guardian." In the urban FGD, it was noted that the increase in the proportion of mixed ethnic group marriages has been a factor that has decreased the sharing of responsibilities between paternal and maternal relatives when death occurs.

Currently, when the death occurs of a male head of household, elders on both sides of the family meet and select a trustee to look after the property and children of the deceased. Paternal relatives are increasingly taking custody of the deceased's property, supposedly to assist in the care of bereaved children. Most of the FGDs noted that there are occasions when the widow is asked to return to her parents' home village with a few personal belongings and her young children, particularly if they are still breast-feeding. Older children are either placed in the care of a trustee or distributed amongst paternal relatives. It is also more permissible now than in the past for the widow to elect to remain in her husband's house with her children. However, should she be suspected to have formed a liaison with another man, she may be asked to leave by her husband's relatives. The widow is most disadvantaged if she has no children, if all her children are young, and if the family lived in rented accommodation.

Because paternal trustees sometimes neglect orphaned children in their care, conflicts often arise when they become adults and demand an account of how their late father's estate was managed. This property is often in the form of assets such as a house or land. The paternal relatives may refuse to hand over these assets once the children have become adults. It has become increasingly common in urban areas for the trustee appointed by elders to legalize the powers invested in him by documenting through a court procedure the estate of the deceased. This documentation ensures that the property in his care is known and can be claimed through a court procedure if necessary. However, informants in the rural FGD reported that such legal approaches rarely occur and that elders were still able to sort out differences when they occurred.

The Regional Social Welfare Officer noted that, increasingly, children who have lost a parent(s) are falling through the traditional safety net which ensured their protection in the past. Accounts of a difficult life with relatives are common. Such children are unable to continue with school, run away from home, and end up on the streets in urban areas where they are vulnerable to behavioral problems, child labor and sexual exploitation. Street children between the ages of 7 - 15 years are starting to appear in the region, although it is unclear what proportion are HIV/AIDS orphans. Many informants felt there was a need to have in place by-laws enforceable at the village government level that ensure that the needs of orphans living with relatives are met and, in this way, regenerate a form of social control and moral obligation for the care of orphans.

Perceived Needs of Female Care Providers in HIV/AIDS-Affected Households

The female care providers in the four households noted the immense difficulties in caring for a person who is chronically ill, understanding what a family member is suffering from, and dealing with concerns regarding the welfare of children left behind. In both of the urban households, the lack of social support networks was very obvious, and this was expressed as a big difficulty.

MS felt that she would have coped better if she had had someone to talk to regarding her daughter's illness as well as someone to advise her on how to take care of her granddaughter. This, for her, was important given the rumors she had started hearing that her daughter had died of AIDS. In all the households, the need to know what a loved one was suffering from was expressed. It was felt this would minimize unnecessary shopping for care—a practice that often happens when health facilities indicate they do not know or could not discover what is wrong with a family member. Shopping for care was reported to deplete meager resources available for the care of the ill family member, and, particularly in urban settings, results in the family being in debt after the death of its ill member.

Many of the care providers felt the public needed to have more information on how to take care of family members with AIDS as well as on protection from infection. More effective medication to alleviate pain and suffering was also suggested, as were policies to ensure that such medications were affordable. Treatment of opportunistic infections was felt to be poor, and one care provider commented:

> "if they could only give medicines to clear the sores in her mouth, she would at least be able to eat, she is dying of hunger." Medical help at times of crisis, it was

felt, would help to decrease stress for care providers as well as alleviate pain and suffering. Most care providers felt health workers made them feel that they would not be welcome to go back to the facility with their chronically ill patient.

Issues Emerging from the Data

Data such as described above cannot be generalized over the whole region, and indeed, this was not the intention at the beginning of the study. However, the narratives of key informants provide information on patterns that relate to the impact of the disease at the household level that can inform areas for further study and develop the potential for intervention.

As has been described elsewhere in Tanzania, household responses to HIV/AIDS in Morogoro are shaped by the socio-cultural contexts within which men, women, and children live (Leshabari *et. al.*, 1996). Women within households remain the major providers of physical care of its ill members, as has been the case traditionally. AIDS, however, provides significant challenges to this lay system of care. We will explore these challenges as they have revealed themselves in the presented data.

Uncertainty regarding cause of illness in a family member and rumors of possible AIDS creates its own challenges for household-based care providers. This could be a reflection of the general level at which HIV/AIDS is understood in the communities where the study was conducted. The current approach of mass media campaigns to provide information on HIV/AIDS appears to have generated awareness of the disease. However, one wonders whether such awareness has moved beyond the simple recall of a health educative message to a more comprehensive understanding of issues such as the mechanisms of HIV transmission, the concept of a long incubation period, and the distinctions between being infected by HIV and suffering from AIDS. During the focus group discussions, though not an adequate measure of knowledge, it was evident that participants were at different levels of understanding the disease and that a majority may have been at a rote learning level of understanding. The importance of specific areas of the country identifying and filling in gaps in knowledge with area specific information, education, and communication programs cannot be over-emphasized. Such programs need to form a part of regional and district development plans given the close links between HIV/AIDS and its ramifications on poverty and development.

Despite concerns regarding the level of poverty in Tanzania, as evidenced by a very low annual per-capita income using macro-economic indices, it appears that the annual per-capita income in the Morogoro region could be even lower than the national average as judged from the reported regional gross domestic product for 1994. The chronic nature of AIDS provides challenges both of a direct and indirect nature for care providers in the household. Direct challenges include decisions regarding the distribution and use of existing resources; more often then not, the needs generated by crisis situations relating to physical ill health results in the purchase of drugs or the seeking of care from a traditional healer taking a priority position. This has implications in terms of resources available to sustain the well-being of other family members (education, food, etc.) in an already poor setting. Indirect implications include time out from productive activities for persons providing care. The stories of neglected farm plots and time away from work for employed persons are compelling and will have long-term implications on increasing levels of poverty in the region.

This poverty is reflected in the scanty services provided within health facilities, not only for HIV/AIDS screening, but also for supplies of drugs relevant to the needs of the population served by the facility. Again, the stories of only simple analgesics being provided and lack of drugs to alleviate suffering caused by oral fungal infections in family members suffering from AIDS are compelling and supported by the accounts from health care providers. It would appear there were different stories from the four households regarding support from health facilities. These ranged from a sense that reporting to a health facility for help with yet another opportunistic infection would not be welcomed by health workers to health workers being prepared to support care providers in the household through visiting the homes and providing health care and advice. Where health workers visited homes, care providers felt supported; where visitation did not occur, a need was expressed for such support. It would appear that issues related to the home-based care of persons with AIDS needs to be addressed so that such care involves an extension of services provided by health-care facilities rather than an abandonment of persons needing services. Focused studies on the feasibility of establishing effective extension home-based care programs in the region would be very welcome at this stage of the epidemic. Health facilities can explore/facilitate other actors in the area such as community-based and non-governmental organizations with whom they could collaborate.

Several issues that could be related to stigma arose in the household interviews. In a country such as Tanzania, with no formal social security systems in place, traditional social-support networks are of immense importance amongst people confronted by misfortune. The reports of a perceived decrease in such support networks within households with an ill family member require more in-depth exploration. From the exploratory data reported, it is clear that female care providers in the home perceive such lack of support as stressful. Possible stigma relating to HIV/AIDS was implied though not explicitly apparent in the data. However, aspects such as avoiding the financial demands generated by caring for a person with AIDS could also have been in operation. It was interesting to note that being visited by an extension community-based HIV/AIDS counselor was useful in facilitating more positive attitudes in households towards an ill member with AIDS. It would appear that being able to provide clear and concise information about HIV/AIDS—about the to take care of an AIDS-affected family member—goes a long way towards decreasing the mysticism that arises out of inexplicable chronic symptomatology. This is another area for exploration and possible service development.

Poverty following the death of a family member with AIDS is common, particularly when one takes into consideration that many who are infected are in the prime of their lives and contributed towards household income. This compounds the economic impact on those left behind, such as single and double orphans. The cultural practices regarding inheritance in such situations of poverty result in AIDS orphans being disadvantaged when choices need to be made regarding their basic needs, including education, over those of biological children of persons entrusted with the estate of the deceased. To a large extent, cultural structures ensuring that guardians meet their cultural obligations towards caring for both orphans and widows has ceased to be relevant in a setting of socio-cultural change, though many of the rituals regarding inheritance are still in place. The AIDS epidemic has precipitated the need to address these changes with clearer and gender-sensitive legislation regarding inheritance practices. The sensitive nature of these issues will perhaps require a bottom-up approach in legislation reform to ensure that new legislation can be implemented.

Conclusion

Health Service Provision

The Morogoro community-based counselors experiment appears to be an important intervention in offering both informational and emotional support to HIV affected families that can extend to communities. Training needs in medical counseling in relation to HIV/AIDS must be identified to ensure disclosure of sero-positive status is given in a clear and sensitive manner allowing for major decisions to be made in terms of risk reduction, living positively with HIV infection, and home-based care. Practical steps to prepare for the care of family members who will be left behind when death occurs is also an important area. In addition to training, supervision of counselors is necessary to ensure that they are able to cope with offering support in an area of high mortality. Community-based counseling is an intervention that has the potential for extension to areas where it does not exist in addition to strengthening and consolidating what counseling services already exist.

The expensive nature of screening for HIV antibodies in a poor country like Tanzania is acknowledged. However, there are less expensive strategies that can be put in place to alleviate the burden currently placed on the shoulders of home-based care providers. This is in the area of treatment of common opportunistic infections that plague persons suffering from HIV/AIDS. There is an urgent need for guidelines to be set out for the identification and management of common AIDS-related opportunistic infections by primary health-care workers. The stories of the pain and suffering of loved ones, as well as the scenes of helplessness amongst care providers in the case studies, suggest an insensitivity on the part of the health system to the plight of persons with AIDS in the home. Though efforts of primary health-care workers are commendable, it is also true that some care providers felt they would not be welcomed again to the health facility should there be yet another health crisis. In order for home-based care to be effective, care providers need the support of health care services in the area. Development of more effective support for care providers in the home is an area that requires more focus, including developing medical counseling and diagnostic skills amongst primary health care workers. The lack of adequate diagnostic facilities and skills also creates a problem in the care of infants and children who have AIDS. The younger children of ill family members in some of the families visited had obvious signs of malnutrition that could as well be manifestations of AIDS (Lesbordes *et. al.*, 1986; Scuerman *et. al.*, 1988).

Supporting Affected Families

A rich culture of social support networks existed particularly in the rural areas. Any attempts at interventions in assisting families should therefore reinforce these networks rather than compromise them. This is a role that can be taken on by community-based counselors. In addition, legislation and structures need to be in place that ensure widows and orphans are taken adequate care of by family members; this may be one method of reinforcing a function that used to be dealt with by elders' councils. The decline in widow inheritance that preceded the AIDS epidemic in the region is welcome given the mode of transmission of AIDS and needs to be reinforced through community participation using the elders' councils where these continue to exist. In addition, legal documentation of properties held in trust by guardians for children of the deceased that has already started to occur needs to be encouraged and supported by local by-laws. The public social work services need to be strengthened so that they can play an important and effective supervisory and monitoring role in the care of orphans by the extended family.

In urban settings, self-sustaining support networks need to be established, including the encouragement of self-support groups amongst affected families and concerned friends which can create a nucleus through which external assistance can be channeled in order to reach those who are affected. Those that exist in rural areas need to be acknowledged and strengthened. These support networks need to be linked closely with poverty eradication activities in the region, given the interrelationship between poverty and the burden of care in households affected by HIV/AIDS. More general interventions such as income-generating activities in communities that focus on gender roles and responsibilities relevant to needs in households will have an impact on decreasing the burden of care in AIDS-affected households. Such activities have to be encouraged at grass-root levels to provide a firm base that will ensure their sustainability. In strengthening the available social support and care-providing networks or interventions, the importance of community involvement and participation in planning and implementing any changes cannot be over- emphasized.

Research and Policy, Evidence-based Interventions

Finally, this preliminary rapid assessment demonstrates the multi-dimensional nature of the impact of HIV/AIDS at the household level and shows that women and persons who are poor appear to bear the brunt of a significant part of this impact due to their lower position within community societal structures. The above findings indicate that approaches towards HIV/AIDS control that focus on prevention of transmission are in themselves insufficient. There is also a need to address the plight of those already affected, the association between social, cultural, and economic factors and HIV transmission risk, as well as care of those with AIDS at the household level.

This calls for in-depth studies to provide policy makers and service providers with adequate information for developing culture- and gender-relevant policies and innovative community-sponsored strategies that substantively promote HIV prevention and support for households affected by HIV/AIDS.

It appears that for programs to be effective they need to promote changes on multiple levels. Although changes at a superstructure level such as underdevelopment, poverty, and gender power differentials are difficult to achieve, changes can be made at social structure levels, which can significantly reduce the burden of care within households. These include by-laws to ensure the security of widows and children and interventions that strengthen traditional social support systems. Community involvement in shaping and implementing such structural change is crucial to their success. For researchers to provide the necessary contextually rich information for such policy decisions, it appears that innovative community participatory data collection methods that include both qualitative and quantitative approaches are important. The multifaceted nature of factors which influence HIV/AIDS transmission and the care of those affected calls for multi- and inter-disciplinary approaches in analyzing the HIV/AIDS situation in communities as well as in planning interventions at various levels.

Chapter Six

HIV/AIDS in Tanzania: The Status of the Epidemic and the National Responses

Saidi H. Kapiga

Introduction

More than 20 years since the first cases of AIDS were recognized, HIV infection has risen to the level of a global pandemic affecting both developed and developing countries. According to UNAIDS, as of 2001, about 40 million adults and children were living with HIV/AIDS worldwide (UNAIDS, 2001). The AIDS pandemic is most severe in sub-Saharan Africa where more than 28 million individuals, almost 10% of people aged 15 - 49 years, are living with HIV/AIDS (UNAIDS, 2001). The prevalence of HIV ranges from under 2% in some West African countries to around 25% or more in southern African countries (UNAIDS, 2000). Countries in central and eastern Africa, which were the first to be affected by the HIV epidemic in the early 1980s, have HIV prevalence between these rates. AIDS has become a leading cause of disease burden and deaths among men and women aged 15-49 years in Africa (WHO, 2000) and is threatening to reverse the economic development in most countries in this region (Piot *et. al.*, 2001).

In this chapter, we describe the status of the HIV epidemic and the evolution of the national responses against HIV/AIDS in Tanzania. Because of limited information about the status of the HIV epidemic in Zanzibar, our discussion will focus on mainland Tanzania. We start by describing the status of the HIV epidemic using data from sentinel surveillance populations and community-based epidemiological studies and examine factors contributing to the expansion of the epidemic in Tanzania. Later, we describe the evolution of national responses against HIV/AIDS and assess its impact on promoting safer sexual practices by using data from five national surveys. Lastly, we discuss the challenges in developing effective national responses and outline potential strategies that could be used to address the challenges.

Status of HIV/AIDS Epidemic in Tanzania

With an area of about 945,000 square kilometers, Tanzania is the largest country in East Africa. Mainland Tanzania is divided into 21 administrative regions, and each region is subdivided into districts. The population of Tanzania was 23.1 million at the last census in 1988, and it is estimated to be more than 33 by the end of 2000. Tanzania was one of the first countries in Africa to be affected by the HIV/AIDS epidemic. The first 3 cases of AIDS were reported in the northwest region of Kagera in 1983 (Fothal *et. al.*, 1986), about one year after AIDS cases had been reported in the neighboring Rakai district in southwestern Uganda (Serwadda *et. al.*, 1985). By 1986, all regions of Tanzania had reported the existence of AIDS cases (United Republic of Tanzania, 2000).

Number of Reported AIDS Cases

All hospitals in Tanzania are required to report AIDS cases to the regional headquarters by using Clinical AIDS Surveillance forms. Each region uses this information to compile quarterly reports that are submitted to the Ministry of Health (MOH). Based on these reports, the cumulative number of AIDS cases in Tanzania increased from 3 in 1983 to 130,386 in 2000 (Figure 1) (United Republic of Tanzania, 2000). The highest number of AIDS cases has been reported in the Mbeya region (21%), followed by Dar es Salaam (12%), Kagera (7%), Mwanza (6%), and the Kilimanjaro (6%) regions. Although the number of AIDS cases can be used to assess the magnitude of the HIV epidemic, there are several factors that make these estimates less helpful in monitoring the status of the epidemic in the general population. First, the number of cases reported is based on patients seen in the hospitals and does not include AIDS cases in other health facilities and cases outside health facilities in the community. As a result, they grossly underestimate the burden of AIDS cases in the general population. Second, the number of AIDS cases is affected by incomplete reporting and lack of a standardized AIDS case-definition in health facilities where HIV diagnostic tests are not routinely performed. Because of these problems, it is estimated that only 1 out of 5 AIDS cases are reported to MOH (United Republic of Tanzania, 2000). Lastly, due to the long incubation period between infection and the occurrence of AIDS, the prevalence of AIDS reflects the level of infection over a long period of time. Hence, the number of AIDS cases may be less useful in monitoring the recent course of the epidemic and in assessing the impact of the interventions.

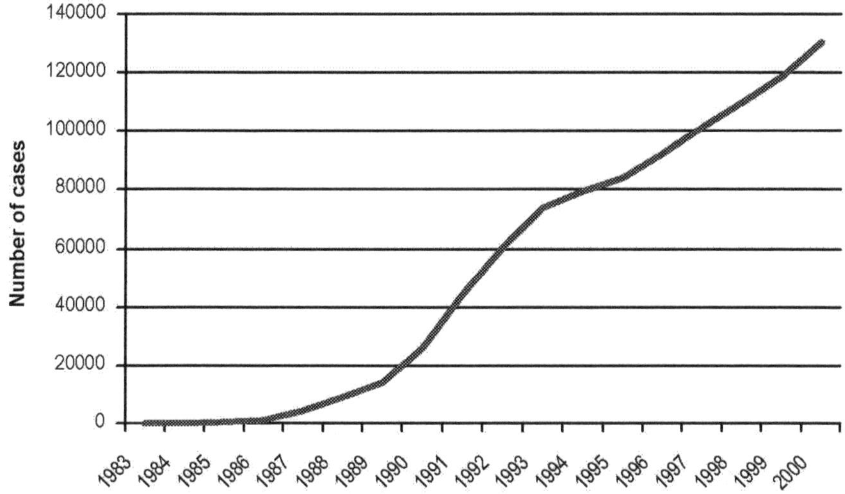

Figure 1: *Reported Cumulative AIDS Cases in Tanzania, 1983-2000*

Source: *United Republic of Tanzania, National AIDS Control Programme. HIV/AIDS/STDs Surveillance Report No. 15, December 2000. Dar es Salaam, Tanzania*

HIV Sero-prevalence Among Blood Donors

As recommended by the World Health Organization (WHO) (WHO, 1988), sentinel surveillance among blood donors and pregnant women was established to monitor the rate of expansion of the HIV epidemic in Tanzania. HIV screening among blood donors was introduced in the regional and referral hospitals in 1987 and was expanded to include all 182 hospitals in 1990 (United Republic of Tanzania, 2000). In most hospitals, the majority of the blood donors (90%) are relatives of recipients of blood transfusions. Between 1990-2000, the prevalence of HIV among donors increased from 5% to 9.2% among men, and from 7.9% to 13.3% among women (Figure 2) (United Republic of Tanzania, 2000). Applying these rates to the general population, more than 1.8 million people aged 15 years and above were estimated to be living with HIV in Tanzania by the end of 2000. This is consistent with UNAIDS estimates of national adult HIV prevalence of 8.1% (Walker *et. al.*, 2001). With the exception of 1994, the prevalence of HIV among blood donors has been consistently higher in women than in men.

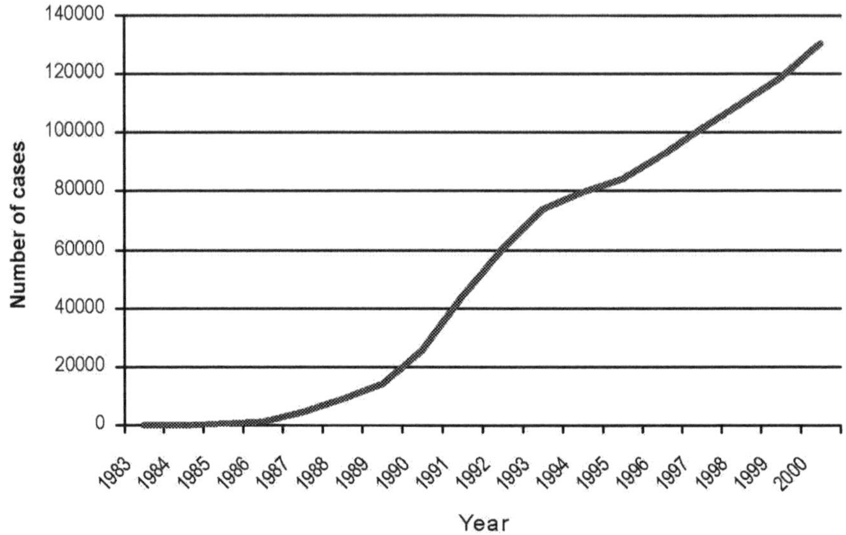

Source: *United Republic of Tanzania, National AIDS Control Programme. HIV/AIDS/STDs Surveillance Report No. 15, December 2000. Dar es Salaam, Tanzania*

The prevalence of HIV among blood donors has also been reported in few epidemiological studies. In a study conducted between 1988-1991 among 4,761 blood donors in a mission hospital in southwest Tanzania, the age-adjusted HIV prevalence among male and female donors was 6.6% and 7.0% respectively (Soderberg *et. al.*, 1994). The prevalence of HIV was positively correlated with the degree of urbanization of the villages where the donors resided. In another study conducted in 1991, the age- and sex-adjusted HIV prevalence among donors in urban and rural areas of the Mwanza region was 12.6% and 3.4% respectively (Borgdorff, et al., 1993). In Dar es Salaam, the prevalence of HIV among blood donors was 8.7% in 1998 (Matee *et. al.*, 1999).

HIV prevalence estimates among blood donors should be interpreted cautiously. In most hospitals, women comprise only a small proportion (20%) of blood donors. Hence, the prevalence of HIV among donors might not be a reliable estimate of the rate of HIV infection among women in the general population. Moreover, there are considerable differences on the HIV screening algorithms used in health facilities, making it difficult to compare results from various geographical areas of Tanzania. Incomplete reporting from the districts is also a major problem. For example, the proportion of districts that submitted screening results to the MOH ranged from 68% in 1990 to 76% in 2000.

Furthermore, potential donors practicing high-risk behaviors are often not allowed to donate blood and may be less likely to volunteer to donate blood. Hence, the rate of infection among blood donors might underestimate the prevalence of HIV infection in the general population.

HIV Sero-Prevalence Among Pregnant Women

HIV sentinel surveillance among pregnant women was established in 24 antenatal clinics (ANC) in 11 regions in 1990 (United Republic of Tanzania, 2000). Most of these clinics, however, are no longer actively involved in this program and have been replaced by other clinics. In Table 1, we present the prevalence of HIV in the ANC sentinel sites for the period 1992-2000. With the exception of 1997-2000, less than a half of the clinics reported HIV prevalence estimates to the MOH. Hence, long-term HIV trends cannot be ascertained in most clinics participating in the sentinel surveillance system. Overall, the prevalence of HIV has been relatively stable in most clinics that have been reporting regularly, with the exception of Isoko and Itete in the Mbeya region. The prevalence of HIV in the Kyela district on the Malawi border has been consistently above 20% since 1996. Results from Bukoba town show a gradual decline of HIV prevalence between 1993-1999, although a relatively higher prevalence estimate was reported in 2000, suggesting that this trend might be changing. Declining HIV trends have also been observed among women, particularly those aged less than 25 years, in the general population in Bukoba town (Kwesigabo *et. al.*, 2000; Kwesigabo *et. al.*, 1998).

There are few other studies that have reported HIV prevalence estimates among pregnant women from health facilities not participating in the sentinel surveillance system. In a study conducted in the Lindi district in southern Tanzania, the prevalence of HIV increased from 0.4% in 1989 to 8.7% in 1993 (Petry and Kingu, 1996). In another study conducted in Dar es Salaam (Mwakagile *et. al.*, 1996), the prevalence of HIV in a random sample of 777 pregnant women was 15.2% in 1993. In a study conducted between 1995-1996 in Dar es Salaam (N=13,876), the prevalence of HIV among women who were screened before the initiation of a large clinical trial was 13.0% (Fawzi *et. al.*, 1998). Overall, results from sentinel surveillance and epidemiological surveys show that HIV is common among pregnant women in Tanzania. HIV sero-positive pregnant women are known to be at increased risk of transmitting the infection to their babies during birth or through

Table 1: *HIV Sero-Prevalence Among Pregnant Women Receiving Antenatal Care at Sentinel Surveillance Clinics, Tanzania, 1992-1999*

Name of the Clinic	*HIV Sero-Prevalence (%) by Year*							
	1992	*1993*	*1994*	*1995*	*1996*	*1997*	*1998*	*1999*
Dar es Salaam Region								
Kasorobo – Temeke		15.3		7.3				15.3
Kigamboni – Temeke								14.1
Sinza – Kinondoni								18.1
Iringa Region								
Mafinga (Roadside)	25.0							20.9
Kagera Region								
Bukoba (Urban)		16.1			13.7			7.0
Kilimanjaro Region								
Umbwe (Rural)	6.4				9.1	10	20	19.2
Mbeya Region								
Mbeya (Rural)	11.1	12.1	20.4	14.2	14.5	15.6	12.3	13.7
Isoko (Rural)					7.2	8.1	10.2	19.1
Itete (Rural)					5.6	14.8	11.8	11.6
Mwambani (Rural)					16.0	13.7	14.5	11.0
Chimala (Roadside)					17.0	15.9	12.5	12.1
Mbeya (Urban)	19.3	17.7	19.8	20.7	18.5	19.6	17.3	18.0
Kiwanjampaka (Urban)	17.0	22.3	19.5		17.0	22.5	20.5	23.0
Meta (Urban)	25.0	13.7	16.0		14.6	17.9	12.5	13.5
Ruanda (Urban)					24.0	18.1	18.8	17.5
Kyela (Border)	26.2	27.5	21.6	33.3	25.9	25.0	24.0	29.5
Morogoro Region								
Morogoro Regional Hospital (Urban)								18.4
Turiani Hospital (Rural)								9.8
Mwanza Region								
Mwanza (Urban)	10.3	11.7	11.7	8.9				
Mkula (Rural)	4.6	5.4		5.4				
Rukwa Region			26.5	17.4				
Namanyere (Rural)	11.3	8.33	19	11.2		11.2		
Sumbawanga (Urban)	12	23.3	31.3	22.2		21.0		
Ruvuma Region								
Songea (Urban)	9.7	16.1	15.7	14.2		11		
Namtumbo (Rural)	3.5	6.7	3.2	5.6		4		
Shinyanga Region								
Shinyanga (Rural)			10.9					

Source: *United Republic of Tanzania, National AIDS Control Programme. HIV/AIDS/STDs Surveillance Report No. 15, December 2000. Dar es Salaam, Tanzania*

breastfeeding. The rate of mother-to-child transmission of HIV in Tanzania has been estimated to be 8.4% at birth (Fawzi et al., 2000; Fawzi *et. al.*, 2001), and about 20-22% between 6 and 26 weeks after delivery (Fawzi *et. al.*, 2000; Fawzi *et. al.*, 2001; Bredberg-Raden *et. al.*, 1995). Because of this, HIV is becoming a major public health problem among children in the general population (Matee *et. al.*, 1995) and among those admitted to health facilities (Kawo *et. al.*, 2000).

The extent to which HIV prevalence among pregnant women receiving antenatal care reflects trends in the general population is influenced by a number of factors including fertility rates in the general population and use of ANC services. As observed in other sub-Saharan African countries, most pregnant women receive antenatal care in Tanzania (National Bureau of Statistics, 2000). Hence, women seen at ANC might be representative of women of reproductive age in the general population. Numerous studies have reported lowered fertility among HIV-infected women in sub-Saharan Africa (Gregson *et. al.*, 1999). Thus, if HIV surveillance is confined to pregnant women, the prevalence of HIV among women of reproductive age in the general population will be seriously underestimated. Several factors have been identified to account for the reduced fertility in HIV-infected women including co-infection with other sexually transmitted diseases (STDs) (Ross *et. al.*, 1999), direct biological effects of HIV disease (Gray *et. al.*, 1998; Zaba and Gregson, 1998), and changes in fertility preferences following HIV post-test counseling (Setel, 1995).

Community-based HIV-1 Sero-Prevalence Studies

In Table 2, we present HIV prevalence estimates from community-based studies in Tanzania. In a study conducted between 1987-88 in the Kagera region, the overall prevalence of HIV in 2,297 adults was 9.6% (Killewo *et. al.*, 1990). The prevalence of HIV was significantly higher in urban areas than in rural areas among both men (16.9% vs. 5.1%) and women (28.6% vs. 4.8%). In another study conducted between 1989-90 among 4,086 adults in the Mara region of northwest Tanzania, the prevalence of HIV was 7.3% (Shao *et. al.*, 1994). In this study, the prevalence of HIV was positively correlated with the degree of urbanization in both men and women. Similar trends have been observed in other studies conducted in the Mwanza (Barongo *et. al.*, 1992; Barongo *et. al.*, 1994; Grosskurth *et. al.*, 1995; Boerma *et. al.*, 1999), Arusha (Mnyika *et. al.*, 1994; Mnyika *et. al.*, 1996), and Kilimanjaro (Klouman *et. al.*, 1997) regions. Studies conducted in Dar es Salaam have reported an HIV prevalence of 11.5% among women receiving family planning services (Kapiga *et. al.*, 1994) and 18.0% and 13.3% among female and male police officers respectively (Bakari *et. al.*, 2000).

Table 2: ***HIV Sero-Prevalence from Community-Based Studies in Tanzania***

Reference	*Year of Data Collection*	*Sample Size*	*Age Range (Years)*	*Place where Conducted*	*Sex*	*Residence*	*% HIV-1 Sero-Positive*
Kilewo, *et.al.* 1990	1987/88	2,297	18-54	Kagera Region	Women	Rural Urban	28.6 4.8
					Men	Rural Urban	16.9 5.1
Shao, *et.al.*, 1994	1989/90	4,086	15-49	Tarime District	Women	Rural Peri-Urban Urban	13.4 7.4 2.6
					Men	Rural Peri-Urban Urban	9.5 4.7 2.6
Barongo, *et.al.*, 1992	1990/91	4,161	15-54	Mwanza Region	Women	Rural Peri-Urban Urban	15.2 8.7 2.8
					Men	Rural Peri-Urban Urban	8.7 5.4 2.4
Barongo, *et.al.*, 1994	1991/92	1,143	15-54	Mwanza Region	Women	Urban	16.6
					Men	Urban	9.8
Grosskurth, *et.al.*, 1995	1991/92	12,500	15-54	Mwanza Region	Women	Roadside Island areas Rural	7.9 1.8 4.2
					Men	Roadside Island areas Rural	7.5 1.8 3.4
Kapinga, *et.al.*, 1994	1991/92	2,285	15-48	Dar es Salaam Region	Women	Urban	11.5
Klouman, *et.al.*, 1997	1991/92	3,239	15-44	Kahe, Kilimanjaro Region	Women	Rural	1.9
					Men	Rural	0.7

Continued

Reference	*Year of Data Collection*	*Sample Size*	*Age Range (Years)*	*Place where Conducted*	*Sex*	*Residence*	*% HIV-1 Sero-Positive*
Mnyika, *et.al.*, 1994	1991/92	1,070	15-54	Arusha Region	Women	Rural Semi-urban and urban	6.5
					Men	Rural Semi-urban and urban	1.7
Mnyika, *et.al.*, 1996	1993/94	862	15-54	Arusha Region	Women	Urban Peri-urban Rural	14.4 6.9 2.3
					Men	Urban Peri-urban Rural	5.7 2.1 0.0
Boerma, *et.al.*, 1999	1994/95	5,820	15-54	Kisesa, Mwanza Region	Women	Urban Peri-urban Rural	12.9 8.7 4.2
					Men	Urban Peri-urban Rural	12.3 6.7 2.8
Bakari, *et. al.*, 2000	1994/95	2,733	18-55	Dar es Salaam Region	Women	Urban	18.0
					Men	Urban	13.3
Boerma, *et. al.*, 1999	1996/97	6,413	15-54	Kisesa, Mwanza Region	Women	Urban Peri-urban Rural	14.9 8.8 4.8
					Men	Urban Peri-urban Rural	11.6 6.7 3.0

**SES, Socio-economic status*

Source: *See various authors cited in the table.*

Community-based HIV-1 Sero-Incidence Studies

In Table 3, we summarize results from prospective studies conducted to estimate the incidence of HIV in Tanzania. In a study conducted between 1987-89 in the Kagera region, the overall HIV incidence among adults was 1.37/100 person-years at risk (Killewo *et. al.*, 1993). The incidence of HIV among men (1.34/100 person-years) was not significantly different from that

Table 3: *HIV Sero-incidence from Prospective Community-Based Studies in Tanzania*

Reference	*Year of Data*	*Sample Size Collection*	*Place Where Conducted*	*Sex*	*Residence*	*IR (95% CI)**
Killewo *et. al.*,1993	1987-89	1,316	Kagera Region	Women	Rural	0.80 (0.3-1.30)
					Urban	5.15 (1.96-8.34)
				Men	Rural	0.85 (0.22-1.48)
					Urban	4.20 (0.84-7.56)
Hugonnet *et. al.*, 2002	1991-95	3,403	Mwanza Region	Women	Rural	0.17 (0.06-0.37)
				Men	Rural	0.45 (0.25-0.74)
Senkoro *et. al.*, 2000	1991-96	2,172	Mwanza Region	Women	Urban	1.92 (1.22-2.89)
				Men	Urban	1.05 (0.72-1.47)
Kapiga *et. al.*, 1998	1992-95	2,471	Dar es Salaam	Women	Urban	3.40 (2.60-4.10)
Boerma *et. al.*, 1999	1994-97	7,609	Kisesa, Mwanza region	Women	Rural	0.84 (0.58-1.17)
				Men	Rural	0.73 (0.48-1.07)
Bakari *et. al.*, 2000	1994-98	2,080	Dar es Salaam Region	Women	Urban	2.24 (1.34-3.36)
				Men	Urban	1.96 (1.12-2.96)

*IR = Number of cases/100 person years; CI = confidence interval

Source: *See various authors cited in the table.*

observed in women (1.39/100 person-years). Among both men and women, the incidence of HIV was significantly more in urban areas than in rural areas. In a retrospective cohort study nested within a community-randomized trial to investigate the impact of STDs control on HIV transmission, the incidence of HIV among couples in stable sexual relationships was 0.17 per 100 person-years in women and 0.45 per 100 person-years in men (Hugonnet *et. al.*, 2002). In a cohort of factory workers and their spouses followed between 1991-96 in the Mwanza region, the incidence of HIV was 1.92/100 person-years among women and 1.05/100 person-years among men (Senkoro *et. al.*, 2000). In another study conducted between 1994-1997 in a rural community in the Mwanza region, the incidence of HIV was less than 1/100 person-years among both women and men (Boerma *et. al.*, 1999). In this study, the incidence of HIV in the trading centers was almost twice that in the rural villages. Two other studies conducted in Dar es Salaam reported the incidence of HIV of 3.40/100 person-years among women using modern family planning methods (Kapiga *et. al.*, 1998) and 2.24 and 1.96 per 100 person-years among women and men police officers respectively (Bakari *et. al.*, 2000).

Molecular Epidemiology

HIV-1 subtypes A and D predominate in the epidemic of East Africa, while HIV-1 subtype C has dominated the rapidly expanding epidemic in southern Africa and Ethiopia (Janssens *et. al.*, 1997). Although information about the distribution of HIV-1 subtypes in various geographical regions of Tanzania is limited, subtypes A, C, and D have been identified since 1988 (Hoelscher *et. al.*, 1998). The proportion of these subtypes, however, varies depending on the geographic area where sampling was done. An analysis of samples collected from 15 patients at the Turiani hospital in the Morogoro region in 1988 showed that 67% envelop V3 sequences belonged to subtype D, while the remaining samples (33%) belonged to subtype D (Zwart *et. al.*, 1993). In another study conducted at almost the same time in Dar es Salaam, *vpu* and *env* sequences from 8 out of 10 AIDS patients (80%) clustered with subtype D viruses and the remaining 2 (20%) with subtype A (Siwka *et. al.*, 1994). Two other studies conducted between 1994-95 in northern Tanzania also clustered with HIV-1 subtypes A and D (Robbins *et. al.*, 1996; Holm-Hansen *et. al.*, 1996).

Relatively recent studies conducted in the Mbeya region of southwest Tanzania and Dar es Salaam city have reported an increasing proportion of subtype C genotypes, including recombinants containing a portion of subtype C (Hoelscher *et. al.*, 1998; Renjifo *et. al.*, 1998; Renjifo *et. al.*, 1999; Hoelscher *et. al.*, 2001). In a study conducted in 1995 among 86 patients in the Mbeya region, the proportion of sub-types was 29% A, 55% C, 15% D, and 1% subtype G (Hoelscher *et. al.*, 1998). In a large clinical trial conducted between 1996-97 in Dar es Salaam, subtype C genotypes, including recombinants containing a portion of subtype C, were found in about 45% of the infected babies born by HIV-1 infected mothers (Renjifo *et. al.*, 1998). The V3 region of subtypes A or C was always selected in A/D and C/D recombinants (Renjifo *et. al.*, 1999). In this clinical trial, mothers infected with HIV-1 subtype A, C, or HIV-1 intersubtype recombinant viruses were more likely to transmit HIV-1 to their babies than mothers infected with HIV-1 subtype D (Renjifo *et. al.*, 2001; Blackard *et. al.*, 2001). A high proportion of unrelated HIV-1 intersubtype recombinants have also been reported in the Mbeya region, where only 22% of the strains were pure C, 22% were subtype A, and 56% were A/C or C/D recombinants (Hoelscher *et. al.*, 2001).

Overall, these studies suggest that subtype D is the most frequent HIV-1 subtype in northern Tanzania. HIV-1 subtype C has existed in the Mbeya region since 1989 and was recently introduced in Dar es Salaam. Although HIV-1 subtype C might have expanded quickly to become one of the major subtypes present in Dar es Salaam city, the relative proportions of subtypes A, C, and D have remained stable since 1989 in the Mbeya region. The existence of HIV-1 subtype C in the Mbeya region might be related to extensive communications existing between residents of this region with southern neighbors in Malawi and Zambia, where sub-type C predominates (Janssens *et. al.*, 1997). The relatively large proportion of HIV-1 subtype C in Dar es Salaam, where only subtypes A and D once predominated, suggests that HIV-1 subtype C might be expanding rapidly and is likely to become a major subtype circulating in Tanzania.

Factors Contributing to the Expansion of the HIV Epidemic

There are several factors contributing to the expansion of the HIV epidemic in Tanzania. The prevalence of HIV has been observed to peak before 25 years of age in women and between 25-34 years in men (Mwakagile *et. al.*, 1996; Shao *et. al.*, 1994; Grosskurth *et. al.*, 1995; Mnyika *et. al.*, 1996; Bakari *et. al.*, 2000). Results from prospective studies show that women get infected at a relatively younger age (Boerma *et. al.*, 1999; Killewo *et. al.*, 1993; Kapiga *et. al.*, 1998) than men (Boerma *et. al.*, 1999; Bakari *et. al.*, 2000; Senkoro *et. al.*, 2000), suggesting that the gender differences in HIV prevalence might be due to age differences at the time of acquisition of new infections. The higher HIV incidence among younger women might be due to the initiation of sexual activity at a relatively earlier age than men. The median age at first sexual intercourse in Tanzania is 16.6 years among women and 17.9 years among men (National Bureau of Statistics, 2000). In various parts of Tanzania, older men have been reported to have sexual relationships with younger and inexperienced women who are perceived to be at lower risk of HIV (Killewo *et. al.*, 1993; Natasha *et. al.*, 1998; Klepp *et. al.*, 1995; Silberschmidt and Rasch, 2001). This practice exposes young women to older men who are more likely to be infected with HIV. In addition, young women have been shown to be at increased risk of STDs that are known to facilitate HIV transmission (Kapiga *et. al.*, 1998; Obasi *et. al.*, 2001).

The associations between other socio-demographic characteristics and HIV have been examined in numerous community-based studies. Unmarried men and women have been reported to be at increased risk of HIV in cross-sectional (Soderberg *et. al.*, 1994; Mwakagile *et. al.*, 1996, Barongo *et. al.*, 1992; Grosskurth *et. al.*, 1995; Mnyika *et. al.*, 1994; Mnyika *et. al.*, 1996; Kapiga *et. al.*, 1994; Kapiga *et. al.*, 2000; Quigley *et. al.*, 1997), and prospective studies (Bakari *et. al.*, 2000; Senkoro *et. al.*, 2000; Kapiga *et. al.*, 1998). Other studies have reported increased risk of HIV among women in polygamous unions when compared with those in monogamous unions (Mwakagile *et. al.*, 1996; Kapiga *et. al.*, 1994; Kapiga *et. al.*, 1998). There are conflicting reports about the association between level of education and HIV. A positive association between the level of education and HIV has been reported in women (Grosskurth *et. al.*, 1995, Kapiga *et. al.*, 1994; Senkoro *et. al.*, 2000; Kapiga *et. al.*, 2000; Quigley *et. al.*, 1997) and men (Grosskurth *et. al.*, 1995), with a dose-response relationship in some studies (Kapiga *et. al.*, 1994; Quigley *et. al.*, 1997). However, HIV was not associated with the level of education in two large studies in northern Tanzania (Mnyika *et. al.*, 1994; Mnyika *et. al.*, 1996). The increased risk of HIV among educated women and men might be due to increased employment-related mobility and residing in urban areas where the prevalence of HIV is high. Numerous surveys have not reported a significantly increased number of sexual partners among educated men and women (National Bureau of Statistics, 2000; Kapiga, 1996; Kapiga and Lugalla, 2002; Mnyika *et. al.*, 1997), suggesting that sexual behavior might not account for the positive association between HIV and level of education. Two cross-sectional studies have reported a positive association between women's risk of HIV and their spouse's level of education (Kapiga *et. al.*, 1994; Kapiga *et. al.*, 2000), although this was not confirmed in a prospective study conducted in the same population (Kapiga *et. al.*, 1998).

Heterosexual contact is the predominant mode of transmission of HIV, accounting for over 80% of all infections in Tanzania (United Republic of Tanzania, 2000). Consequently, sexual behavior is a major determinant of HIV transmission. Studies that have examined the associations between sexual behavior and HIV have used different measures of sexual behavior with varying recall periods. For this reason, the differences across studies need to be interpreted cautiously. In general, the number of sexual partners has been observed to be positively associated with increased risk of HIV infection (Barongo *et. al.*, 1992; Boerma *et. al.*, 1999; Mnyika *et. al.*, 1994; Mnyika *et. al.*, 1996; Kapiga *et. al.*, 1994; Senkoro *et. al.*, 2000; Kapiga *et. al.*, 1998; Quigley *et. al.*, 1997;

Mwakagile *et. al.*, 2001), although the number of sexual partners reported varies across studies. Other sexual behaviors associated with increased risk of HIV include pre- and extra-marital sexual relationships (Kapiga *et. al.*, 2000), casual sexual partners (Killewo *et. al.*, 1990; Kapiga *et. al.*, 1998; Quigley *et. al.*, 1997), and the initiation of sexual activity at an early age (Mnyika *et. al.*, 1996; Kapiga *et. al.*, 1994; Kapiga *et. al.*, 1998; Kapiga *et. al.*, 2000; Mwakagile *et. al.*, 2001). These high-risk sexual behaviors have been shown to be more common in men than in women (National Bureau of Statistics, 2000; Mnyika *et. al.*,1997; Grosskurth *et. al.*, 1995; Konings *et. al.*, 1994; Munguti *et. al.*, 1997), suggesting that men's sexual behavior might be associated with an increased transmission of HIV in Tanzania. Other studies have shown that the male partner's sexual behavior was a major predictor of HIV in women not practicing high-risk sexual behaviors (Kapiga *et. al.*, 1994; Munguti *et. al.*, 1997).

Other groups more likely to practice high-risk sexual behaviors include unmarried men and women (National Bureau of Statistics, 2000, Kapiga, 1996; Kapiga and Lugalla, 2002), persons aged less than 24 years (National Bureau of Statistics, 2000, Kapiga, 1996; Kapiga and Lugalla, 2002), and residents of urban, peri-urban, and trading centers (National Bureau of Statistics, 2000, Boerma et al., 1999; Kapiga and Lugalla, 2002; Mnyika *et. al.*, 1997). High-risk sexual behaviors are also common among women working in the bars and hotels (Kapiga *et. al.*, 2002; Kapiga *et. al.*, 1995; Outwater *et. al.*, 2000; Mgalla and Pool, 1997) and long-distance truck drivers (Laukamm-Josten, *et. al.*, 2000; Mwizarubi *et. al.*, 1997). These population groups have been identified to be at increased risk of HIV and associated with increased sexual transmission of HIV in Tanzania (Kapiga *et. al.*, 1994; Kapiga *et. al.*, 2002; Mhalu *et. al.*, 1991; Laukamm-Josten, *et. al.*, 1993). Because of increased geographical mobility, long-distance truck drivers have been associated with increased transmission of HIV in the urban centers and roadside villages along major truck routes in Tanzania (Laukamm-Josten, *et. al.*, 2000; Mwizarubi *et. al.*, 1997). Various studies have shown that female bar and hotel workers not only serve beer and drinks, but also attend to their customers sexually to augment their salaries outside working hours (Kapiga *et. al.*, 2002; Mgalla and Pool, 1997; Mhalu *et. al.*, 1991). In most parts of Tanzania, bars and hotels are often the only places for recreational activities, and most men with disposable income tend to visit these sites. Thus, women working in these settings are in contact with a large number of men and may be responsible for the continued expansion of the HIV epidemic in the general population.

A significantly increased risk of HIV has been observed among subjects with non-ulcerative (Klouman *et. al.*, 1997; Kapiga *et. al.*, 1994; Kapiga *et. al.*, 1998) and ulcerative (Barongo *et. al.*, 1992; Grosskurth *et. al.*, 1995; Klouman *et. al.*, 1997; Rodriguez *et. al.*, 2002) STD, indicating that STDs are an important determinant of HIV in Tanzania. Other studies have reported an increased risk of HIV among people with STD-related symptoms (Grosskurth *et. al.*, 1995; Quigley *et. al.*, 1997) and in those with disturbances of vaginal flora and bacterial vaginosis (Kapiga *et. al.*, 2002). Results from sentinel surveillance populations and epidemiological studies show that STDs are a major public health problem in Tanzania. According to the MOH, more than 149,000 patients with new STD syndromes were managed in health facilities in 17 regions of Tanzania between January and December of 2000 (United Republic of Tanzania, 2000). The most common causes of STDs were Genital Discharge Syndrome (44.3%), followed by Genital Ulcer Syndrome (23.3%).

Results from community-based studies show that STDs are common in the general population in Tanzania. The prevalence of active syphilis in adults ranges from 7.8%-9.4% in the Mwanza region (Barongo *et. al.*, 1992; Barongo *et. al.*, 1994; Grosskurth *et. al.*, 1995; Mosha *et. al.*, 1993; Mayaud *et. al.*, 2001; Newell *et. al.*, 1993), 2.3%-4.5% in Dar es Salaam region (Matee *et. al.*, 1999; Mwakagile *et. al.*, 1996; Kapiga *et. al.*, 1994; Bakari *et. al.*, 2000; Kapiga *et. al.*, 1998; Mwakagile*et. al.*, 2001), 5.9% in the Kagera region (Killewo *et. al.*, 1993), and 5.2% in the Mara region (Shao *et. al.*, 1994). The incidence of active syphilis was reported to be 1.2/100 person-years in Kagera (Killewo *et. al.*, 1994), 0.9/100 person-years in the Dar es Salaam region (Bakari *et. al.*, 2000), and 1.8% in the Mwanza region (Todd *et. al.*, 2001). The prevalence of other STDs ranges from 1%-8.1% for gonorrhea (Mwakagile *et. al.*, 1996; Klouman *et. al.*, 1997; Kapiga *et. al.*, 1994; Kapiga *et. al.*, 1998; Mayaud *et. al.*, 2001; Klouman *et. al.*, 2000; Mayaud *et. al.*, 1995), 6.7% - 9.6% for chlamydia (Klouman *et. al.*, 1997, Kapiga *et. al.*, 1998; Mayaud *et. al.*, 2001; Klouman *et. al.*, 2000; Mayaud *et. al.*, 1995), 12.9%-27.4% for trichomoniasis (Mwakagile *et. al.*, 1996; Kapiga *et. al.*, 1994; Kapiga *et. al.*, 1998; Mayaud et al., 2001; Mayaud *et. al.*, 1995), and 23.7%-43.5% for herpes simplex virus type 2 infection (Kapiga *et. al.*, 2002; Rodriquez *et. al.*, 2002; Obasi *et. al.*, 1999; Langeland *et. al.*, 1998).

Evolution of the National Responses against HIV/AIDS

Two years after the first cases of AIDS were reported in Tanzania, a national AIDS Task Force was formed to coordinate a short-term plan for training health workers on the clinical aspects of AIDS and developing blood transfusion safety procedures. In 1987, the National AIDS Control Program (NACP) was formed to develop a national response to HIV/AIDS and to mitigate the socio-economic impact of the AIDS epidemic. The NACP was established as a vertical program under the directorate of preventive services in the MOH. Between 1987-91, the first five-year medium-term plan (MTP-I) was developed with the support of the WHO Global Program on AIDS. The main HIV/AIDS prevention strategies during this phase were mass campaigns to raise general awareness about AIDS and promotion of safer sexual practices, including condom use. AIDS information was distributed widely by using printed materials (such as pamphlets and posters), newspapers, and radio and television programs.

In a 1991 program evaluation, limited participation of other sectors outside the MOH and lack of community involvement in the planned activities were identified as the major weaknesses of MTP-I. Between 1992-96, the second five-year plan (MTP-II) was developed and implemented. The main thrust of MTP-II was to increase multisectoral involvement, including the participation of non-governmental organizations (NGOs) and other community-based organizations; the decentralization of NACP activities to the district level; and increased community involvement and mobilization. To increase multisectoral involvement, the National AIDS Committee (NAC) was formed with representation by principal secretaries from eight key ministries. The NAC was chaired by the Principal Secretary in the Prime Minister's office. Furthermore, AIDS technical committees were formed in the key ministries to coordinate AIDS control activities. In 1993, a five-year USAID-supported Tanzania AIDS Project (TAP) was developed in 10 regions. The main objectives of TAP were to build the capacity of indigenous NGOs and other community-based organizations to develop HIV prevention activities and support families affected by the epidemic (Tanzania AIDS Project, 1997). In all regions participating in the TAP, a network of NGOs and community-based organizations working on HIV/AIDS was established to coordinate their activities. To increase access of male condoms, a condom social marketing program was developed as part of TAP, with technical support from Population Services International (PSI). Condoms were marketed under the local brand name, *salama*, in pharmacies, grocery stores, and non-traditional outlets ranging from bars and hotels to street newspaper stands, hair salons, photo studios, and gas stations. Through TAP, a bilateral grant was availed to strengthen the capacity of the NACP in coordinating AIDS control activities and to improve the condom distribution system in the public health facilities.

Under MTP-II, access to AIDS information increased and the condom distribution system was improved (United Republic of Tanzania, 1995). The number of male condoms distributed each year doubled from 22 million in 1993 to 46 million in 2000. With the exception of 1995, the number of male condoms distributed by the government remained around 20 million each year. The number of male condoms distributed by the social marketing program increased from 3.7 million in 1994 to 19.3 million in 2000. Female condoms were recently introduced in Tanzania. The number of female condoms sold increased from 51,358 in 1999 to 85,530 in 2000. Despite these successes, there were several problems encountered during the implementation of MTP-II. Members of the NAC and AIDS technical committees failed to meet regularly because of other competing demands on their time. As a result, NAC failed to play its leadership role in the program, compromising the ability of NACP to coordinate and mobilize effective multisectoral initiatives. The major barrier in the successful implementation of MTP-II was lack of strong political support and commitment on the part of the government. As a consequence, AIDS prevention was not given the highest priority at all levels of the political structure. Lack of political support and commitment resulted in limited financial resources being allocated for AIDS control activities. Only about 20% of the program's budgeted funds were mobilized in MTP-II. As a result, efforts to curb the HIV/AIDS epidemic largely depended on external resources.

The third five-year plan (MTP-III) was implemented between 1998-2002. The main goal of this plan was to develop an expanded multisectoral national response to reduce high-risk sexual behaviors and more distal determinants of HIV/AIDS vulnerability (United Republic of Tanzania, 1998). Because of the disproportionate impact of the AIDS epidemic on disadvantaged groups, prevention of HIV infection among the most vulnerable populations was one of the specific aims of MTP-III. Members of these groups were identified to be women, youths, and highly mobile populations including sex workers, petty traders, migrant workers, military personnel, and long-distance drivers. This plan was designed to take advantage of the existing local community structures to mount effective interventions in these populations and develop long-term strategies to reduce HIV/AIDS vulnerability. Provision of HIV/AIDS education as part of the curriculum in primary and secondary schools and teacher training colleges was developed to reach increasing numbers of in-school youths. The implementation of the planned activities was expected to involve various sectors outside the MOH, including local government, NGOs, community-based organizations, and people living with HIV/AIDS. To increase political support and commitment, representatives of the six co-sponsors of UNAIDS formed a UN Theme Group. This group, together with other donor organizations, has been working very closely with the government of Tanzania to increase political support of the ongoing HIV/AIDS prevention activities.

TRENDS IN HIV/AIDS KNOWLEDGE AND AWARENESS, SEXUAL BEHAVIOR AND CONDOM USE

Five cross-sectional surveys conducted between 1989-1999 provide data that can be used to determine trends in AIDS knowledge and awareness, sexual behavior and condom use, and assess the impact of the HIV/AIDS prevention activities in Tanzania. These surveys involved national representative samples of men and women aged 15-59 and 15-49 years respectively. The 1989/90 Knowledge, Attitudes, Beliefs and Practices (KABP) Survey (Carael *et. al.*, 1995) was conducted by WHO as part of a multi-country study to assess AIDS-related knowledge, attitudes, and sexual behaviors in developing countries affected by the HIV/AIDS epidemic. The 1991/92 (Bureau of Statistics and Macro International, 1993) and 1996 (Bureau of Statistics and Macro International, 1997) surveys were standard Demographic and Health Surveys (DHS) carried out by Macro International and the Tanzania Bureau of Statistics. The DHS have been conducted at regular intervals in many developing countries since the early 1980s to assess fertility and maternal and child health in women from nationally representative samples. Beginning in the late 1980s, these surveys were expanded to include men, and additional questions about AIDS knowledge and sexual behavior were included. The 1994 Tanzania Knowledge, Attitudes and Practices Survey (TKAP) (Bureau of Statistics and Macro International, 1995) and 1999 Reproductive and Child Health Survey (RCHS) (National Bureau of Statistics, 2000) surveys were conducted by Macro International and the Tanzania Bureau of Statistics by using the DHS sampling frame. These surveys collected more detailed information about reproductive health knowledge and sexual behavior than the standard DHS. In all the surveys, three out of four respondents were living in the rural areas, while about two-thirds of women and slightly less than 60% of men were married or cohabiting at the time of data collection. In Table 4, we present trends in HIV/AIDS knowledge and awareness and sexual behavior and condom use in Tanzania for the period 1989-99.

Table 4: *Trends in HIV/AIDS knowledge and Awareness, Sexual Behavior and Condom Use in Tanzania, 1989 – 1999*

	1989/90 KABP[1]	*1991/92 DHS*[2]	*1994 TKAP*[3]	*1996 DHS*[2]	*1999 RCHS*[4]
HIV/AIDS knowledge and awareness					
Total sample (# of subjects)					
Women	2341	9238	4225	8120	4144
Men	1511	2114	2097	2256	3812
Has heard of AIDS (%)					
Women	91	93	98	97	97
Men	94	98	99	99	99

	1989/90 KABP[1]	*1991/92 DHS*[2]	*1994 TKAP*[3]	*1996 DHS*[2]	*1999 RCHS*[4]
Knows HIV can be avoided[5] (%)					
Women	N/a	n/a	64	62	82
Men	N/a	n/a	80	76	89
Knows infected person can appear healthy[5] (%)					
Women	28	57	67	68	69
Men	37	66	78	78	77
Knows HIV can be transmitted from mother to child[5] (%)					
Women	78	77	77	75	81
Men	80	77	82	77	81
Knows that HIV cannot be transmitted by mosquitoes[5] (%)					
Women	35	61	70	50	54
Men	40	56	71	53	59
Knows that HIV cannot be transmitted by sharing food or eating utensils[5] (%)					
Women	44	70	72	57	59
Men	48	69	73	61	64
Knows AIDS can be avoided by having one partner[5] (%)					
Women	n/a	n/a	80	77	68
Men	n/a	n/a	83	82	79
Knows AIDS can be avoided by using condoms[5] (%)					
Women	n/a	n/a	59	62	66
Men	n/a	n/a	70	69	77
Knows someone with HIV or who has died of AIDS[5] (%)					
Women	n/a	n/a	49	48	65
Men	n/a	n/a	52	52	69
Sexual behavior					
Had premarital sex during the past year[6] (%)					
Women	n/a	31	28	29	41
Men	n/a	66	61	45	61
Had one or more non-regular partners in the past year[7] (%)					
Women	n/a	n/a	6	4	25
Men	n/a	n/a	25	20	48
Had sex with someone other than spouse in the past year[8] (%)					
Women	n/a	n/a	3	2	8
Men	n/a	n/a	18	13	28
Condom awareness and use					
Aware of condoms (%)					
Women	60	45	67	81	83
Men	70	65	79	92	90
Knows where to get condoms (%)					
Women	45	45	45	46	53
Men	50	58	63	69	72
Has ever used condoms[7] (%)					
Women	5	4	7	12	13
Men	10	17	18	34	32
Used condoms during last					

Source: [1] World Health Organization's Knowledge, Attitudes, Beliefs and Practices Survey, quoted from Carael M. *et. al.* AIDS 1995: 9:1171-5.

[2] 1991/92 Tanzania Demographic and Health Survey, 1993.

[3] 1994 Tanzania Knowledge, Attitudes and Practices Survey, Bureau of Statistics and Macro International, 1995.

[4] 1999 Reproductive and Child Health Survey (RCHS): National Bureau of Statistics (Tanzania) and Macro international Inc. 2000.

[5] Includes people who have heard of AIDS.

[6] Includes never-married individuals aged 15-24 years.

[7] Includes sexually active individuals.

[8] Includes individuals who were married or cohabiting.

[9] Includes those individuals who reported having at least one non-regular partner during the last year who have also heard of condoms. Non-regular partners were those with whom the individual had sex but who were not spouses or in cohabiting unions.

n/a = not applicable, p-value, test for linear trend

HIV/AIDS Knowledge and Awareness

After the first AIDS cases were reported in early 1980s, AIDS awareness increased rapidly in Tanzania. About 91% of women and 94% of men had heard about AIDS in 1989/90. By 1999, AIDS awareness was almost universal among both men and women. Overall, women and residents of rural areas were relatively less knowledgeable than men and urban residents respectively, indicating that AIDS knowledge was not uniform in Tanzania. Among respondents aware of AIDS, the proportion who knew that AIDS could be avoided increased from 64% in 1994 to 82% in 1999 among women and from 80% to 89% among men. Specific knowledge about AIDS also increased over time. The proportion of respondents who mentioned using condoms and having one faithful partner as ways to reduce their risk of HIV increased between 1994 and1999. In 1989/90, there were only 28% of women and 37% of men who knew that a person infected with HIV could appear healthy, compared with 69% of women and 77% of men in 1999.

Although AIDS awareness was high, misconceptions about HIV/AIDS were also common. In 1999, only 54% of women and 59% of men thought it was not possible to get AIDS from mosquito bites, while 41% of women and 36% of men thought that sharing food or eating utensils with an AIDS patient could transmit HIV. Consistent with increasing HIV prevalence in the general population, the proportion of respondents who knew someone living with HIV or that had died of AIDS increased from about a half in 1994 to 65% of women and 69% of men in 1999. Although personal experience with

HIV/AIDS is increasing, risk perception has not changed significantly since 1994. The proportion of men who perceived themselves at high risk of HIV was 37% in 1994 and 46% in 1999, while for women it was 40% in 1994 and 43% in 1999.

Sexual Behavior

Studies conducted between 1991 and 1999 show limited changes in terms of the age at first sex and pre-marital sexual activity. During this period, the median age at first sex among women and men ranged between 16-17 years. Most women got married about 2 years later, while men got married at age 24 or 25. Premarital sexual activity has been measured by collecting information about the sexual behavior of never-married adolescents (15-24 years old). In 1999, 41% of women and 61% of men in this age group had a sexual encounter during the past year. Information about non-regular (defined as non-marital and non-cohabiting partners) and extra-marital partnerships could be used to measure sexual behaviors related to HIV/AIDS in the general population. In 1999, 25% of women and 48% of men reported sex with at least one non-regular partner during the past year. This proportion was much higher than in 1994 and 1996 where 4-6% of women and 20-25% of men reported such behaviors. Similarly, the proportion of married women and men reporting extra-marital sexual relationship was relatively higher in 1999 (8% for women and 28% for men) than in 1994 (3% for women and 18% for men) and 1996 (2% for women and 13% for men).

Although these results suggest an increase in the proportion of men and women reporting multiple sexual partners and extra-marital relations in more recent years, these differences could be due to improved reporting and changes in the way information about sexual behavior was collected in these surveys. In 1994 and 1996, respondents were first asked information about the last sexual encounter with their spouse or cohabiting partner. Later, they were asked more sensitive questions about sexual encounters with any partner other than their spouse or cohabiting partner. In the1999 survey, detailed questions were asked about the last sexual encounter with each partner during the last 12 months. These questions did not directly ask about extramarital relationships and might have elicited a more complete reporting of the number of partners. This is supported by results from other surveys that have not shown an increased reporting of high-risk sexual behaviors among men and women in Tanzania (Kapiga, 1996; Kapiga and Lugalla, 2002).

Condom Use

Condom awareness has been increasing steadily since 1989. The proportion of women who were aware of condoms increased from 60% in 1989 to 83% in 1999. During the same time period, condom awareness among men increased from 70% to 90%. Similarly, reported condom use has been increasing among both men and women, although the proportion of people using condoms remains low. Between 1989 and 1999, the proportion of respondents who had used condoms increased from 5% to 13% among women and from 10% to 32% among men. Most people who had used condoms report to have done so only occasionally. These results indicate that despite the increasing number of condoms distributed in Tanzania since 1993, only a small proportion of people report to having used condoms. Although it is difficult to provide precise reasons to account for the discrepancy between condom distribution/sales figures and reported condom use, there are several potential factors that could explain these differences. Distribution and sales figures are based on the number of condoms supplied from the central stores to the retailers and other distribution points. Thus, some of the condoms reported to have been distributed might be in these outlets waiting to be purchased. It is also possible that some of the condoms purchased by the customers have not been used. Lastly, information about condom use might be less reliable because of potential over-reporting in the community surveys.

Discussion

Overall, results from sentinel surveillance populations and community-based studies show that Tanzania is experiencing a generalized HIV epidemic, although the prevalence of HIV varies considerably in different geographical areas. In most parts of Tanzania, the prevalence of HIV is significantly higher in urban centers than in rural communities. Within rural areas, considerable differences in HIV prevalence estimates exist between rural agricultural villages, roadside settlements, and peri-urban or trading centers. The highest prevalence estimates are in peri-urban and trading centers, indicating that the risk of HIV is positively correlated with the degree of urbanization within rural communities. Thus, effective HIV prevention programs in urban and peri-urban or trading centers are likely to have a major impact on the course of the epidemic in Tanzania. Relatively high HIV incidence has been reported in some rural communities of the Mwanza region (Boerma *et. al.*, 1999), indicating that additional efforts are needed to strengthen prevention programs in less urbanized areas where potential future expansion of the epidemic is likely to occur.

The prevalence of HIV was considerably higher in women than men, although the actual differences vary across studies. Similar findings have been reported in other African countries (Carael, 1997). In all studies that included a sample from urban populations, the prevalence of HIV among women was above 11%, while most studies report less than 10% prevalence estimates among men. The relatively increased risk of HIV among women might be due to biological as well as socio-cultural factors. Male-to-female transmission has been shown to be more efficient, mainly because of a relatively larger female genital tract surface area exposed to seminal ejaculate (Royce *et. al.*, 1997). Other factors that could account for the increased prevalence of HIV in women include early age of initiation of sexual activity and younger women engaging in sexual relationships with older male partners who are more likely to be HIV-infected than younger men (Glynn *et. al.*, 2001). The differences in HIV prevalence between men and women were most pronounced in urban and peri-urban areas and almost disappeared in rural communities, suggesting that social and behavioral factors rather than biological vulnerability could account for the gender differences in HIV prevalence in Tanzania.

Results from prospective studies show that new HIV infections continue to occur in various parts of Tanzania, indicating that the epidemic is expanding rapidly in the general population. Most new infections are concentrated in young people, particularly young women. This suggests that the HIV epidemic in Tanzania can be controlled only if the prevalence of HIV in young women falls. Hence, development of effective HIV intervention programs targeted at this population should be given the highest priority. Although the full impact of the epidemic is yet to be realized, the devastating effects of AIDS are being experienced in Tanzania. AIDS has become a leading cause of hospital admissions and deaths among men and women aged 15-49 years in many regions (Adult Morbidity and Mortality Project, 2000). In Mwanza, 65% of male and 60% of female deaths were attributable to HIV infection among factory workers and their spouses (Senkoro *et. al.*, 2000). AIDS-associated mortality is also increasing in rural areas where the prevalence of HIV is still low. For example, the proportion of adult deaths attributable to AIDS in the rural populations in the Mwanza region ranges from 35% to about 50% (Todd *et. al.*, 1997; Urassa *et. al.*, 2001). In addition, the HIV epidemic is having a major impact on the occurrence of smear-positive tuberculosis (TB) cases. The TB case notification in Tanzania increased from 38 per 100,000 population in 1983-1987 to 69 per 100,000 population in 1993-1997 (Range *et. al.*, 2001). Between 40-67% of this increase was attributable to the HIV epidemic (Range *et. al.*, 2001; Van Cleeff and Chum, 1995; Van den Broek *et. al.*, 1993; Chum *et. al.*, 1996). The increasing number of TB cases poses a major burden on the existing health services in Tanzania.

Since most HIV infections in Tanzania are transmitted through heterosexual contact, HIV/AIDS control activities have focused on increasing general AIDS awareness and the promotion of safer sexual practices. Although these efforts have been successful in raising AIDS awareness and knowledge, results from community-based studies show that this awareness has not resulted in significant changes in sexual behaviors. Multiple sexual partnerships continue to be common, although trends from various studies are difficult to assess due to both changes in the wording of survey questions and the potential for changes over time in reporting bias. As observed in other African countries (Buve *et. al.*, 2002), multiple sexual partnerships were common in Tanzania, particularly among men residing in urban areas. These results highlight the importance of developing HIV intervention programs targeted at men in urban centers.

Promotion of barrier methods such as condoms has been a central theme of the HIV/AIDS prevention efforts in Tanzania. This aspect of the national response has also been less successful. Only a small proportion of men and women report to having ever used condoms, indicating that most sexual encounters were not protected by condoms in Tanzania.

Condoms were more likely to be used by people who are less than 25 years of age and among men and residents of urban areas (Kapiga, 1996; Kapiga and Lugalla, 2002). Increased condom use in urban areas, where most HIV/AIDS control activities have been implemented, might be due to relatively high AIDS awareness associated with improved condom availability and acceptability. Condom use has been reported to increase with increasing levels of education and among men and women practicing high-risk sexual behaviors (Kapiga, 1996; Kapiga and Lugalla, 2002; Kapiga e*t. al.*, 1995). Increased condom use among people engaged in high-risk sexual behaviors might be indicative of some success in the efforts to promote condoms in populations at highest risk of HIV/AIDS (Kapiga *et. al.*, 1995). It is also possible that due to perceived HIV/AIDS protection, availability of condoms and willingness to use them may increase the tendency to engage in high-risk sexual behaviors (Konde-Lule *et. al.*, 1997).

As the HIV epidemic continues to evolve rapidly in Tanzania, there is an urgent need to take stock of the experience that has been gained and develop strategies to increase safer sexual practices. Perhaps a major lesson that has been learned during the past two decades is that efforts to raise general awareness about HIV transmission and prevention are necessary but not sufficient to induce widespread changes in sexual behaviors. Thus, HIV prevention efforts should go beyond increasing awareness by addressing the broader societal factors that reinforce high-risk sexual behaviors in the general population. Analysis of the major social, political, and economic changes that have occurred in Tanzania during the last four decades might help to provide a deeper understanding of the social context of the HIV epidemic and form a basis for a more comprehensive national response. Following an agreement with the World Bank in 1986, Tanzania adopted the structural-adjustment policies (SAPs). These policies advocated the devaluation of the local currency to stimulate foreign investments, privatization, liberalization of the economy, retrenchment of workers, reduced spending on non-productive sectors, and the introduction of user fees in the social services such as health and education.

Although SAPs have helped to improve fiscal discipline in the government institutions, there is evidence to suggest that these policies have resulted in the further deterioration of the living conditions in the general population (Lugalla, 1995; Lugalla, 1995; Mlawa and Green, 1998). The devaluation of the local currency has been responsible for the increased prices of both locally produced and imported commodities. Reduced budgets have adversely affected the ability of the government to provide social services and the availability of employment opportunities in the public sector, while privatization of the public institutions and retrenchment of workers have contributed to increased unemployment. Furthermore, the abolition of government subsidies on agricultural inputs has increased the cost of production in the agricultural sector leading to increased prices of foodstuffs in urban areas. All these changes have resulted in reduced real wages, increased poverty, and rising inflation and cost of living for the majority of people in Tanzania.

These social changes have created conditions that increase personal and societal vulnerability and might contribute to the rapid expansion of the HIV epidemic in Tanzania. In conditions of poverty, the risk of HIV assumes a low priority to people's daily concerns. Increasing cost of living thus poverty have contributed in increasing existing gender inequalities and enhancing the economic dependence of women on men. Lack of employment opportunities in the formal sector has resulted in an increased number of young men and women migrating to urban areas to seek low-paying jobs in the informal sector. Migrants leave their families in rural areas and enter an urban environment where sexual risk-taking is common. Some women who fail to get employment in the informal sector may be forced to practice commercial sexual activities to survive and support their family (Silberschmidt and Rasch, 2001; Buve *et. al.*, 2002; Lugalla *et. al.*, 1999). Furthermore, the introduction of user fees in the health facilities and schools is likely to make these social services inaccessible to a substantial proportion of people who are unable to make these payments.

Strategies to address these underlying factors that increase personal and societal vulnerability to HIV should be developed as part of the broader national response against HIV/AIDS in Tanzania. Such strategies should include efforts to improve living conditions and reduce poverty, programs to increase employment opportunities for young people in both rural and urban areas, and the empowerment of women and other marginalized groups. Furthermore, since HIV is likely to contribute to increased poverty, HIV prevention efforts should become an integral part of the national strategies to tackle economic underdevelopment and increase human development.

Despite the gravity of the HIV epidemic in Tanzania, it took more than 15 years for the top political leaders to engage more openly in AIDS prevention activities. This is mainly because of the denial and stigmatization that accompanied the disease. Political support and commitment has significantly increased in more recent years mainly because of persistent pressure from the UN Theme Group and other members of the donor community and increased awareness about the devastating effects of the AIDS epidemic in the general population. As a result of these changes, senior government officials have started using political meetings to discuss AIDS and to be more actively involved in AIDS prevention efforts. In December 2000, the Tanzania AIDS Commission (TACAIDS) was formed in the Prime Minister's office to provide strategic leadership for and coordinate the implementation of, a national multisectoral response to HIV/AIDS. Following intensive consultations with stakeholders in various sectors, a national policy for HIV/AIDS prevention and control was launched in November 2001. These favorable changes have helped to bring AIDS to the top of the national agenda and increase the openness and visibility of ongoing HIV prevention activities. The main challenge now is to sustain these efforts and maximize social support for HIV/AIDS prevention efforts.

Much of the international "best practices" worldwide have been driven by the civil society and community-based NGOs. Although there has been a gradual increase in the number of NGOs and other community-based organizations working on AIDS in Tanzania during the last decade, most HIV prevention activities have been implemented by the government institutions. Most NGO activities cover limited geographical areas, mostly in major urban centers. While NGO activities have been instrumental in mobilizing community AIDS-control activities in some areas of Tanzania, strong partnerships between these organizations and government institutions involved in HIV prevention is required to strengthen the national responses to HIV/AIDS. The government of Tanzania needs to reach out to NGOs working on AIDS, as well as to people living with AIDS, and to include them routinely in program planning and implementation. Since most Tanzania government institutions have limited experience working with the private sector, involvement of NGOs and other community-based organizations in a national HIV prevention program is not going to be easy.

Lastly, the weakest part of the national response to HIV in Tanzania is the lack of programs for provision of care and support for people living with HIV/AIDS. In a few parts of Tanzania, NGOs have mobilized volunteers to provide home-based care and support for people living with HIV/AIDS. As in other parts of Africa, the prices of antiretroviral drugs have dropped significantly in most major urban centers of Tanzania, resulting in a gradual increase in the number of people using combination therapies, including HAART. However, the prices of the drugs are still high for most people, and only few relatively well-to-do patients can afford these therapies. In April 2002, the MOH produced the first national guidelines for the clinical management of HIV disease in Tanzania (United Republic of Tanzania, 2002). This document provides MOH guidelines on universal medical precautions, counseling and HIV testing, prevention of mother-to-child transmission of HIV, community-based care, management of opportunistic infections, and treatment of HIV diseases by using antiretroviral drugs. Although widespread provision of antiretroviral drugs is not feasible at this point in Tanzania, the government needs to develop a comprehensive plan that will allow an increasing number of individuals living with HIV/AIDS to gain access to care and support for HIV disease and opportunistic infections. This is likely to pose many challenges as a delicate balance between HIV prevention activities and provision of care and support for HIV-infected individuals will be required.

Chapter Seven

Decline in Prevalence and Incidence of HIV infection in Kagera: Analysis of Socio-Demographic and Behavioral Factors

Gideon Kwesigabo, Willy Urassa, Japhet Z.J. Killewo, Joe L.P. Lugalla, Maria Emmelin, Aldin Mutembei, Lars Dahlgren, Anita Sandstrom

Introduction

The problem of HIV/AIDS in Kagera dates back to 1983 when the first three AIDS cases in Tanzania where first reported. Since then the disease has continued to spread in the general population in various parts of the country, mainly through heterosexual contact, which accounts for over 90% of the infections (Caldwell and Caldwell, 1994). In order to understand the dynamics of spread and to assess the social response to this epidemic in Kagera, various studies have been conducted over a period of time (Killewo, 1994, Kwesigabo, 2001). These studies, among other things, have enabled the investigation of HIV infection trends and the associated factors in the region. This has been important because disease trends provide information about the past and present and may help to predict future patterns of diseases that are needed for planning future health needs and the formulation of public health policy (Dondero *et. al.*, 1988.)

When reviewing HIV infection trends since the beginning of the epidemic in the early eighties, various patterns have been reported in the general as well as in specific population groups. Most have been reported as either stable or increasing, and a few have been reported as decreasing (Mbizvo *et. al.*, 1996, UNAIDS, 1999, Wilkinson *et. al.*, 2000). Findings indicating a downward trend in the prevalence of HIV infection have been reported from countries such as Uganda, Thailand, Guinea Bissau, and Tanzania - to mention just a few (Kwesigabo *et. al.*, 1998, Larsen *et. al.*, 1998, Mason *et. al.*, 1995, Mulder *et. al.*, 1995). In some places like Kagera, the downward trend in prevalence has also been reflected by a similar downward trend in incidence. In other places, however, this pattern has not been observed. Studies carried out in Uganda have indicated a downward prevalence trend that did not reflect corresponding trends in incidence (Kamali *et. al.*, 2000, Wawer *et. al.*, 1997.) Most downward trends, on the other hand, have been observed in areas which had originally experienced high prevalence or incidence rates that were associated with so-called maturation states of the epidemic (Wawer *et. al.*, 1997). In these areas where prevalence decline does not reflect a corresponding decline in incidence, several factors could be responsible. These include excessive mortality among HIV-positive individuals, non-random migration, temporary absenteeism of the infected, and differential or selective refusal to participate in the intended studies. However, in areas where these explanatory factors can be ruled out, behavioral change has been singled out as being the most consistent explanation for the observed decline in prevalence (Kamali *et. al.*, 2000, Kilian *et. al.*, 1999). This write-up presents the HIV infection disease trends in the Kagera region for the period of 1987 to 2002 and explores the possible behavioral factors which could have modified the pattern of the epidemic in this region. Information used in this report is a result of research work conducted in the region by the Kagera AIDS Research Project.

Kagera Region: Administrative Structure and Intervention Activities

The Kagera region is situated on the western side of Lake Victoria and is divided into six administrative districts, namely Bukoba urban, Bukoba rural, Muleba, Karagwe, Ngara and Biharamulo. According to projections from the 1988 population census (Government *et. al.*, 1988), the total population of the region is about 1.8 million of which 63,000 are residents of Bukoba urban. Districts in the region are further divided into divisions, wards and villages, or streets. Villages are mainly rural and are further subdivided into *vitongoji* which are the smallest administrative units in the country with households varying between 25 and 200. In the urban setting, streets may have a similar number of households. The majority of the people in the region are Christians by religion followed by Moslems and traditional religions, while Buddhists and Hindus are the minority.

Intervention Activities in the Area

In Kagera, the earliest organized activities aimed at controlling the AIDS epidemic were initiated as early as 1987. By 1993, there were more than 13 governmental and non-governmental organizations providing interventions in various parts of the region. The nature of activities, the target population, methods, and coverage have varied from one organization to the other. Activities carried out included: IEC strategies, spiritual and moral strengthening, condom distribution, material support to orphans and schools, vocational training for the youth, and agricultural promotion. In health care settings, they included: training of traditional birth attendants and providing them with supplies to conduct home deliveries, immunization against communicable diseases, counseling of patients and people living with AIDS, provision of home-based care for AIDS patients, and improvement of diagnostic and treatment facilities. These activities were targeted at the general population and other specific groups namely, in and out of school children; teachers and their supporting staff; post primary and secondary school students; orphaned children and their families; fishermen, bar, guest house as well as hotel workers; and health care workers. In about a third of the organizations, their activities covered the whole region while the rest covered one or several districts, mainly Bukoba urban, Bukoba rural, and Muleba (Killewo *et. al.*, 1993, Lugalla *et. al.*, 1997).

Background to the Kagera AIDS Research Project

The Kagera AIDS Research Project (KARP) is one of the components of the bilateral collaborative research project between Tanzania and Sweden coded TANSWED HIV Programme initiated in 1986 and originally called the HIV Bilateral Programme. This collaboration has involved various disciplines drawn from various institutions both in Tanzania and in Sweden after having developed the understanding that the problem of AIDS cannot be investigated/solved from a single perspective alone. The program has been made possible by long-term technical, material, and financial support from Sida/SAREC and the Government of Tanzania. The original aim of the collaboration was to investigate the HIV/AIDS problem in Tanzania and to strengthen the research capacity of the Tanzanian participating institutions. TANSWED has expanded from the original seven projects developed and funded in 1986 to the current 13 projects altogether. Specifically for KARP, at inception, the major aim of the project was to investigate the epidemiology, dynamics, and spread of HIV infection in the region in order to arrive at appropriate entry points for intervention. Following a regional cross-sectional study in 1987, subsequent project activities have been developed over time, with results from previous studies influencing further planning. This has resulted in a series of population-based epidemiological and socio-anthropological studies enabling, among other things, the monitoring of trends in the study area. The project has so far collected and analyzed a large amount of data aimed at addressing a series of objectives developed at each study phase. Findings from the project have been disseminated through various avenues including conferences, seminars, and publications (Emmelin *et. al.*, December 1997, Emmelin *et. al.*, 12-16 September 1999, Killewo, 1994, Killewo *et. al.*, 1994, Killewo *et. al.*, 1990, Killewo *et. al.*, 1998, Killewo *et. al.*, 1993, Killewo *et. al.*, 1994, Killewo *et. al.*, 1993, Kwesigabo *et. al.*, 1998, Kwesigabo *et. al.*, 1996, Kwesigabo *et. al.*, 1999, Kwesigabo *et. al.*, 2000, Kwesigabo *et. al.*, June 28-July 3rd 1998, Lugalla *et. al.*, 4/1997, Lugalla *et. al.*, 1999, Lwihula *et. al.*, 1993, Urassa *et. al.*, 1999). Inter-disciplinary co-operation as well as collaboration between the biomedical and applied sciences has, from the beginning, been a basic trait in the project. The multiplicity in methodology on different levels has been emphasized both in methods of data collection and analysis. This strategy has been based on a joint venture between the disciplines of epidemiology, sociology, linguistics, clinical medicine, and microbiology/immunology. As part of feedback at regional level, the project has been working closely with the Kagera regional health administration. Workshops and general meetings have been organized from time to time as a means of disseminating of research results to the policy makers and the general population (Killewo *et. al.*, 1993). At the study population level, the service and feedback component activities included the IEC with distribution of AIDS educational materials and condoms, as well as provision of treatment for patients with syphilis and their sexual partners (Killewo, 1994).

Methods Used for Data Collection, Management and Analysis

Selection of Study Areas

From the six administrative districts, three were selected in the following manner: The initial study for estimation of prevalence and associated factors was carried out in 1987. In order to obtain a representative sample for this region-wide cross-sectional study, the region was divided into 4 zones on the basis of presumed contrasting HIV infection rates as reflected by the differing number of reported AIDS cases from the region. Findings from the 1987 regional survey varied between the zones, as had been predicted (Killewo *et. al.*,

1990). The prevalence was 24.2% in the Bukoba urban district, 10% in Bukoba Rural and Muleba, 4.5% in Karagwe and 0.6% in the Ngara/ Biharamulo districts. For the purpose of monitoring HIV infection trends, Bukoba urban was selected to represent a high prevalence area, while Muleba and Karagwe were selected to represent medium and low-prevalence areas respectively.

The Cross-Sectional Studies

Following the regional baseline cross-sectional study in 1987, subsequent cross-sectional studies were carried out in the Bukoba urban district in 1993 and 1996, in the Muleba district in 1996 and 1999, and in the Karagwe district in 1999. All studies involved new samples obtained through probability sampling strategies. Details of implementation of the 1987, 1993, and 1996 cross-sectional studies have been reported earlier (Killewo *et. al.*, 1993, Kwesigabo *et. al.*, 1998, Kwesigabo *et. al.*, 2000). The cross-sectional studies conducted in the Muleba and Karagwe districts in 1999 used the same sampling methodology as was used in the earlier studies.

The Incidence Studies of Bukoba Urban and Muleba Districts

HIV sero-negative individuals who were identified during the cross-sectional studies formed the population at risk for follow-up studies designed to measure incidence of HIV infection. Consequently, the study population recruited in Bukoba urban in 1993 was followed up in 1996; the population studied in Muleba in 1996 was followed up to the year 2000. The number of individuals becoming HIV positive during the interim period divided by the respective total number of person years of observation formed the basis for calculation of incidence estimates.

HIV Serology

All samples from this series of studies were tested using two Enzyme Linked Immunoabsorbent Assays; discordant sera to the two tests where subjected to the Western Blot test. Accordingly, HIV testing was supervised and validated by microbiologists/immunologists from the Swedish Institute for Infectious Disease Control (WHO Reference Laboratory) and/or from the Muhimbili University College of Health Sciences (A Tanzania National HIV reference laboratory). During the whole process of conducting these studies, internal quality control was strictly adhered to.

Behavioral Studies

While the cross-sectional population studies have been going on, the socio-anthropological component of the project has been carrying out studies that address social as well as behavioral issues associated with HIV/AIDS. At the beginning, the social scientists focused on the social, economic, and cultural factors that facilitate the rapid transmission of HIV/AIDS in Kagera (Lugalla *et. al.*, 1999). Through these we have managed to explain the factors that led to the quick spread of the AIDS epidemic in the Kagera region. By bringing these factors out into the open, we have been able to provide a variety of non-governmental organizations with data and information that is important in formulating policies on AIDS and AIDS intervention. KARP has also managed to carry out studies on existing interventions as well as people's accessibility to and acceptance of interventions that are available in the region. We have also been able to assess the impact of these interventions. In order to explain the observed declining trends of HIV/AIDS interventions that currently exist in Kagera, KARP carried out in-depth studies on behavioral changes in (2001). KARP is currently initiating studies on sexuality and education in order to understand how the nature and pattern of education on sexuality can either facilitate or hinder the spread of HIV/AIDS.

Data Management and Analysis

Using EPIINFO, Quest, and Cohort computer software packages, data were entered, cleaned, and analyzed. Differences between proportions were assessed using Chi square tests; the Fisher's exact test was used where the expected value in the cell was less than five. Trends over time were assessed using the Chi square test for trends. Incidence estimates were calculated using person years of observation as the denominator. Where the exact dates of birth were missing, the 1st of July was used as an approximation. Seroconversion was assumed to have occurred any time between the date of entry and end of follow-up. Confidence intervals around the incidence estimates were calculated using the Poisson method. Changes in the age of first sexual intercourse over time were assessed by plotting cumulative frequency of age at first sex for each five-year study cohort for the urban cross-sectional study during 1996.

Findings

Prevalence Estimates

In the *high* prevalence area of the Bukoba urban district, a total of 553, 653, and 1276 individuals was studied during the cross-sectional studies of 1987, 1993, and 1996, with corresponding response rates of 86%, 66%, and 74% respectively. The overall response, i.e. individuals participating fully and giving a blood sample, for all the cross-sectional studies combined was 82.2%. Ten percent were not found at home after up to four visits, 6.3% responded to the questionnaire but did not give a blood sample, and 1.6% refused to be interviewed. The overall age-adjusted prevalence for the *high* prevalence area declined from 24.2% in 1987 to 18.0% in 1993 and to 12.8% in 1996 ($p<0.001$). The decline was more pronounced among females (from 29.2% in 1987 to 18.7% in 1993 and to 14.4% in 1996 ($p<0.001$)) as compared with males (17.1% in 1987, 17.1% in 1993 and 10.4% in 1996 ($p=0.01$)). For both sexes, the decline was more pronounced in the age group 15-24 years (table 1).

In the *medium* prevalence area of the Muleba district, a total of 538, 1728, and 1639 individuals was studied during 1987, 1996, and 1999, the corresponding response rates being 90.1%, 70.0%, and 95.6% respectively. The age adjusted prevalence declined from 10.0% in 1987 to 6.8% in 1996 and to 4.3% in 1999 ($p<0.001$). Similar to the high prevalence area, the decline in the medium prevalence area was also more pronounced among females - from 10.1% in 1987 to 7.6% in 1996 and to 3.7% in 1999 ($p<0.001$) - as compared with males - 9.9% in 1987, 5.7% in 1996 and 5.5% in 1999 ($p=0.05$). Further details are shown in table 2. In the *low* prevalence area of the Karagwe district, a total of 670 and 1,341 individuals was recruited in 1987 and 1999, with corresponding response rates of 98.5% and 93.2% respectively. The age adjusted prevalence declined from 4.5% in 1987 to 2.6% in 1999 ($p=0.01$). The downward trend was also more pronounced among females—from 5.3% to 2.6% ($p=0.02$) (Table 3). However, the decline observed among males was not statistically significant (3.3% to 2.7% $p=0.6$).

Figure 1 shows the sex-specific prevalence trends in the three studied areas. In all sites, the prevalence of HIV-1 infection had a downward trend regardless of its magnitude at baseline in 1987. Tables 1, 2, and 3 show trends in the prevalence of HIV infection for various socio-demographic variables in the three areas. Females aged 15-24 years show a significant decline in prevalence in all the three areas; a significant decline was also seen across the three areas among Christians by religion and peasants by occupation. Individuals who had attained education levels of primary class five and above, as well as those married monogamously, also showed a significant decline, but this observation was limited to the high and medium prevalence areas.

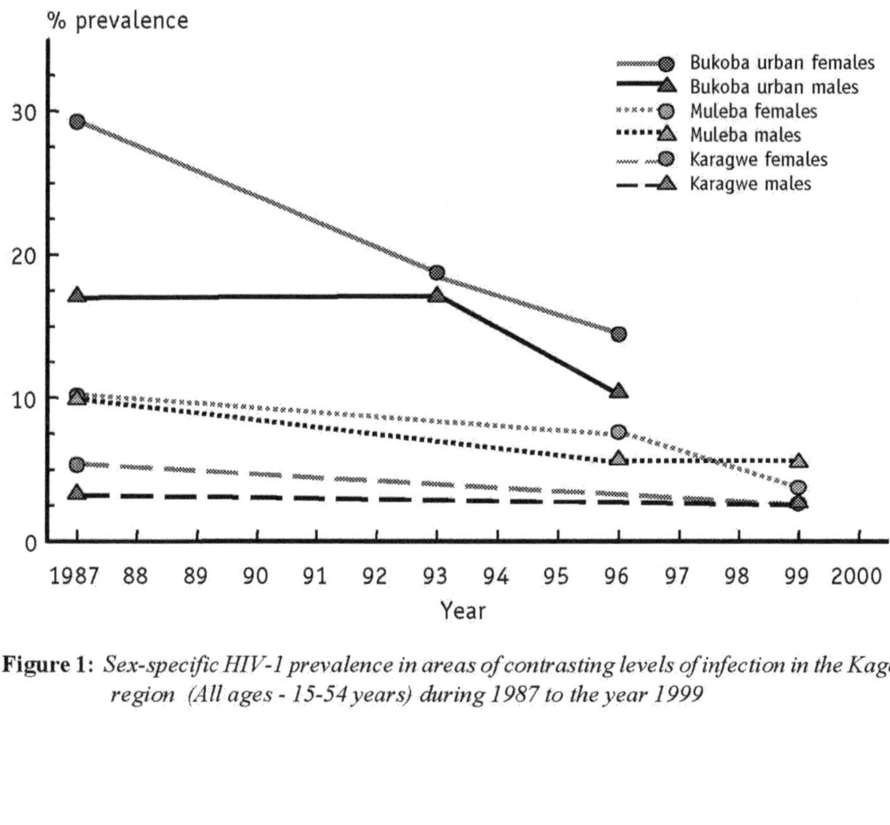

Figure 1: *Sex-specific HIV-1 prevalence in areas of contrasting levels of infection in the Kagera region (All ages - 15-54 years) during 1987 to the year 1999*

Table 1: *Trends in the prevalence of HIV-1 infection by selected socio-demographic characteristics during 1987, 1993 and 1996 for Bukoba Urban District*

	1987			1993			1996			
Socio-demographic characteristics	*Number Tested*	*Number HIV pos*	*Prev (%)*	*Number Tested*	*Number HIV pos*	*Prev (%)*	*Number Tested*	*Number HIV pos*	*Prev (%)*	*p-value Trend Test*
Age: Males										
15-24	90	10	11.1	92	6	6.5	185	3	1.6	**
25-34	76	17	22.4	90	17	18.9	146	24	16.4	
35+	62	12	19.4	76	21	27.6	158	24	15.2	
Age: Females										
15-24	127	35	27.6	170	19	11.2	344	25	7.3	**
25-34	134	48	35.8	127	42	33.1	262	56	21.4	
35+	64	12	18.8	98	13	13.3	181	32	17.7	
Religion										
Christian	386	103	26.7	510	96	18.8	980	133	13.6	**
Moslem plus other	167	31	18.6	143	22	15.4	295	31	10.5	
Occupation										
Peasant	80	25	31.3	114	22	19.3	242	36	14.9	**
Govt. or parastatal	158	37	23.4	127	22	17.3	301	35	11.6	**
Business	138	41	29.7	103	31	30.1	212	34	16.0	**
Other	177	31	17.5	309	43	13.9	521	59	11.3	
Education										
None/Adult	41	10	24.4	71	13	18.3	78	11	14.1	
Primary 1-4	64	23	35.9	92	19	20.6	125	22	17.6	
Primary 5-7	344	89	25.9	406	74	18.2	817	111	13.6	**
Secondary plus	104	12	11.5	84	12	14.3	252	20	7.9	
Marital Status										
Single	176	18	10.2	180	13	7.2	402	21	5.2	
Monogamous marriage	234	55	23.5	333	64	19.2	562	69	12.3	**
Polygamous marriage	60	28	46.7	53	10	18.9	96	16	16.7	**
Separated/Divorced	64	25	39.0	57	19	33.3	152	36	23.7	
Widow/Widower	19	8	42.1	30	12	40.0	59	22	37.3	
Total	553	134	24.2*	653	118	18.0*	1276	164	12.8*	**

* Age-adjusted

** Significant at p<0.001

Source: Kagera AIDS Research Project Findings

Table 2: *Trends in the prevalence of HIV-1 infection by selected socio-demographic characteristics during 1987, 1996 and 1999 for Muleba Rural District*

	1987			1996			1999			
Socio-demographic characteristics	*Number Tested*	*Number HIV pos*	*Prev (%)*	*Number Tested*	*Number HIV pos*	*Prev (%)*	*Number Tested*	*Number HIV pos*	*Prev (%)*	*p-value Trend Test*
Age: Males										
15-24	70	2	2.8	227	0	0.0	205	3	1.5	-
25-34	64	9	14.1	211	19	9.0	240	15	6.3	
35+	67	9	13.4	258	21	8.1	258	21	8.1	
Age: Females										
15-24	124	12	9.7	383	12	3.1	302	4	1.3	**
25-34	97	14	14.4	326	31	9.5	295	23	7.8	
35+	116	8	6.9	323	35	10.8	339	8	2.4	**
Religion										
Christian	457	50	10.9	1473	106	7.2	1444	69	4.8	**
Moslem plus other	81	4	4.9	255	12	4.7	195	5	2.6	
Occupation										
Peasant	441	42	9.5	1396	106	7.6	1527	64	4.2	0
Other	97	12	12.4	332	12	3.6	112	10	8.9	
Education										
None/Adult	114	9	7.9	378	29	7.7	469	16	3.4	
Primary 1-4	146	13	8.9	352	23	6.5	347	16	4.6	
Primary 5-7	252	27	10.7	950	63	6.6	775	42	5.4	
Secondary plus	26	5	19.2	48	3	6.3	48	0	0.0	**
Marital Status										
Single	140	2	1.4	338	8	2.4	277	2	0.7	
Monogamous marriage	264	36	13.6	942	52	5.5	1023	43	4.2	**
Polygamous marriage	67	5	7.5	190	9	4.7	140	6	4.3	
Separated/Divorced	47	7	14.9	165	23	13.9	118	15	12.7	
Widow/Widower	20	4	20.0	93	26	28.0	76	8	10.5	
Total	538	54	20.0*	1728	118	6.8*	1639	74	4.3*	**

* Age adjusted

** Significant at p<0.001

Source: Kagera AIDS Research Project Findings

Table 3: *Trends in the prevalence of HIV-1 infection by selected socio-demographic characteristics during 1987 and 1999 for Karagwe Rural District*

	1987			1999			
Socio-demographic characteristics	*Number Tested*	*Number HIV pos*	*Prev (%)*	*Number Tested*	*Number HIV pos*	*Prev (%)*	*p-value Trend Test*
Age: Males							
15-24	119	1	0.8	187	3	1.6	
25-34	56	3	5.4	193	7	3.6	
35+	95	5	5.3	207	6	2.9	
Age: Females							
15-24	153	8	5.2	252	4	1.6	
25-34	143	8	5.6	267	7	2.6	
35+	104	5	4.8	239	9	3.8	
Religion							
Christian	630	27	4.3	1256	32	2.5	**
Moslem plus other	40	3	7.5	89	4	4.5	
Occupation							
Peasant	583	25	4.3	1222	31	2.5	**
Other	88	5	5.7	123	5	4.1	
Education							
None/Adult	154	4	2.6	365	8	2.2	
Primary 1-4	161	10	6.2	232	7	3.0	
Primary 5-7	278	8	2.9	648	17	2.6	
Secondary plus	74	8	10.8	100	4	4.0	
Marital Status							
Single	161	7	4.3	229	3	1.3	**
Monogamous marriage	335	13	3.9	750	18	2.4	
Polygamous marriage	112	4	3.6	188	5	2.7	
Separated/Divorced	37	4	10.8	109	3	2.8	**
Widow/Widower	18	2	11.1	69	7	10.1	
Total	670	30	5.5*	1345	36	2.6*	**

* Age adjusted

** Significant at $p<0.05$

Source: Kagera AIDS Research Project Findings

Incidence Estimates

A total of 535 HIV sero-negative individuals was eligible for follow-up from 1993 to 1996 in the high prevalence area of the Bukoba urban district. Of these, 238 individuals was fully followed up until 1996. The corresponding figure of eligible individuals for the medium prevalence area of the Muleba rural district in 1996 was 1610. Of these, a total of 1193 individuals were fully followed up until 2000. Reasons for non-participation varied between the urban and rural settings. In the urban setting, those responding fully were 45.5%, 9.4% answered the questions but did not give a blood sample, 3.8% refused to participate, 5.7% were not found, 8.3% were presumed dead, and 27.4% had migrated. For the rural area, 74.1% responded fully, 16.6% answered the questionnaire but did not give a blood sample, 0.9% refused to answer, and 8.4% were not found. Table 4 shows sex-specific incidence of HIV-1 infection in the Bukoba urban and Muleba districts for the respective follow-up periods during 1987 to 2000. In the Bukoba urban district, the overall incidence declined significantly from 47.5/1000 person years at risk (PYAR) in 1989 to 9.1/1000 PYAR in 1996. Compared with males, females showed a significant decline. For the medium prevalence area, the Muleba district, the overall incidence declined from 8.2 per 1000 PYAR in 1989 to 3.9 per 1000 PYAR in 2000.

Table 4: *Incidence of HIV-1 infection in Bukoba urban district during the periods of 1987-89 and 1993-1996 and Muleba District during 1987-89 and 96-2000*

	No followed up	*Person years of follow-up*	*No HIV pos*	*Incidence***	*95%CI*
Bukoba Urban (High prevalence area)					
1987-1989*					
Male	95	143.0	6	42.0	15.5-91.6
Female	127	194.0	10	51.5	25.6-95.4
Total	222	337.0	16	47.5	24.2-77.8
1993-1996					
Male	71	230.4	2	8.7	1.0-31.2
Female	167	542.3	5	9.2	3.0-22.1
Total	238	772.7	7	9.1	3.6-19.0

	No followed up	*Person years of follow-up*	*No HIV pos*	*Incidence***	*95%CI*
Muleba District (Medium prevalence area)					
1987-1989*					
Male	438	822.4	7	8.5	3.4-18.0
Female	656	1246.3	10	8.0	3.8-15.0
Total	1094	2068.7	17	8.2	4.8-13.1
1996-2000					
Male	482	1955.8	7	3.6	1.4-7.4
Female	703	2852.9	12	4.2	2.2-7.3
Total	1185	4808.8	19	3.9	2.4-6.7

* Adopted from Killewo et al. 1993 (Killewo, *et. al.*, 1993) (CI have been recalculated assuming a Poisson distribution)

** Incidence per 1000 person years at risk.

Source: Kagera AIDS Research Project Findings

Behavioral Factors – Sexual Risk

Sexual behavior, such as the number of sexual partners per year, condom use, marriages, and age at first sex were analyzed for trends. KARP has also been able to confirm the association between poverty, gender inequality, economic crisis, political instability, prostitution, traditional practices of widow inheritance, and others with HIV/AIDS. Our recent studies on behavioral trends reveal that some of these harmful risk practices are fading away.

Average Number of Sexual Partners and Condom Use

The average number of sexual partners per year was analyzed for the Bukoba urban district in 1993 compared with 1996. There was no significant change in the average number of sexual partners when the 1993 result was compared with that of 1996 i.e. 1.2 (1.1-1.3) compared to 1.3 (1.2-1.3) respectively. However, there was a significant rise in condom use (regardless of type of sexual partner) from 23.1% (N=546) in 1993 to 30.9% (N=1291) in 1996 (p=0.0001). Among the religious groupings having a significant rise in condom use were the Christians as compared with other religious groups (21.2% to 30.2%, p=0.01).

Over 80% of the studied individuals in the three areas of differing levels of infection reported having one sexual partner at the time of the latest round of studies, regardless of marital status.

*=p<0.001

Source: Kagera AIDS Research Project Findings

Age Group	*1987*			*1993*			*1996*			*1999*			*Trend text p value*
	Total	*Married*	*%*	*Total*	*Married*	*%*	*Total*	*Married*	*%*	*Total*	*Married*	*%*	
Bukoba Urban District													
15-24	217	49	22.6	262	97	37.0	524	173	33.0				*
25-34	210	116	55.2	217	152	70.0	408	260	63.7				*
35*	126	84	66.7	174	124	71.3	338	224	66.3				
Total	553	249	45.0	653	373	57.1	1270	657	51.7				*
Muleba District													
15-24	194	65	33.5				610	300	49.2	506	285	56.3	*
25-34	161	132	82.0				537	447	83.2	534	436	81.6	
35*	183	134	73.2				581	421	72.5	594	442	74.4	
Total	538	331	61.5				1728	1168	67.6	1634	1163	71.2	*
Karagwe District													
15-24	269	122	45.3							465	262	56.3	*
25-34	196	158	80.6							487	378	77.6	
35*	197	166	84.3							470	352	74.8	*
Total	662	446	67.4							1422	992	69.8	

Table 6: *Trend in percentage of married individuals in areas of varying levels of HIV-1 infection in Kagera Region*

Proportion Married

Analysis of marital status information (categorized as either monogamous or polygamous marriages) revealed that the proportion of married individuals increased with time, and they were marrying at an earlier age than before. This proportion also increased as people moved away from high to low prevalence areas. This information is shown in Table 6 which also shows that this increasing trend was significant in the age group 15-24 years in all three areas.

Age at First Sexual Contact

In assessing whether there has been a change in the age at first sexual act, a cumulative curve of age at first sexual act was constructed for each 5-year age cohort of the studied Bukoba urban population of 1996. For both sexes, a decrease was noted regarding age at first sexual act, the majority of individuals now aged 15-19 having started sex at an earlier age in comparison with the rest of the cohorts. These are followed by age groups 20-24 and 25-29 years. See figures 2 and 3.

Fig 2: *Cumulative distribution for age at first sexual contact for 5 year cohorts of the studied population in Bukoba Urban District during 1996 (Females)*

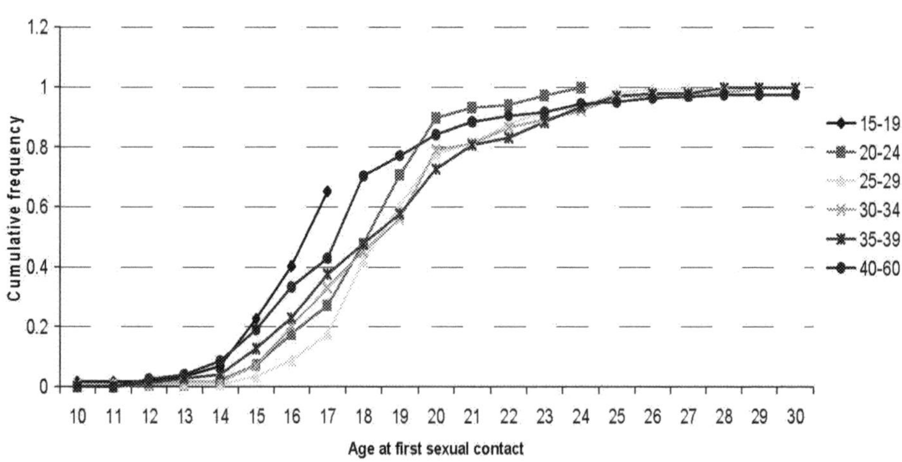

Source: Kagera AIDS Research Project Findings

Fig 3: *Cumulative frequency curve of age at first sexual contact for 5 year cohorts of the studied population in Bukoba Urban District during 1996 (Males)*

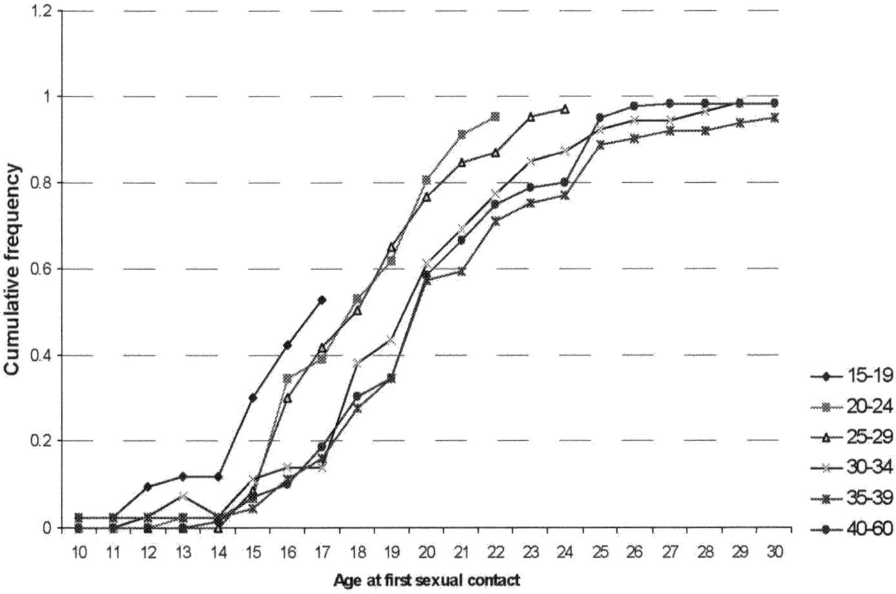

Source: Kagera AIDS Research Project Findings

General Reporting of Precautions Taken

When the study population members were asked as to whether they took any precaution to avoid being infected with the HIV virus, over 96% indicated that they took some form of precaution. The major precautions mentioned included sticking to one partner - described as no sex outside marriage; condom use for casual sex; and for individuals who are still single, abstinence coupled with premarital voluntary counseling and testing (VCT) when they want to get married.

Lessons Learnt and Implications for the Future

Studies conducted in Kagera over a period of 13 years in the general population have indicated a downward trend in overall HIV-1 prevalence which was also reflected by a downward trend in incidence. This downward trend was noted in areas with contrasting levels of infection classified as high, medium, and low HIV-1 infection prevalence areas, the decline being observed regardless of the initial level of infection. Analysis of the age specific prevalence trends showed that the decline was significant among young women aged between 15 and 24 years in all the three areas, as well as in men of the same age in the high prevalence area. Analysis of behavioral factors indicated that over 80% of individuals had one sexual partner, there was a rise in condom use, a rise in the proportion of individuals getting married, and marriage at an earlier age than before. However, the average number of sexual partners remained the same (1.2), and age at first sex decreased with time.

The purpose of the cross-sectional studies was to estimate the magnitude and spread of HIV-1 infection through a representative probability sample of the population. This representative sample yielded response rates varying from 66-95.6%. The overall response, however, (defined as all individuals participating fully by answering questions and consenting to a blood test at recruitment and at the end of the follow-up period) for all the cross-sectional studies combined was 82.2%. Reasons for non participation included, not found at home after up to four visits (10.0%), responded to the questionnaire but did not give a blood sample (6.3%), and refused to answer the questionnaire (1.6%). No significant differences were found when the demographic characteristics of individuals responding fully were compared with the non-respondents. However, behavioral characteristics of non-respondents were not available for comparison with those of respondents.

Cross-sectional studies can provide point estimates and trends of HIV infection in the general population. To understand changes in prevalence within a population, stratification into age, sex, and other socio-demographic factors is essential to help identify particular patterns of change within population sub-groups that may be masked by a reliance upon a general sample of the population (Batter *et. al.*, 1994). In addition, serial age specific sero-prevalence may unmask the age structure of the epidemic and its evolution over time (Ades, 1995). Age, sex, and other demographic characteristics were incorporated in the research instruments used in the Kagera studies right from the time the studies were initiated. The availability of these variables and the involvement of larger sample sizes over time have enabled stratified analysis despite the decreasing prevalence.

In an area where over 90% of infections are acquired through heterosexual contact, a decrease in the number of new infections mainly implies behavioral change. This could be a result of a diminished compensatory increase in the supply of new susceptibles with a high risk or lack of increase in the risk behavior of others in the population. This will lead to a fall in the average level of risk that, in turn, will lead to a reduced incidence of infection (UNAIDS, 1999).

One of the possible explanations for the observed decline could be the study participants modifying their behavior positively as a result of receiving testing and counseling during the cross-sectional and follow-up studies which may be translated as a form of intervention. For cross-sectional studies, this is unlikely because at all times when the studies were being carried out, new samples were drawn - samples which had no prior exposure to research VCT. However, this phenomenon may not be ruled out in the case of incidence studies. The series of studies in Kagera has shown an overall and specific decrease in prevalence among young people. A study in Uganda showed slightly different findings: despite a decline among people in the young age groups, no change was observed in the overall prevalence (Mulder *et. al.*, 1995).

Prevalence trends may not reflect incidence trends. Studies in Uganda have demonstrated a reduced prevalence of HIV infection in men and women not reflected by a similar decrease in incidence (Kamali *et. al.*, 2000, Wawer *et. al.*, 1997). This may imply that excess mortality or migration could be possible explanatory factors for the observed decline in prevalence in these areas. It is worth noting that prevalence data from young people reflect infections that had occurred recently (Mertens *et. al.*, 1994). For this reason, differential mortality may not be of major concern to this age group (Fabiani *et. al.*, 2001).

Findings from incidence studies carried out in Kagera have indicated a downward trend in incidence from 47.5/1000 PYAR in 1989 to 9.1/1000 PYAR in 1996 in the Bukoba urban district and from 8.2/1000 PYAR in 1989 to 3.9/1000 PYAR in 2000 in the Muleba district. These findings therefore confirm the downward trend demonstrated in cross-sectional studies.

Behavioral change can alter the course of the epidemic at an early stage, averting its disastrous consequences if left to grow. The low prevalence area in Kagera experienced this. In the high and medium prevalence areas, behavioral change has been shown to alter the course of the epidemic towards a downward trend. Over 80% of individuals reporting to have had one sexual partner at the time of the study and a rise in condom use are some of the factors which have been observed in these populations. In addition, the proportion of individuals getting married (1987-99) was found to rise, and each time most age cohorts got married earlier than the preceding one.

However, the average number of sexual partners remained the same. There was a tendency for age at first sexual contact to decrease, especially for the 15-19 years age group for both sexes.

These findings may partially explain the observed decline in prevalence and incidence. It is important that these behavioral findings are not over-interpreted due to the nature of the methodology used in their collection. There were difficulties in establishing trends in behavioral factors due to the variability and sometimes absence of consistent questions in cross-sectional surveys that could be compared over time to elicit any behavioral changes. In addition, factors other than patterns of marriage were not available in all the studied areas except the Bukoba urban district. Misinterpretation and failure to differentiate between the number of current sexual partners and serial monogamy could also result in individuals reporting a fewer or higher number of current sexual partners than the true number. This would make comparisons over time invalid. Although a rise in condom use over time was demonstrated, it may not have reflected consistent use. All these knowledge gaps require approaches that will further elucidate these changes in behavior. In addition, the role contributed by changes in the virulence of the virus in the area is unknown.

In investigating the reasons for a the observed decline in HIV infection in one area of Uganda, it was found that there was a delay in the onset of sexual intercourse among youths and that condom use was found to rise in the same groups. It was then hypothesized that the observed declining trends were a result of behavioral change (Asiimwe-Okiror *et. al.*, 1997). A similar study in the same country detected an increase in condom use, marriage at later ages for girls, later sexual debut for boys, and a fall in fertility especially among unmarried teenagers (Kamali *et. al.*, 2000). This study also demonstrated the role of behavioral change in the decline in prevalence.

How much reduction in HIV prevalence and incidence can be attributed to intervention activities may be difficult to answer. Studies in Thailand have indicated a possible association between intervention activities and a fall in HIV prevalence (Nelson *et. al.*, 1993, UNAIDS, 1999). On the other hand, it has been noted that prevalence may fall without the direct effects of interventions (Bouckenooghe and Shandera, 1999). This calls for further studies to determine what other factors may explain the changes.

In Kagera, upon recognition that there was a problem, the government, non-governmental organizations, and individuals instituted interventions in the area. The type, nature, frequency, magnitude, mode of delivery, and coverage varied from one area to another and from organization to organization. Although it may be difficult to link the observed changes and the respective interventions, clearly all these interventions must have had an influence on people's behavior. Many years of condom promotion and distribution, for example, have led to an increased use as reflected by a rise even among Catholic Christians, who according to their teaching, believe condoms should not be used. On the other hand, grief and agony concretized by personal experiences of caring for the sick and increased mortality due to AIDS may have influenced people to mould their behavior afresh. Marrying at an early age and probably sticking to those partners reduces the rate of premarital and extramarital sexual exposure respectively thereby reducing the risk of infection.

In conclusion, despite possible limitations, these sets of studies have provided evidence that there has been a decline in the prevalence and incidence of HIV-1 in the general population of the Kagera region, most significantly among females in the age group 15-24 years, and to a lesser extent, among males of the same age. This decline was observed in all the three areas classified as high, medium, or low prevalence, implying that prevalence declined regardless of the baseline magnitude of infection documented by the 1987 study. Behavioral change at the individual level may alter the course of the epidemic and can result in a decline or prevent the epidemic from rising to saturation point before a decline is noted.

These findings are encouraging for other parts of the country, and indeed for other countries in that it is possible for HIV epidemic trends to be reversed through behavioral change. However, the general population still remains at risk of HIV infection, and all efforts to bring the magnitude down should continue unabated. Otherwise, laxity in the intervention activities may result in a resurgence of the epidemic.

PART THREE

MENTAL HEALTH

Chapter Eight

Depressive Illness and Primary Health Care in Sub-Saharan Africa: With Special Reference to Tanzania

Sylvia F. Kaaya and Melkizedeck T. Leshabari

Introduction

Epidemiological Evidence on Mental Disorders: A Global Perspective

It is estimated that about 450 million people world wide suffer neuro-psychiatric conditions that include unipolar depressive disorders, bipolar affective disorder, schizophrenia, epilepsy, alcohol and selected drug use disorders (WHO, 2001). Recent quantification of the "burden of disease" that measures the impact of premature death and disability on a population combined in a single measure provides a balanced approach to assessing health needs and priorities. The DALYs (disability-adjusted life years) that expresses the years of life lost due to premature death and years lived with a disability of a specified severity and duration is a sensitive measure of burden of disease that better accommodates chronic and disabling conditions than measures of incidence, prevalence and mortality.

Mental and neurological conditions contribute to 10.5% of the total DALYs lost due to all diseases and injuries globally, accounting for five of the top ten leading causes of DALYs as summarized in Table 1. Unipolar depressive disorder that accounts for 4.4% of the total DALYs, can affect individuals at any stage of the life span. Though the incidence of unipolar depression increases with age, it is increasingly recognized as a condition that also occurs in adolescence and young adulthood (Lewinsohn *et. al.*, 1993), and is one of the common mental disorders seen at primary levels of health care systems (Goldberg and Lecrubier, 1995). While the overall prevalence of mental illness is about the same amongst men and women world wide, unipolar depression, is twice as prevalent in females compared to males.

Table 1: *Leading Causes of Disability-adjusted Years Globally (DALYs) in 15-44 Year-Olds Estimates for 2000*

Disease/injury	*% total DALYs*
HIV/AIDS	13.0
Unipolar depressive disorders	8.6
Road traffic accidents	4.9
Tuberculosis	3.9
Alcohol use disorders	3.0
Self inflicted injuries	2.7
Iron deficiency anaemia	2.6
Schizophrenia	2.6
Bipolar affective disorder	2.5
Violence	2.3

Source: *WHO, 2001*

Conditions of poverty with associated unemployment, low educational level, deprivation and homelessness common in the developing world are important determinants of depressive disorders. These observations make it important to consider depressive disorders in a developing context. This chapter will explore what is known about the extent of depression at primary healthcare levels in Sub-Saharan Africa (SSA), and use Tanzania as a window to discuss possibilities for integration of recognition and treatment of depression primary levels of care.

Mental Disorders in the Developing World: Sub-Saharan Africa

The centralized and custodial nature of allopathic mental health services before the 1960s, and poor availability and accessibility of services in SA resulted in over-representation of psychotic forms of mental disorders in healthcare facilities (Carothers, 1947; Gordon, 1936). However, with expansion of allopathic medical services to rural areas, there is increasing evidence that mood disorders are highly prevalent at primary levels of allopathic healthcare, approach the level found in industrialized countries (German, 1987), and categories of mental disorders recognized in the West are also identifiable in Africa (Odejide *et. al.*, 1989; Westermeyer, 1985; Ben-Tovim, 1985).

Table 2: *DALYs Among 15-44 Year-Olds by Cause Group in Sub-Saharan Africa*

Rank	*Disease or Injury*	*Total DALYs (thousands)*	*Percent of Total DALYs*
1.	**All causes**	**76,637**	
	Infections and parasitic disease	21,873	28.5
	Tuberculosis	(2,773)	(12.7)
	HIV	(2,474)	(11.3)
2.	Intentional injuries	12,926	16.9
	Violence	(4,908)	(38.0)
	War	(4,171)	(32.2)
3.	Unintentional injuries	10,935	14.3
4.	Neuro-psychiatric conditions	9,452	12.3
5.	Maternal conditions	9,115	11.9
6.	Cardiovascular diseases	3,052	4.0
7.	Respiratory diseases	2,080	2.7
8.	Other conditions[1]	1,904	2.5
9.	Digestive diseases	1,725	2.3
10.	Malignant neoplasm's	1,564	2.0
11.	Nutritional deficiencies	1,127	1.5
12.	Respiratory infections	884	1.2

Source: Cohen, 1998.

The top twelve causes of DALYs for adults aged 15-44 years in Sub-Saharan Africa summarized in table 2, indicate a different pattern from what is observed in developed regions of the world. Infectious and parasitic diseases account for more than one quarter of the disease burden, whereas neuro-psychiatric conditions account for only 12 per cent. The DALYs attributable to infectious disease though high need to be given some further scrutiny. DALYs attributable to HIV/AIDS and tuberculosis that are closely related diseases, hide an unrecognised psychological burden. Kilonzo *et. al.* (1999) in Tanzania, report the impact of widespread loss of significant family members from HIV/AIDS that curtails grieving and mourning practices, though the emotional toll on

[1] Other conditions include: musculoskeletal diseases, endocrine disorders, sensory organ diseases, congenital anomalies, diabetes mellitus, oral conditions, peri-natal conditions and others.

persons affected by such losses is unclear. Many families and communities are stretched beyond their capacity to cope with illness and grief and these impacts of HIV/AIDS go far beyond that of related disease conditions and death. It is unlikely co-morbid psychopathological condition in persons attacked by HIV/AIDS and other debilitating physical conditions will be reflected in future DALY's if they are not considered.

Relatively few wide scale prevalence studies on the extent and determinants of neuro-psychiatric morbidity at primary care health levels have been conducted in Sub-Saharan Africa. However, several small scale studies summarized in Table 3 indicate morbidity amongst children, adolescents and adults is equal to or perhaps exceeds that found in more developed regions of the world. Prevalence rates for mental disorders range from 12% to 19% amongst children and adolescents and 11% to 32% amongst adults when both a screening and diagnostic instrument is used.

Table 3: *Prevalence of Mental Disorder in Primary care Populations in SSA - Some Findings 1980-1999*

Authors	*Country*	*Sample*	*Age (years)*	*N*	*Instrument*	*Prevalence %*
Children/Adolescents						
Broughton (1986)	RSA	Urban	5-15	137	RCQ	71.0
Diop *et. al.* (1982)	Senegal	Rural	5-15	545	RCQ	16.9
Giel *et. al.* (1981, 1988)	Sudan	Rural	5-15	250	RCQ/SSI	12-19
Adults						
Harding *et. al.* (1980)	Sudan	Rural	?18	360	SRQ/PSE	10.6
Diop *et. al.* (1982)	Senegal	Rural	Adults	933	SRQ	16.2
Dhaphale *et. al.* 1982)	Kenya	Rural	18-55	186	SRQ/SPI	25.8
Dhaphale *et. al.* (1983)	Kenya	Rural/SU	18-55	200	SRQ/SPI	29.0
Dhaphale and Ellison (1983)	Kenya	Urban	18-55	200	SRQ/SPI	32.0
Hall & Williams (1987)	Zimbabwe	Urban	?16	448	SRQ	10.5
Kortamann (1990)	Ethiopia	Urban	?18	30	SRQ	27
Thom *et. al.* (1993)	RSA	Urban	16-60	301	SRQ/PSE	10.3-14.3

Source: *Extracted from Parry, 1996, Table 1.*

The use of difference methodologies and sample size perhaps accounts for the observed wide variations in rates of psychiatry morbidity. The choice of what screening and diagnostic instruments to use in a primary care population may also influence observed rates. Parry (1996), notes the risk of under-estimating prevalence when the Present State Examination (PSE), (developed for use in mentally ill populations) is used as a diagnostic tool in community and primary care samples, where minor morbidity is more prevalent. When screening instruments are utilized alone without re-calibration of cut-off scores against a "gold-standard" on the other hand, there is risk of morbidity being over-estimated. The cultural adaptation of instruments developed outside the African context, is a potential area of risk to the validity of research results due to difficulties in transfer across cultures of concepts related to the experience and expression of suffering and emotional worlds. A standard translation, back-translation and adjustment sequence was utilized in most of the studies in Table 1 where instruments were translated to local languages. The use of indigenous translators sensitive to the nuances of local languages and with experience in working with mentally ill populations is a strategy used in some studies to reduce threats to validity (Orley and Wing, 1979; Giel and Van Luijk, 1969); as is physical examination to assess possibility of physical disorders causing the mental disturbance (Dhaphale *et. al.*, 1983).

Despite the methodological issues noted above, the reported studies do demonstrate that a high proportion of attendees at primary health care facilities present with psychiatric morbidity. Several African studies reveal that a large proportion of the psychiatric morbidity presenting at primary care levels comprises anxiety and depressive disorders, as has been found in the West (Blacker and Clare, 1987; Katon, 1982). Ndetei and Muhangi (1979) noted that most patients present with anxiety and depressive states. Almost 63% of a Gambian sample were found to be suffering from psycho-neuroses as defined by the International Classification of Diseases, version 9 (ICD-9) (De Jong, 1987), while about 63% of Kenyan primary care attendees with psychiatric morbidity were either suffering from anxiety or depression as defined by the ICD-8 (Dhaphale, 1989). Gureje (1992), using the Diagnostic and Statistical Manual Version III revised edition (DMS-IIIR) criteria, estimated that 23.5% of 787 primary care attendees seen had depressive or generalized anxiety disorder represented a large proportion of those identified with psychiatric morbidity.

Many of the studies carried out at primary care levels in Africa report a tendency for patients with psychiatric morbidity, especially depressive illness, to present with somatic symptoms (Abiodun, 1989; Climent *et. al.*, 1980; Ndetei and Muhangi, 1979; Holmes and Speight, 1976; Giel and Van Luijk, 1969). More recent studies in the region, however, indicate that though symptoms, as recognized in the West, may not be voluntarily reported they could be elicited on inquiry (Odejide *et. al.*, 1989; Dhaphale *et. al.*, 1989). The tendency for psychosocial distress to present in the form of physical symptoms is termed somatisation. Somatised presentations of psychological distress have been reported in other cultural settings (Goldberg and Bridges, 1988; Kleinman, 1980), and have been viewed by some as a basic universal mechanism which the human species have for responding to stress and experiencing affective symptoms (Bridges and Goldberg, 1991). In addition, patients may believe that doctors expect to hear physical complaints, and would therefore present more physical than psychological manifestations of psychosocial distress.

Difficulties in the recognition of psychiatric morbidity at primary care levels have been noted in many western studies (Johnstone and Goldberg, 1976; Kessel, 1960). In two African studies, less than a third of patients with psychiatric morbidity were found by some researchers to be correctly identified by primary health care workers (De Jong, 1987; Climent, 1980). Recognition of psychiatric morbidity also appears to present difficulties at tertiary levels of care. Kigamwa (1991) identified 22% of such morbidity in 200 medical inpatients at a consultant hospital, of which 59% comprised affective disorder and very little (9%) of the total psychiatric morbidity was recognized by attending physicians. Evidence from the West has demonstrated that skills required by primary care physicians for recognition of psychological distress can be identified and effectively taught (Kaaya *et. al.*, 1991; Goldberg, 1990; Gask *et. al.*, 1988; Davenport *et. al.*, 1987; Goldberg *et. al.*, 1980)

Recognition and effective management of non-psychotic psychiatric morbidity result in a shorter duration of the illness for some patients and avoidance of illnesses running a chronic course (Freeling et al., 1985; Johnstone and Goldberg, 1976). Dhaphale *et. al.* (1983) noted that 64% of patients identified with psychiatric morbidity reported symptoms lasting more than three months, while an almost equal proportion of those with no psychiatric morbidity reported their symptoms as lasting less than a month. Of those identified with psychiatric morbidity by Giel and Van Luijk (1969), 62% had attended the health facility more than once, while 35% had been seen at another primary care facility with complaints relating to the current episode of illness. The risk of chronicity in the African setting is accompanied by needless use of limited medical resources in terms of medical time, investigations and medication chronicity also results in increased patient suffering, frustration for the patient and the attending primary healthcare workers and a vicious cycle of continuous somatic complaints, needless investigations and frustration that are not conducive to a therapeutic environment.

There is little retrievable evidence on the determinants of depressive disorders in sub-Saharan Africa. Population based studies from both developed and developing countries suggest that poverty and common mental disorders exacerbate each other (WHO International Consortium of Psychiatric Epidemiology, 2000; Abas and Broadhead, 1997; Todd *et. al.*, 1999; Patel *et. al.*, 1999). Patel *at. al.* (1999), demonstrated in cross-national surveys in Brazil, Chile, India and Zimbabwe that common mental disorders are twice more frequent among the poor as among the rich. While mental disorders can lead to catastrophic costs for the individual/family that could tip them into poverty; poor people are also more likely to have symptoms of mental distress (Narayan *et. al.*, 2000). A prospective study associated poverty with and incidence of common mental disorders; 30% of subjects who had experienced hunger in this study developed a CMD as compared to 12% who had not (Todd *et. al.*, 1999). There is also evidence from the West to suggest that the course of mental disorders is influenced by the socio-economic status of the individual (Kessler *at. al.*, 1994, Saraceno and Barbui, 1997). This may be the result of service related factors such as poor access to mental health services that may be of particular relevance to the poor.

Studies in the African context suggest psychiatry morbidity measured at community and primary care levels may be more prevalent in women compared to men, female to male ratios ranging from 1.6:1 to 2-3:1 (Orley and Wing, 1979; Hollifield *et. al.*, 1990; Tafari *et. al.*, 1991; Gureje, 1992), though some studies have demonstrated relatively similar rates (Dhaphale et al., 1983; De Jong, 1987). The mental health of women raises concern given evidence that suggests role stress may increase vulnerability to conditions such as depression. Broadhead and Abas (1998) in Zimbabwe, note that that the majority (44%) of severe life events reported by an urban sample of women involved marital or other relationship crises. Further more, stressful life events occur more frequently in women's lives then men and women are more likely to be exposed to specific and common types of violence such as violence in intimate partnerships and sexual violence in times of conflict than men. The women in the African context hold multiple roles in biological and social reproduction as well as in maintaining family cohesion. Given her lower status relative to men, the current changes towards a market-oriented economy in Africa are bound to add to rather than decrease her roles with consequent risks to mental health.

Depressive Illnesses In Tanzania

In recent decades there has been no systematic documentation of the extent of psychiatric morbidity in Tanzania, but using WHO estimates of a point prevalence of 1% of the general population, it was estimated that in 1979, Tanzania had about 100,000 severely mentally ill adults (Schulsinger and Jablenski, 1991). However, this estimate does not take into account the less severe forms of mental illnesses which may present at primary care facilities and cause not only various levels of social incapacitation for the sufferer but also inappropriate utilization of meagre health resources if not correctly recognized.

Although data is minimal, there is no reason to suppose that rates for depression in Tanzania will be any different from those observed in other countries in Sub-Saharan Africa. Much of what is known on the prevalence of depressive illness in Tanzania is derived from clinical and community surveys of general psychiatric morbidity, few that utilized standardized criteria for case identification or definition. A survey of treatment practices was carried out within 33 peripheral public health services in two regions of Tanzania. Health workers were requested to fill in an evaluation form for each patient seen; out of 703 patients with psychiatric disorders, 22.3% met criteria for non-psychotic mental disorder broadly categorized as neurotic (Bloch, 1991). The investigator noted that most of these patients (83%) tended to somatise their psychological distress. It is not evident from the report what proportion of these patients met criteria for depression. A more recent study in a primary care populationindicated from factor analysis of a depression and anxiety symptom checklist that a depression anxiety construct is discernible (Kaaya *et. al.*, 2002). From a cross-sectional study, 24% of 178 clients recruited from two primary care facilities and 48% of 176 from eight randomly selected traditional healers were classified as having a common mental disorder on the Clinical Interview Schedule Revised Version (CIS-R) (Ngoma *et. al.*, 2003).

The extent of recognition of psychiatry morbidity at primary care levels in Tanzania has not been systematically explored. However,

Kempinski (1991), in a survey of 4,615 consecutive attendees at rural health centres and dispensaries, noted that while 7% had psychiatric complaints, only 3.9% were given a psychiatric diagnosis. Of those with a psychiatric diagnosis, 41.7% were diagnosed as neurotic while only 2.8% were reported to be depressed. The high prevalence of the diagnosis of neurotic illness is noted by the author to perhaps reflect difficulties in accuracy of diagnosis at primary health care level, where depression associated with somatisation is often erroneously labelled as neurosis. Holmes and Speight (1975) studied patients in Tanzania who were first time referrals to medical clinics. They noted 48% of patients with physical complaints were primarily suffering from a psychiatric disorder, a significant proportion being depressed. These patients had been extensively investigated in primary care health facilities and treated for other conditions, partly because the underlying psychopathology was not recognized.

A community-based survey conducted in two regions revealed that many respondents did not recognize depression as a condition of sadness in the absence of apparent external cause (Whyte, 1991). In many cases, sadness was attributed to tangible aversive life situations such as loss or financial problems. Respondents recognized the idea, however, that worries could be a direct cause of illness. Using case vignettes based on bio-medical conceptualisations of depressive disorders, the investigators were able to demonstrate that 41.6% of 202 respondents were familiar with depression. However, it was the least recognized of the psychiatric conditions studied.

Framework for Understanding Access to Mental Health Services

In the settings of both developing and developed countries, there is increasing evidence those individuals who identify themselves as ill use a variety of available pathways to health care. Illness behaviours are defined as activities and beliefs exhibited by an individual and his or her social circle in response to bodily indications perceived as symptoms (Mechanic 1962). Illness behaviours therefore include, the definition of symptoms, body monitoring for symptom change or progress and remedial action by making use of lay or professional help. The activities aimed at securing treatment for the illness experienced are what have been termed "help-seeking behaviours" (Kleinman, 1980).

Local explanatory models of illness influence illness behaviours. These refer to the patient's and family's perceptions of the nature of a particular illness, its causes and effects, expected and/or desired treatment, and apprehensions about the outcome (Ware *et. al.* 1992). Explanatory models are grounded in culturally defined systems of meanings given to illness experiences. These systems of meanings originate from local epistemologies about the nature of the body, of suffering, and of the person. Cultural categories organize various types of illness and methods of treatment, which also inform explanatory models. Ware *et. al.* (1992) note that explanatory models find expression in illness episodes and rationalize decisions about what is most at stake and what sort of treatment action should be undertaken.

With special reference to affect, Kleinman (1980) viewed affects in individuals as "fundamental psychological phenomenon engendered by external (e.g. interpersonal) and internal stimuli (e.g. intra-psychic or somatic)." Stimuli, which may be environmental, social, psychological or physiological, and which give rise to intense affects, are viewed as stressors. Culture, in this model, determines the evaluation of stimuli as stressors and provides a cognitive framework in which the experience and expression of affect is shaped. Schieffelin (1985) argues further that as culture provides the cognitive and social environment to which an individual learns to accommodate, it also provides appropriate behavioural models and defence mechanisms for copying with the stressors.

The above conceptual approach tends to offer insights to individual and community factors motivating one to consult for perceived changes in self that may be defined as illness. Perhaps linked to the above individual perspectives, studies using a pathways approach to psychiatric care give additional scope for consideration of other factors, particularly as they relate to health care services which influence the recognition and management of psychiatric morbidity (Goldberg and Huxley, 1980). Such studies have reviewed factors that relate to four points along the referral pathway; which include; the decision to consult, the detection of psychiatric illness by the doctor, referral to psychiatry outpatients and admission to psychiatry in-patient beds. An important contribution of such studies has been summarized by the description of a schematic model with five levels demonstrating different stages of the help seeking process among patients with psychiatric morbidity (ibid.). Level one is represented by psychiatric morbidity detected in the community. Level two refers to morbidity among patients presenting at primary care facilities irrespective of whether the attending primary care worker/physician has detected the illness. Conspicuous psychiatry morbidity (this is morbidity detected by primary health care workers) is demonstrated by level three, while level four and five represent psychiatry morbidity treated by psychiatrists at outpatient clinics and in-patient units respectively. Whether or not an individual in the community presents with psychiatric morbidity, thus passing through the first filter to 'level two' morbidity, is determined to a large extent by illness behaviours of the patient, which in turn are to a large extent socio-culturally determined. Passage through the second filter to conspicuous psychiatry morbidity at level three is largely determined by the ability of primary healthcare workers to recognize such morbidity.

Integration of Mental Health in Primary Health Care Services: Focus on Tanzania

A summary report of mental health services in ten eastern and southern African countries (South Africa, Botswana, Swaziland, Zimbabwe, Zambia, Eritrea, Kenya, Tanzania, Uganda, Mozambique), revealed that the number of psychiatrists in these countries (except South Africa) ranged from one to 50, serving populations of between one to 29 million. The numbers of clinical psychologists were even lower, though nurses with specialization in psychiatry ranged from seven to 1,232. Qualified mental health professionals in much of eastern and southern Africa, except for South Africa, were few, and those available predominately worked in urban settings (Sartorius, 1996). All but two of these countries had in place mental health legislation and only two had mental health policies. Despite the lack of qualified personnel, specific mental health care policies and legislation, mental health services that take into consideration the meagre resources available are being developed at primary care/community levels.

In Mozambique, where in 1996 there was one psychiatrist and one psychiatry nurse for example, the Mental Health Section of the Ministry of Health was in the process of initiating a pilot psychosocial programme. The programme was multidisciplinary in nature involving health workers, teachers, and volunteer social welfare community workers supported by 34 medical assistants trained in psychiatry and a mental health programme. The psychosocial programme represented a shift from a traditional hierarchical mental health service delivered from four asylum-like psychiatric hospitals to community based mental health interventions. The interventions were informed by needs assessments that took into consideration a capacity building component and evaluation (Mandlhate, 1996).

Eritrea, with just one psychiatrist, a psychologist and seven psychiatric nurses, serving an estimated population of three million, approached the development of mental health services through drawing up a mental health policy. The policy focused on establishment of a mental health unit in the Ministry of Health, as well as regional units that would monitor and evaluate mental health programmes in their jurisdiction. The country currently offers services at one psychiatry hospital, but hoped to decentralize mental health services to tertiary and regional health units (Gabgrenegus, 1996). Similar moves towards decentralizing mental health services through the establishment of mental health units at provincial and regions levels are reported from Zambia (Haworth, 1996), Zimbabwe (Chikara, 1996), Botswana (Mambwe, 1996), Uganda (Nakasi, 1996) and Kenya (Omar, 1996). In many of the reported countries mental healthcare capacity building of health care workers as well as the development of a core of mental health workers at various echelons of health care delivery hierarchies are areas of focus. These examples demonstrate initial positive steps towards intergration of mental health in primary healthcare services, if the broadest definition of primary health care is used. In order to have a clearer understanding of the tasks required to integrate mental health services with primary healthcare in sub-Saharan Africa, the health care system in Tanzania will be used as an illustrative example.

Integration of mental healthcare into primary health services can be viewed as a process with historical underpinnings. In Tanzania, wide-ranging strategies have been used since the country's independence in 1960 to develop peripheral health care services. The guidelines for primary health care issued by the Tanzanian Ministry of Health (MOH, 1983), stressed the importance of primary healthcare as the key to the overall goal of health for all members of the population. Though emphasis on development of rural health services had been a national policy since independence in 1961, it was only between 1971 and 1981 that an increase in health budget allocations to rural health services occurred. This was evidenced by an impressive increase in rural health facilities, an increase in medical auxiliary staff and staff deployment to rural health facilities (Table 4).

Health services are administered at national, regional and district levels and delivered at consultant hospitals, regional hospitals, district hospitals, health centres, dispensaries and village health posts. Services are provided to a large extent by the government and to an increasing extent by voluntary and private for profit agencies. Since the deregulation of private practice in the country in the early 1990s, the private health care delivery sector is in its infancy. In addition to allopathic medical services, traditional medical services are provided by a variety of healers and traditional birth attendants.

Table 4: *Rural/Urban Government Health Expenditures, and Increase in Health Facilities and Personnel 1971-81*

	Year	*1971/72*	*1975/76*	*1977/78*	*1980/81*
Health Expenditure (%)					
	Urban	80	62	60	58
	Rural	20	8	40	42
Doctors					
	Urban	418	487	513	598
	Rural	216	399	479	547
Medical Auxiliaries					
(MA/RMA)	Urban	208	456	624	910
	Rural	605	1363	2166	2800
Nurses	Urban	2606	2760	2868	3570
	Rural	1653	2060	3322	4705
H/Centres, Dispensaries					
	Rural	1600	-	-	2600

MA=Medical Assistants, RMA=Rural Medical Aides

Source: *Heggenhougen and Magari, 1992.*

It was envisaged that each village in the country would have a village health post, manned by one or two community health workers (CHW); each dispensary would serve a population of 10,000 people; and a health centre would serve as a referral point for five dispensaries (MOH, 1983). Some progress was made in achieving these goals as evidenced by the distribution of health facilities within various administrative levels in the country by 1992 as demonstrated in Table 5.

Basic health service delivery points were expected to be the epicentre of primary health care (PHC) activities with a major focus on preventive services. Dispensaries are manned by Rural Medical Aides (RMAs), who received three years training in diagnosis and prevention of basic health problems at village level, after having completed seven years of compulsory primary education. The health centres are under the leader-ship of a Medical Assistant (currently, Clinical Assistant), who is a secondary school graduate (four years post primary school) trained for four years in a government paramedical institution. Maternal and child health services in both dispensaries and health centres have a strong preventive care emphasis. Medical assistants are expected to handle patients referred by RMAs, as well as to refer patients they cannot treat to district hospitals, which are the first health service delivery points with a medical doctor on staff.

Table 5: *Type of Health Facility in Tanzania According to Administrative Areas by 1981*

Administrative area		*Type of Health Facility*	
Area	*No.*	*Type*	*No.*
Village	8300	Village Health Post	1500*
Ward	1963	Dispensary	2600
Division	360	Health Centre	239
District	104	District Hospital	126
Region	20	Regional Hospital	17
Zone	6	Consultant Hospital	3
		Special hospitals	2

* This figure is an estimate

Source: *Heggenhougen and Magari, 1992.*

Districts have a primary responsibility for the administration, supervision and support of health services within the district under the leadership of the District Medical Officer (DMO). District hospitals provide both curative and preventive services and serve as referral centres for peripheral units. They also serve as training centres for community health workers, and provide in-service training for various other health workers within the district. At this level, there is a District Health Management Team (DHMT) that increasingly in a reforming process of the health sector, performs most if not all of the health planning activities for the district; providing relevant information to local governments for resource allocation. Patients requiring the attention of medical specialists are referred from the district to regional hospitals, while consultant services are available at four consultant hospitals in the country. The geographical distribution of consultant hospitals is such that arbitrary zones are created so that each consultant hospital is a referral points for various regional hospitals. Through this approach the services of the few medical doctors available are maximized by providing a screening system that allows specific problems to be handled at various echelons of the healthcare delivery system.

MENTAL HEALTH SERVICES

Allopathic Services

During the early post independence period, there was severe lack of facilities for the treatment of the mentally ill in Tanzania. Except for 11 holding beds in Dar es Salaam, most of the mentally ill were treated at four mental hospitals, with a total bed capacity of 1,332, under the control of the central government (Titmuss, 1963). These hospitals treated long and short-term stay voluntary patients as well as patients referred for treatment through the courts. As the only acute mental hospitals in Tanzania they accepted referrals from all over the country and they were invariably overcrowded. There were only two psychiatrists in the country by 1963, who in addition to clinical and administrative duties in their own hospitals, also held outpatient clinics in Dar es Salaam, and clinical and forensic consultations all over the country.

The appropriation of funds for feeding, clothing and treating mentally ill patients, though in line with what was available for other long-stay government hospitals did not take into consideration the expenses involved in acute management of the mentally ill. Due to the high prevalence of infectious diseases and malnutrition, a considerable portion of the drug budgets of mental hospitals was spent on vitamins and antibiotics. The hospitals had no contact with most of their patients following discharge and no welfare services were available for the mentally ill. In 1963, a committee set up to define health needs that were in line with the country's policies recommended continued medium and long term institutional mental healthcare in facilities located close to general hospitals (Titmuss, 1963). Furthermore, there was an emphasis on the establishment of psychiatric units in general hospitals for the initial assessment of mental illness and management of many short-stay patients and those with psychoneuroses. The committee also recommended increasing the mental health component in the training of doctors and nurses, and an allocation of four percent of the health budget for mental health services. Decentralization of mental health services was viewed as feasible through general hospitals taking on the role of managing the mentally ill, with support from consultants and specialists in psychiatry for consultation and advice.

Table 6: *Mental Health Facilities in Tanzania in 1964 and 1981*

Type of Facility	*Year*			
	1964		*1981*	
	No	*Beds*	*No.*	*Beds*
Government mental hospitals	2	992	2	1,320
Missionary mental hospitals	2	340	0	0
Psychiatric units	0	0	5	300
Rehabilitation villages	0	0	9	>275*
Total	**4**	**1,332**	**16**	**1,895**

* Information not available for 4 rehabilitation villages.

Source: Schulsinger & Jablensky, 1992; Kilonzo, 1992

With the establishment of a medical school, the first psychiatric unit was established in Dar es Salaam in 1965, followed by four psychiatry units at three regional general hospitals (Mwanza, Mbeya and Tabora) and at a district hospital in the Kilimanjaro Region. Drawing inspiration from innovations in Nigeria in the management of psychiatric patients in a therapeutic village environment, where patients and relatives were housed and treated (Lambo, 1961), Tanzania developed its first psychiatric rehabilitation villages in the late 1960's. Patients resided in rehabilitation villages that served as half way homes prior to being discharged to their home villages. The villages have increasingly been used not only for social and occupational rehabilitation of patients with more acute mental disorders but also in the rehabilitation of patients with alcohol and drug dependence (Kilonzo, 1992). The villages provide a less restrictive environment than hospitals, discourage dependency and regression, and provide training in agricultural work and artisan skills as a component of occupational therapy. There are currently nine operating villages, distributed in six regions of the country, while an additional three are in various stages of completion.

Despite developments in primary healthcare (PHC), services for mental health care lagged behind those for physical healthcare and were not integrated within the development of the primary healthcare services. Between 1964 and 1981, there was neither a substantial increase in mental health facilities (Table 6) nor in mental health care personnel. There were only two active psychiatrists in the country by 1981, and 40 grade B nurses had been trained for a year as psychiatric nurses. Care for the mentally ill remained largely concentrated in psychiatric hospitals while mental health units in regions provided treatment for an overwhelming number of patients referred from all over the region.

The National Mental Health Program (NMHP) project was initiated by the Government, jointly with the Danish International Development Agency (DANIDA) and the World Health Organization (WHO), from 1979-1980, as a long-term plan to integrate mental health in primary healthcare services. The NMHP drew heavily on the recommendations of the WHO expert committee on Mental Health (1975) that advocated basic mental healthcare provision by PHC workers. The program's primary aim was to decentralize mental healthcare by developing community psychiatry care integrated within primary healthcare. A psychiatric unit and a psychiatric rehabilitation village would backed these services in each of the 20 administrative regions of the country (Schulsinger and Jablenski, 1991).

In order to achieve the program's objectives, an emphasis was on the establishment of peripheral organization for the performance of specific outpatient tasks at the regional level rather than on the establishment and equipping of in-patient facilities, which would have been more costly. A selective strategy was employed to guide the development of a conceptual framework for the program. This included identification of conditions on which management efforts were to focus, and the definition of the scope of psychiatric work to be assigned to the primary health worker (first echelon) and to the mental health worker (second echelon). The skills that were required at each of these levels were developed in order to define the tasks in operational terms. These aspects were fitted into a medical model framework within which most primary healthcare workers had been trained. Common emotional problems were amongst the five target conditions selected for the program. A pilot project, in which regional mental health teams were established, headed by a Regional Mental Health Coordinator (RMHC), was successful in the training of nursing staff. The trained staff took on the role of therapists and trainers and the establishment of district mental health teams, based in district hospitals patterned after the regional teams (Schulsinger and Jablensky, 1991).

District and regional mental health teams continue to function in the two pilot regions (Morogoro and Kilimanjaro) despite logistical and financial constraints within the program. These constraints have stalled the second phase of extending the program to other regions in the country. However, a series of training seminars have been carried out aiming at primary healthcare workers (first echelon), which have resulted in the appointment of mental health coordinators in all the regions and districts in the country. These coordinators are medical doctors, assistant medical officers, medical assistants or mental health nurses at regional level, and medical assistants and mental health nurses at district level. Due to the influence of some of these coordinators, despite the absence of psychiatric units, patients are provided with beds in medical wards when hospitalisation is necessary.

However, mental health services in different regions are operating at different levels of efficiency; most of those outside the pilot area are operating less than optimally. Anecdotal observations and discussions with mental health coordinators have revealed difficulties in supervision of activities at the first and second echelons of care. Data on the types of patients seen by the mental health teams are not integrated in existing health management information systems and are not regularly sent to the regional or national level, making it difficult to assess needs. Until recently, a match between target mental health problems to be addressed at different levels of care and care level specific essential drugs available had not been made, with resultant poor availability of necessary drugs at district and regional level that often results in inappropriate referrals. An insufficient number of assistant medical officers have been trained in psychiatry, and it is unclear how many of them have been deployed to district hospitals. The lack of psychiatrits perhaps contributes to inadequate supervision of mental health services, poor development of training programmes for primary healthcare staff and poor needs assessment to ensure adequate drugs and other resources are available at district and regional levels.

Traditional Healers and Mental Illness in Tanzania

Despite the lack of comprehensive studies of the role of traditional healers in the recognition and management of psychiatric morbidity, evidence points to the fact that much of such morbidity is catered for by a wide range of lay and traditional healers (Gureje *et. al.*, 1992; Kilonzo, 1992; Assen, 1991; Asuni, 1991; De Jong, 1987; Swantz, 1990). Ngoma *et. al.* (2003), notes in a survey of common mental disorders amongst attendees at traditional healing facilities, that healing practices could be classified in four main categories with some overlap that includes diviners, herbalists, herbalists-ritualists and faith healers. They also note healers tend to have lighter clinic caseloads compared to that at primary care facilities. The use of traditional healing services is related not only to their better availability, but also to their cultural relevance for the populations they serve (Patel et al., 1995). Heggenhougen and Wilson (1997) note in Tanzania, that traditional healers incorporate their knowledge of community life and the cultural milieu into their practice, and may be particularly effective with psychosomatic problems by mobilizing the patients own psychic energies. One traditional healer, when interviewed in a survey on attitudes towards mental illness recognized the value of listening and encouraging problem solving in such situations (Whyte, 1991). The psychological efficacy of traditional medical practices is widely recognized (Edgerton 1980), but has not been systematically investigated in the Tanzanian context.

A significant proportion of persons with psychiatric morbidity tend to access traditional healing services in Tanzania. Whyte (1991) demonstrated that 45% of rural respondents felt that traditional healers should treat depression. Over a third of primary care attendees with psychiatric symptoms or diagnoses were reported to have seen a traditional healer prior to attendance at a primary care facility (Kempinski 1991; Bloch, 1991). Ngoma *et. al.* (2003) noted in an urban locality that most common symptoms presented by clients of traditional healers and patients at primary care facilities included somatic symptoms of depression reported by 25% of all and 64.3% of CIS-R cases and 35% of all and 55.3% of CIS-R cases respectively. Clients with common mental disorders attending traditional healers were twice as likely to say they were unable to say what was wrong with them, more likely to attribute illness to supernatural causes, more likely to have had symptoms for a longer duration, more likely to have consulted several biomedical practitioners for the same problem and were less likely to present with distinct physical symptoms than patients seen at the primary care facilities. These observations support an over-representation of persons with psychiatry morbidity in clients of traditional healing services; but also suggest "missed" diagnosis of common mental disorders at primary levels of care allopathic.

Though traditional healers play a major role in treating psychiatric disorders and constitute an important healthcare resource in Tanzania, there are difficulties in establishing how best to make use of this resource in terms of collaboration with the allopathic health service. Traditional healers in the Tanzanian setting practice folk medicine rather than formal traditional medical practices. There is a large variety of traditional healers and little standardization in their recruitment and training that ranges from apprenticeship to those who believe they have the ability to heal following experiencing visions (Heggenhougen and Gilson, 1997; Swantz, 1990). For traditional healers to be considered as health agents in primary mental healthcare, the challenging task of defining the process and parameters for collaboration with allopathic services needs to be addressed. The traditional and allopathic health services differ in very basic aspects such as; what is considered ethical; how does one identify an authentic healer; views regarding body functioning, causal models for illness and disease and treatment. There are efforts in Tanzania to encourage the community of traditional healers, to formalize their healthcare system as a primary step towards gaining official recognition, in addition to involving and collaborating with such healers in provision of specific primary healthcare services.

Discussion and Future Directions

While there have been dramatic improvements in physical health and reductions in mortality rates of populations in most countries of the world over the past decade, the same cannot be said for mental, behavioural and social health problems. Projections indicate that the burden of mental disorders will increase by 15% in the year 2020 (Murray and Lopez, 1996). Several reasons exist for the anticipation of increased burden from these conditions including the increased life expectancy of those with mental and neurological disorders and a larger number of people reaching adolescence leading to a greater absolute number of those that develop conditions of young adulthood such as schizophrenia. It is important that mental health is addressed due to the undefined and hidden burden of mental health problems.

The undefined burden of mental health problems refers to the economic and social burden of mental disorders for families, communities and countries. This burden is difficult to efficiently measure due to lack of quantitative data and difficulties in measuring and evaluating. Measurable wide-ranging and long lasting economic impacts of mental disorders include health and social service needs. Studies from countries with established economies indicate mental disorders consume 20% of all health services costs; in the US for example, the aggregate yearly costs of mental disorders in 1990 was US$ 148,000 million (Rice *et. al.*, 1990). Mental disorders are disabling and last for many years, having an emotional toll and diminishing socio-economic capabilities on care providers who are often family members. This is particularly the case where the health system is unable to offer treatment and support at an early stage of illness. Indirect costs arising from productivity loss account for a larger proportion of overall costs than direct costs in settings such as Sub-Sahara Africa where there is low availability and coverage of mental healthcare (WHO, 2001). There is a hidden burden of mental illness that refers to the burdens associated with stigma and violations of human rights and freedoms of those affected by mental illness. Stigma and discrimination associated with mental illness increases the toll of illness by generating unease, low confidence, self-esteem and general alienation from society for both those affected and their families. These effects are often irreversible even after symptoms are controlled or the illness cured. Social rejection takes many forms such as lost opportunity for education, employment and a normal social life for both the ill person and the family. Such lost opportunity costs to individuals and families are usually not taken into consideration in computations of the economic impact of mental illness.

It is evident that psychiatric disorders at primary care levels in Tanzania are common, poorly recognized by healthcare providers and hence not treated promptly resulting in both the risk of chronicity of symptoms as well missed opportunities for mental healthcare interventions. A lingering emphasis on treatment of psychotic disorders, which are described by the Swahili term for mental illness "*Kichaa*" (mad), results in non-psychotic disorders more common at allopathic primary care levels receiving less recognition than physical health problems. While many common mental disorders are addressed by traditional healing systems, no systematic enquiry into the efficacy of treatments offered has been conducted. Further, there is a strong cultural influence on both experience and presentations of psychological distress that provide challenges for measuring psychopathology. This discussion will focus on implications for mental health research, training, health resource allocation and structural aspects of mental healthcare.

Research

There is a need for more studies to establish the magnitude of depressive disorders in particularly high-risk groups such as women and adolescents. Such quantitative research needs to take into consideration not only adequate transfer of conceptual meanings inherent in standardized psychiatry epidemiological instruments, but also recalibration of cut-off scores far development of screening tools that can be used by both mental health care and primary care workers. Increasing capacities in psychiatry epidemiology in Tanzania will be important for gaining a better understanding of cultural influences on/and core manifestations of psychological morbidity.

The influence of culture on experience, expression and local causal models for psychopathology, particularly where changes in affect are concerned makes it important for illness behaviours of affected individuals to be understood. Kleinman (1980) points out the importance of explanatory models of illness in determining illness behaviours.

To develop programs aimed at improving recognition and treatment of depressive disorders, it is important to build a knowledge base on how individuals experience, categorize and respond to such morbidity. In contrast to the utility of quantitative research methods in understanding the magnitude and determinants of mental disorders, formative qualitative research better serves answering questions regarding experience and expression of mental disorders in various cultural groups of Tanzania. Such a knowledge base will allow not only an understanding of help seeking behaviours in lay, traditional and allopathic health services; and treatment responses for various illness categories, but also idioms used to express various types of psychopathology. Generated information can be utilized in the development of teaching material for the training of primary and mental healthcare workers in the recognition and management of common mental disorders.

Mental healthcare at primary levels of care in both traditional and allopathic healthcare systems should ideally be informed by what works in context. Supervision of services should be supported by in built monitoring and evaluation tools for mental healthcare delivery packages at primary care levels that allow for rapid feedback and utility of information for service improvement.

Training and Capacity Building

Difficulties in the supervision of primary and mental healthcare workers at the first two echelons of the NMHP have been alluded to earlier. The goal of having psychiatric units run by psychiatrists in every region who would provide a large part of this supervision is far from being reached. Experiences from Kenya and other African countries indicate that developing post-graduate training programs within country, achieves a greater number of psychiatry specialists in a shorter time period, with culturally relevant skills than relliance on overseas scholarships and training. Tanzanian mental health services would be better served by increasing the number of psychiatry specialty training opportunities in country. Given the very few medical doctors available in the country and the diverse health needs of the population, however, transfer of mental health care knowledge and skills to frontline health care providers will for a long time to come have to be a priority. Mental healthcare professionals have an important role to play with this regards and need to be equipped with the ability both to train and monitor mental healthcare provision at different levels of care.

While in-service training of primary healthcare workers is an important need, for a sustained process of integration of mental healthcare in PHC, review of medical and other health training curricula to improve mental health components is essential. There is a need to develop culturally relevant teaching materials, is augment existing traditional textbooks, for use in medical and paramedical and nursing training institutions in the country. In addition, raising awareness of mental health problems encountered at primary healthcare levels is especially important for the community and health planners who make important resource allocation decisions at District and Regional levels of the healthcare delivery system.

In the current health sector reform process and the decentralization of the nexus for decision-making for resource allocation to district healthcare levels, budget allocations at the district level will increasingly depend on how well

District Mental Health Coordinators and mental healthcare teams can assess and articulate needs for mental healthcare provision at the district and lower echelons of care. In order for mental healthcare agendas to achieve recognition, skilled representation of mental health services at district level is required. District mental health coordinators will require in-service training in management of mental healthcare services.

Allocation of Resources for Mental Healthcare

It is unclear what proportion of the health budget in the country is allocated to mental health services. It could well be that the figure of 4% of the total health budget set by the Titmuss Committee in 1964 is still operational at the national level. However, the limited data available indicates that at least a fifth of primary health care attendees suffer primarily from psychiatric morbidity. There is therefore a large discrepancy, between the budget allocation and the proportion of patients seen who require mental health services. Appropriate budget allocation and political good will appears to have been instrumental in increasing rural health services in Tanzania. By the same token, unless serious consideration is given to increasing the budget allocation for mental healthcare, it is unlikely that a significant increase in mental health services at the local level will occur.

Infrastructure and human resourceneeds will become meaningly evident on knowledge and skills for mental healthcare are transferred to primary levels of care. For an effective supportive referral system and the DMHC to have adequate supervision, it is important that a goal of having a psychiatrist and a well staffed psychiatry unit or adequate psychiatry beds in medical wards at district levels in densely populated urban settings and at regional level in rural settings be realized.

Structural Issues

At the national level, very recently the coordination of the NMHP has shifted from a desk manned by a psychiatry nurse to a section headed by a psychiatrist housed in the curative services directorate of the Ministry of Health. These are indeed positive advances in a direction intended to not only address current mental health needs, but also to address anticipated escalation of mental health care needs in the future. Strategies are in place to increase the recognition of the contribution of mental health problems to the national burden of disease. However, a reorientation is also required in the health sector to broaden the conceptualisation of mental health care from a purely psychiatric disorder and curative perspective to one that encompasses a broader mental health promotion and prevention agenda. Perhaps an appropriate broad definition of mental health is one put forward by the Canadian Health and Welfare Report (Health and Welfare Canada, 1989), where it is defined as:

> The capacity of the individual, the group and the environment to interact in ways that promote subjective well-being, optimal development and use of mental abilities and achievement of individual and collective goals consistent with justice and the attainment and preservation of conditions of fundamental equality.

In addition to direct clinical care, support from sections outside health will be important in the development of a mental health promotion and prevention agenda. This is not limtied to, but includes supporting elements such as policy, legislation frameworks, support from social welfare services and users' organizations for the protection of the rights to treatment and other services of person's with mental disorders that is balanced objectively against the protection of communities. Mental health needs to be considered with other preventive health service agendas given the rapid socio-economic and cultural changes Tanzania is experiencing. Such changes have been documented to herald "health transitions" in developing countries with attendant increases in behavioural pathology (Christakis *et. al.*, 1993; Sugar *et. al.*, 1991).

In conclusion, for primary healthcare services to meet the comprehensive mental health needs of the communities they serve in Tanzania there is a need for health and development planning and management to put mental health in its broadest definition on the agenda. This can best be achieved through the development of mental health programs into comprehensive country based mental health policies that allow for informed planning and implementation of mental health activities at individual, community and service provision levels.

Chapter Nine

The Challenges of Psychiatry Amidst Economic Deprivations and Social Change in Dar es Salaam City, Tanzania

Noah K. Ndosi

Introduction

Within three decades, urbanization in Dar es Salaam city has grown by a factor of nearly twenty, and it continues to grow unabated amidst economic deprivations. Ensuing social changes are shrouded by diverse problems which impact mental health negatively by meager financial allocations. Rapid urbanization has led to overcrowded housing and the emergence of squatter-settlements, poor sanitation, unemployment, poverty, and stresses which cumulatively not only affect mental problems and services adversely but also increase social stress and the risks of significant mental problems. Available mental health facilities are inadequate, and the only official psychiatric unit at Muhimbili is often congested with clinically-demanding and costly patients who suffer from intercurrent organic diseases, predominantly infections. As shown in Table 1, in a six-year period, 36,329 out-patients were attended to in the unit and 10,424 patients were admitted of whom 184 died. Due to limited awareness of mental health at the primary level, inadequate provisions for in-patients, lack of psychotropic drugs, and insufficient supervision of mental patients at home, vagrant chronic mental patients (schizophrenia in particular) are not unusual along the streets of Dar es Salaam. The main diagnostic categories of psychiatric morbidity include schizophrenia, affective disorders, organic mental syndromes, neurosis, and alcohol and drug abuse. From limited available data, the number of patients treated in the psychiatric unit at Muhimbili and in the three catchment areas is inadequate for the at least five percent prevalence of significant psychiatric morbidity among 2.8 million people in the city. The innovative rehabilitation of chronic mental patients in Mwera and Vikruti villages is a challenge demanding skilful planning and more financial resources to sustain gainful rehabilitation.

Urbanization

Rapid urbanization in Africa over the last three decades has become part of the process of under-development leading to considerable poverty. Both lack of sustainable economic growth and rapid population increase have led to inadequate control of the rate of urbanization. Within three decades, the population of Tanzania has trebled from 9 million in 1961 to 30 million people currently. While the urban population of Tanzania was 6 percent in 1967, it had risen steeply to 18 percent by 1988 and to about 30 percent currently. By the year 2000, it is estimated that over 50% of the population of Tanzania will be urban inhabitants (Mwaluko *et. al.*, 1991; Haub & Yanagishita, 1992). Rapid urbanization is partly attributed to urban migration and the natural increase of populations as a result of low family planning awareness. Burdensome social consequences of a high annual population growth rate of 2.8% are aggravated further by the inadequate maintenance of infrastructure including poor housing, contaminated water supply, poor waste disposal and inadequate sanitation in poor city communities, malnutrition, infectious diseases, accidents, substance abuse, and significant psychopathology associated with the above factors. Due to the prevailing overcrowding, the city is ill-prepared to accommodate the influx of people from rural areas into the urban centers.

Tanzania underwent a severe economic crisis from 1970 to 1996 as a result of declining gross domestic product and poor agricultural performance. Scarce foreign exchange has triggered increased internal borrowing, which in turn has eroded both the standards of the mass population and the level of social services provision. Despite government strategies to alleviate poverty, per capita income of Tanzania in 1990 was only 110 US dollars and a life expectancy at birth of 51 years (World Bank, 1993). Although the total health expenditure amounts to 109 million US dollars, the government can afford a mere 4.7 % of the GDP for the health sector which amounts to a very low health budget per capita of four US dollars. Mental health is allocated a meager 4% of the annual health budget because of Tanzania's poor socio-economic development (Desjarlais *et. al.*, 1995).

Dar es Salaam, the biggest city and the commercial capital of Tanzania, has an estimated population of 3 million inhabitants. In the mid 1980s, 50 percent of all Tanzanians lived in poor households while 36 percent lived in households classified as hard-core poor according to The World Bank. Nearly sixty percent of people living in rural villages were then considered to be poor, and a considerably lower proportion of residents in Dar es Salaam were poor (World Bank, 1993). However, rapid growth of population and a continuous exodus of rural populations into the city have led to social transformations of wide inter-generational changes which affect all age groups adversely. More people in the city are now getting poorer with time.

Since health is related to income, poverty is inevitably the most important factor which affects health. Although 90% of the people in Dar es Salaam city are literate, the health condition of most residents is still very poor because they live in congested industrial and non-industrial city squatters and slums which suffer from a higher incidence of various diseases. Currently, the majority of urban dwellers in Dar es Salaam live below the poverty line, and the government planning and resources are unable to keep pace with the population growth. Often, city authorities lack power, resources, and trained personnel to meet their obligations of providing social services and facilities. The lack of adequate comprehensive care facilities for the mentally ill renders them more susceptible to relapses and even greater disability.

Social Factors

In the last three decades, tremendous socio-economic and cultural changes have taken place in Tanzania. A cash economy with emphasis on individual rather than collective needs, increased cultural mixing, and social services with prolonged life expectancy at birth have occurred. In urban Dar es Salaam, the family is progressively moving towards a conjugal, nuclear, and neo-local residence pattern of living. Whereas the extended family provided a safety-net in the traditional societies, more people are now becoming more exposed to psycho-social stresses. Consequent changes of social norms and loosening of the family-bonds have led to a decline of social and moral values, especially among urban dwellers. The extent of crime, alienation, bewilderment, insecurity, breakdown of traditional values, weakening of social control of the individual, matrimonial disharmony, child neglect, prostitution, and mental illnesses are increasingly becoming more conspicuous in urban populations, especially in the overcrowded quarters of Dar es Salaam city.

During 1990/91, half of the 172,904 unemployed youths in Tanzania were in Dar es Salaam (Tungaraza & Ndosi, 1995), and it is currently estimated that at least a third of the population in the city are either unemployed or underemployed. Despite a relatively higher household expenditure (of 2.9 percent) on health in Dar es Salaam, (average 2.6 percent) health service provisions are both poor and inadequate (World Bank, 1993). Moreover, the speed of urbanization, social change, and the growing disparity between social groups relate considerably to mental health (Nianfeng, 1993). Most mental disorders have their highest prevalence rate in the lowest socio-economic class, and the poor are more than twice as likely as others to complain of poor health (Robert Wood Johnson Foundation, 1987).

Although it is widely known that mental disorders have enormous costs in terms of suffering, disability, and resource loss in the community, the burden of mental illness cannot easily be assessed since it usually does not produce dramatic death rates like motor accidents along the roads. There are indicators that the Disability Adjusted Years caused by mental problems are greater than that caused by tuberculosis, cancer, or heart disease (Desjarlais *et. al.*, 1995). For example, in adults aged between 15-44 years, neuropsychiatric diseases are estimated to account for at least 10 percent of the national burden of diseases, but the mental health budget allocation of only 4 percent of a meager total health budget clearly undermines initiatives to sustain or to expand mental health services. The launching in the 1970s of a sound National Mental Health Programme to extend mental health services to the community at the grassroots level and integrate them into general medical services (Schulsinger & Jabensky, 1991) has particularly been undermined by a scarcity of financial resources.

Mental Health Facilities

In Tanzanian communities, infectious diseases, family planning, and child health carry more active programs than mental illnesses. Although mental illnesses and psychosocial disorders, particularly in urban areas, are more conspicuous than in the rural communities, they do not receive the attention they deserve. Due to inadequate psychiatric facilities, lack of education, and pervading strong cultural beliefs, the majority of mental patients with psychiatric disorders in Dar es Salaam continue to be treated by traditional healers who attend to them with compassion and cultural power. It is estimated that the ratio of physicians to the population is 1 to 20,000 while that of traditional healers is 1 to 25. A considerable proportion of mental patients are also treated by rural medical aids, medical assistants, and general practitioners who frequently refer them to the psychiatric unit at Muhimbili hospital. From clinical experience, a third of mental patients seeking hospital treatment have usually consulted traditional healers prior to hospital consultation.

The psychiatric unit at Muhimbili hospital is the only official and reliable mental health facility in Dar es Salaam. The unit serves the majority of mental patients within Muhimbili hospital and services 146 dispensaries, 6 health centers, and 13 hospitals (with 504 hospital beds) from the city (MOH, 1994).

The unit was established in 1965 to provide for mental health services in the Eastern region. Later on, it was converted to a specialized Department of Psychiatry under the Faculty of Medicine, University of Dar es Salaam in 1977 (Bugaisa & Rugeiyamu, 1991). Initially, it had an admission capacity of 35 male and 15 female patients at any one time. Currently, the psychiatric unit admits at least 1,200 adult patients annually and serves about seven times as many out-patients. Due to the rising number of mental patients in Dar es Salaam, about 100 patients are sometimes admitted into wards experiencing stressful congestion. Many in-patients share beds or sleep on the floors. The unit has eight psychiatrists—a favorable number considering that Tanzania has a mere score of psychiatrists. There are three psychologists and about fifty psychiatric nurses and social workers.

Mental health services are often constrained by limited therapeutic facilities, inadequately trained personnel, sporadic availability of drugs, unhygienic conditions due to overcrowding, the presence of active intercurrent physical illnesses like TB, HIV-infections, malaria, worms, as well as malnutrition, and injuries. These factors complicate the treatment of underlying mental problems since only a few patients can afford to pay for the needed hospital treatment.

Table 1: *Number of Out-patients, In-patients, New Cases and Deaths During 1990-95 at the Muhimbili Psychiatric Unit*

Year	*Outpatients*		*Inpatients*		*New Cases*		*Deaths*	
	Male	*Female*	*Male*	*Female*	*Male*	*Female*	*Male*	*Female*
1990	4,124	2,691	1,009	452	199	130	21	9
1991	4,254	2,591	1,164	591	188	106	17	10
1992	3,324	2,236	1,217	575	169	93	22	5
1993	2,984	2,092	1,111	514	156	96	13	7
1994	3,593	2,371	855	428	159	109	26	16
1995	3,551	2,518	1,751	757	139	108	26	12
S/TOTAL	21,830	14,499	7,107	3,317	1,010	642	125	59
G/TOTAL	**36,329**		**10,424**		**1,652**		**184**	

Source: *Muhimbili National Hospital*

From 1990 to 1995, the department catered for a total of 36,329 out-patients. Most of these patients needed psychiatric assessment, initial treatment, and maintenance drug-therapy. As shown in table 1 above, a total of 10,424 adult in-patients, of which males twice out-numbered females, were admitted into the psychiatric unit between 1990 and 1995. A total of 184 patients died. On average, the hospital stay of an in-patient was two weeks. Recently, more than half of the death cases in the department were mental patients suffering from recurrent psychotic episodes. These deaths were primarily attributed to infections (Ndosi & Kisesa, 1997).

On average, 50 new patients are referred to the psychiatric unit at Muhimbili monthly from other hospitals, health centers, dispensaries, and the prisons within the city. Although annual statistics indicating the nature of psychological problems and patient load are inadequate, a recent study on 205 case referrals to the unit found that 43 percent of the referrals were from Muhimbili hospital. This high proportion of case referrals is accounted for by the large number of more seriously ill in-patients with physical illnesses who often develop significant psychiatric illnesses during the course of their treatment at Muhimbili hospital (Matuja, Ndosi & Collins, 1995).

Child psychiatric services started in 1990, and the number of children seeking psychiatric expertise is increasing gradually. In 1995, 1063 children aged up to 17 years were attended to in the out-patient child psychiatric service. The majority of these children suffered from mental subnormality, seizures, and behavioral disturbances. Moreover, the provision of liaison psychiatric services to other departments in the Muhimbili hospital is an important obligation of the department. Mentally ill offenders are frequently referred to the unit from the police and courts of law for forensic assessment and management.

Community Psychiatry

The psychiatric unit tries as much as possible to closely follow up discharged patients and to monitor clinical progress as well as to supervise compliance of drug-treatment at home. This is achieved by creating community mental health centers in the three districts of Dar es Salaam and by collaborating with health personnel from the city council. The community psychiatric team, which comprises a psychiatrist of the catchment area, together with psychiatric nurses and social workers, pay domiciliary visits to needy families who can afford their patient's needed maintenance medication including transport expenses for the visitors.

For example, from July 1993 to November 1994, 705 mental patients were attended to and 55 domiciliary visits carried out in the Temeke district (a catchment area of 20 km radius), while Ilala district (15 km radius) had the highest number of patients (769) and only 50 visits. Kinondoni, the largest of the three districts (a catchment area of radius 30 km), had 761 attendances, and 91 home visits were paid. Although Ilala is the smallest district, patients live closer to the mental health providing facility at Muhimbili, and it is more accessible by road than Kinondoni district, whose population is greater but has a poorly developed road-network to the services. Community education concerning mental health in Kinondoni needs to be strengthened because of its large size and highest number of out-patient attendances at the psychiatric unit.

Major Mental Problems

In developing countries, the nature and prevalence of psychiatric disorders is broadly similar to that in developed countries, but there is more psychiatric morbidity associated with untreated or inadequately treated physical illness (German, 1987). Mental patients *(wagonjwa wa akili)* suffer impairment directly due to psychiatric illness, such as persistent hallucinations, social withdrawal, under-activity, and slowness. Additional disadvantages like unemployment, poverty, and homelessness, as well as stigma attached to chronic psychiatric illness are secondary social problems. The main categories of admission diagnosis include schizophrenia and paranoid states, affective disorders, organic psychoses, neurosis, drug abuse, epilepsy, and mental subnormality.

Schizophrenia

Schizophrenia is locally known as *wazimu*— literally meaning one who is possessed by evil spirits. Whereas patients suffering from schizophrenia are usually more tolerated and supported in rural areas, in urban areas they are often more easily isolated, neglected, and even publicly abused. Even in urban populations, the majority of patients who suffer from schizophrenia initially seek help from traditional healers *(waganga)* who are locally believed to have power over the causative agents. Since many of these patients delay in seeking hospital help, many of them tend to develop symptoms of chronicity relatively early. Moreover, wage labor tends to affect schizophrenic patients more negatively with respect to occupational and economic stress as well as consequences of unemployment (Kleinman, 1987). In urban areas, chronic schizophrenic patients tend to develop more conspicuous symptoms of depression, apathy, irritability, negativity, emotional over-dependence, social withdrawal, isolation, loneliness, loss of self-esteem, loss of identity, and disorientation with regard to time. At least three out of ten patients admitted to the psychiatric unit suffer from schizophrenia while twice as many are regularly seen in the out-patient clinic at Muhimbili hospital. At least two out of three patients undergoing rehabilitation at Mwera and Vikruti suffer from recurrent psychoses, predominantly chronic schizophrenia (Ndosi, 1991).

Depression

Psychiatric literature in Africa indicates that 20 to 33 percent of the general out-patient attendants suffer from depression (Ovuga, 1986). Despite the high prevalence of depression, only a minority of depressed patients receive appropriate treatment because depression among African patients is frequently somatized and less likely to be recognized. The expression of personal and social distress in an idiom of bodily complaints and medical help-seeking behaviour in depression is a culturally more acceptable explanatory model of illness-behavior. In the wake of economic deterioration, lack of supportive social services, and increasing social despondency, which affects women more severely, especially in urban populations, depression is affecting greater numbers of females among urban dwellers. These factors create a vicious circle by progressively weakening the individual and devastating family and community social support which acted as buffers against mental health-related stressors and mental problems within traditional African communities. The worst consequence of depression is deliberate self-harm; the risk of self-harm among those with affective disorders has been estimated to be 30 times that of the general population (Kupfer *et. al.*, 1992). A recent study on parasuicides in Dar es Salaam found that 9% of the 300 attempters (the majority being women aged 22) suffered from major depression. The attempts were found to be embedded within socio-economic deprivations and recent acute interpersonal conflicts often aggravated by ill health and the mood-altering effect of alcohol (Ndosi & Waziri, 1997).

Organic Mental Disorders

Organic mental disorders result from demonstrable structural diseases of the brain or from dysfunction which is clearly caused by disease outside the brain. The acute or chronic impairment of psychological functioning is usually generalized or specific. Rapid increases of viral infections, tuberculosis, cerebral abscess, malaria, malnutrition, and anemia—so common in urban populations—have lately contributed heavily to organic psychiatric disorders. Organic mental disorders among patients attending urban hospitals in Zambia and Kenya were found to be 40% and 28% respectively (Rwegellera & Mwambe, 1977; Acuda & Ovuga, 1985). Although organic brain syndromes among adolescents in Dar es Salaam constituted 22% of a study cohort in 1979 (Mbatia, 1979), more recently, 36.7% of adult mortality cases at the Muhimbili psychiatric unit were found to be a result of organic brain syndromes predominantly caused by infectious diseases (Ndosi & Kisesa, 1997). Organic brain syndromes tend to be more frequent where physical illness abounds in poorer socio-economic settings. Of the 100 children treated at the psychiatric unit monthly, at least half of them suffer from a form of mental subnormality often accompanied by seizure disorders and accompanying behavioural disturbances. Of the 205 first-case referrals to psychiatric unit, only 4 patients (2.4%) were found to be demented (Matuja, Ndosi & Collins, 1995). Dementia in a few elderly patients occurs mostly due to trauma to the brain, severe physical illnesses like meningitis, encephalitis, alcoholism, and malnutrition related to vitamin B deficiency. The majority of patients suffering from dementia in Tanzania do not seek medical help because culturally, dementia is believed to be an illness of old age for which there is no cure.

Stress and Psychoneurosis

Stress and psychoneurosis are psychobiological forms of human distress in which the psychological and biological vulnerability of an individual combines with social pressures to create syndromes of distress common to vulnerable people living in poor third world cities like Dar es Salaam. In both the inner city and poor urban settlements, congestion and under-planning are clearly visible. About a third of the population live in highly, challenging are stressful situations often aggravated by either unemployment or under-employment. Chronic and multiple experiences of stress combined with meager social resources places an increased psychological burden on people, associated with more serious somatic as well as social ill-health. In his study of the breakdown of adaptation in psychological trauma, Janet delineates a biologically based trauma resulting in fragmentation of mental cohesion causing a biological, behavioural, cognitive and emotional residue of past experience which continues to govern current behavior (Van de Kolk & Van der Hart,

1989). Anxiety is typically characterized by exaggerated worries or fears, somatization, and avoidance behavior. It is caused by environmental factors and personal experience. Individuals alienated from extended family care, especially the unemployed living in congested squatters in the city where hardships abound, are particularly vulnerable to neurotic anxiety. Holmes and Speight (1975) found that 48 percent of patients attending general out-patient services in Dar es Salaam accounted for neurosis (Holmes & Speight, 1975), while among adolescents attending the out-patient clinic at Muhimbili in 1979, 38% were diagnosed as neurotic (Mbatia, 1979). Among recent first-case referrals to the psychiatric unit, only about one patient in every five was found to be suffering from neurosis (Matuja, Ndosi & Collins, 1995). From personal clinical experience, hysteria among girls attending boarding schools is common in Tanzania.

Drug Abuse

Drug abuse is a delinquent activity which leads to the maladaptation of an individual in society. Despite on-going campaigns against substance abuse, the use of drugs and alcohol by adolescents and young adults in urban Tanzania continues to be a public health issue for the nation and is strongly associated not only with morbidity and mortality, but also with economic costs. Lately, Dar es Salaam harbour has become a transit route of mandrax, cocaine, heroin, cannabis, analgesics, and benzodiazepines from the Far East to Southern and Central Africa. A retrospective study of drug-related admissions in Dar es Salaam (1991) found out that the majority were single, unemployed, or underemployed males below the age of 30 years (Ndosi & Yongolo, 1991). These patients were commonly concomitant or simultaneous multiple drug-abusers (especially alcohol/ cannabis) and were likely to exhibit psychotic symptoms. Moreover, driving under the influence of alcohol is one of the strongest factors contributing to loss of many lives through accidents. Between 1983 and 1990, there were 92,948 accidents countrywide in which 11,223 Tanzanians died (Rutazamba, 1991), and of the 1,913 injuries which occurred in Dar es Salaam during 13 months (1988/89), a quarter were under the influence of alcohol while almost a third of traffic injuries involved alcohol use (Kilonzo & Pitkaenen, 1992).

Epilepsy

Epilepsy, locally known as *kifafa,* is among the first five priorities of the national mental health program because of its high prevalence and grossly lacking established neurological services, together with the fact that over half of patients with epilepsy suffer from psychological disturbances needing interventions (Kempinski, 1991). Moreover, cultural notions surrounding its etiology consider epilepsy to be a mental illness. The commonest causes of febrile convulsions *(degedege)* among children in Dar es Salaam include central nervous system infections and head injuries—especially during parturition (Matuja, 1990). Among the first-case referrals to Muhimbili hospital, epilepsy constituted 16.6% (Matuja, Ndosi & Collins, 1997). Over half of the epileptics had partial seizures and suffered from interictal psychotic changes with significant disturbances of mood which needed psychiatric intervention.

Rehabilitation

During the late 1980s, increasing numbers of vagrant psychotic patients along the streets of Dar es Salaam aroused public concern because of their deteriorated self-neglect, acts of aggression and violence, walking naked, begging along the ways, and their picking up and carrying about heaps of rubbish. The government reacted by organizing law-enforcement operations which rounded up 124 male and 38 female patients (average age 38 years) who later were rehabilitated through the psychiatric unit at Muhimbili. Ninety percent of these patients were from Dar es Salaam, half of them single, and a third were either divorced or separated from their spouses. A third were illiterate while another third were unemployed (Kilima *et. al.*, 1990). Wandering psychotic patients are also not uncommon in other major Tanzanian towns.

Two rehabilitation villages, Mwera and Vikruti, cater for selected mental patients who initially undergo treatment at the psychiatric unit at Muhimbili. The main objective of rehabilitation is to create a natural and stimulating environment for chronic mental patients who constitute a big proportion of those served by the national mental healthcare system. Between 1980 and 1989, a total of 514 mental patients (316 males and 198 females) underwent rehabilitation at Mwera. The diagnostic categories of these patients were: schizophrenia (84.2%), depression (6.2%), epilepsy (3.9%), and others (5.6%), including drug and alcohol abusers and mentally retarded individuals (Ndosi, 1991).

Mwera rehabilitation village had 21 patients during 1987/88 and 31 patients during 1991/92. The number of patients rehabilitated here is smaller compared with the number of patients in Vikruti—29 in 1987/88 and 59 in 1991/92. Mwera is remotely located, its soil sandy, and the weather dry most of the year. The village has a higher level of dependence than Vikruti which can accommodate more patients and has a higher turnover with a greater focus on occupational therapy. Mwera admits more socially disabled patients whose rehabilitation focuses more on restoration of social skills. Both rehabilitation villages are run by psychiatric nurses, agricultural experts, nurse auxiliaries, and security guards (MUCHS, 1996). The rehabilitation of mental patients in the villages is a great challenge facing mental health services because of the delicate balance between gainful rehabilitation and meager financial resources available. This innovative care of the mentally ill needs greater support and more commitment from the health sector to sustain it because of the potential influence it carries for the care of chronic mental patients countrywide.

What Can Be Done?

Solutions to problems affecting mental healthcare and services in Dar es Salaam cannot be tackled in isolation, but countrywide. Foremost, Tanzania needs more active family planning programs nationally to decrease its current annual population growth of 2.8 percent. Improving the quality of life for rural populations through provisions of clean water, energy, better roads, schools, and health facilities would considerably reduce the rate of urbanization which has contributed to unprecedented overcrowding and congested living conditions with poor housing and sanitation in urban areas. Strengthening the economy through the diversification of production through modernized agriculture and industry can provide the basis for improving the health of people by acquiring more resources for health per capita. Undoubtedly, sound mental health programs are more likely to succeed where the people have better basic education, higher public health awareness, and an active system of primary healthcare.

The effective delivery of mental health services at the primary health level in communities—using an integrative approach into the existing formal health delivery system—needs to be strengthened. The misdirection of meager available resources and the significant deterioration of the established infrastructures have plagued the mental health sector, and the poor economic crisis experienced amidst the pressure of the structural adjustments of the World Bank is likely to remain unchanged for a long time. Moreover, mental health is politically not likely to receive an appropriate budget, partly due to the stigma attached to mental illness and the attitude of administrators.

Nevertheless, to address mental health problems in the city with limited resources more effectively, it is essential to comprehensively assess the burden of mental health problems first and then identify priorities of psychiatric emergencies, chronic major diseases, psychiatric problems associated with physical conditions, and specific high-risk groups like drug and alcohol abusers. Since integration or prevention is not enough, personal and community-wide efforts in the three districts have to be directed towards the maintenance and improvement of health, treatment of diseases, and human development. More linkages between the non-formal and the formal systems will be beneficial. On the whole, the quantity, type, and structure of services to be provided—and the period of accomplishment—will largely depend on the availability of resources, political will, foresight, and diligence of the city administration.

Since awareness on the part of decision-makers of the importance of mental health is insufficient, it is advantageous for mental health experts to campaign more vigorously about the pressing plight of the mentally disabled while making use of the indigenous knowledge and practices with innovative perspectives. In particular, the high threshold of community tolerance in Tanzanian communities ought to be exploited so that the ultimate aim of the national mental health program to ensure the availability and accessibility of basic mental healthcare can be realized.

Chapter Ten

Development of Mental Health Services in Tanzania: A Reappraisal for the Future

Gad P. Kilonzo and N. Simmons

Abstract

The article traces the historical development of mental health services in Tanzania from traditional practices through custodial institutions during the colonial period; efforts towards decentralization, including the development of innovative agricultural rehabilitation villages during the 60s; and the introduction of primary mental healthcare during the 1980s right up to the present. Available resources in Tanzania, including the traditional healing system, the family, and ample arable land were examined in terms of how these might be used in the care of mental patients and the promotion of mental health in general. The article points to real opportunities and a possible course of action for the future.

Introduction

Mental health is undeniably one of our most precious possessions. We need to be nurtured, promoted, and preserved as best we can. It is that state of mind in which the individual can experience sustained joy of life while working productively, interacting with others meaningfully, and facing up to adversity without losing the capacity to function physically, psychologically, and socially. It is undoubtedly a vital resource for a nation's development, and its absence represents a great burden to the economic, political, and social functioning of that nation. This pivotal position of mental health, however, is not often reflected in the allocation of national resources, resulting in insufficient attention being paid to the research and promotion of mental health. Moreover, the low level of economic development in Tanzania, as in much of Africa, puts limits on the financial and human resources that can be made available. Given such meager financial resources, innovative approaches for the provision of mental health services and the promotion of mental health are called for.

Country Description

Tanzania is located on the eastern part of the African continent immediately south of the Equator. It encompasses 945,000 km² with a population of 27 million people. A significant proportion of the population (45.8%) is below age 15 (Bureau of Statistics, 1991). With a per capita income of US$ 180, it ranks amongst the poorest countries of the world.

Profound transformations have taken place in the country over the past 30 years such as "villagization," the creation of planned communal villages inspired in 1967 by Nyerere, Tanzania's first president; urbanization; and industrialization, all of which have been accompanied by changes in the social fabric.

In 1894, Dar es Salaam, the commercial capital of Tanzania, was a minor settlement of 10, 000 people. By 1957, it had grown to 128, 742 and by 1969, to 315, 000 (Flanagan, 1977). Today, the city boasts more than 1,500,000 inhabitants. The urbanization of Tanzania occurred very quickly. In 1965, only 5% of the population lived in urban areas. By 1987, this had increased to 29%, half of whom lived in Dar es Salaam (World Bank, 1989). The average annual growth rate of the urban population is 8.87% compared with the general population growth rate of 2.8% (Bureau of Statistics, 1991). This accelerated rural-to-urban migration only partially parallels the pace of industrial expansion.

Over the past 30 years, industrial output has grown from 5% of the GNP to more than 25% with some fluctuations. Tanzania's rapid urbanization mirrors much of Africa and is fuelled not only by a growth in industrial production, but more importantly perhaps by other factors, such as the growth of the informal sector, the allure of the cities, and influences of extended family networks (Flanagan, 1977; Kortteinen, 1989).

The process of urbanization weakens the social fabric, in much the same way as when men migrate to towns. These men leave their families behind to live off the land while they engage in low-paying jobs. The resulting dislocation from traditional family ties to more heterogeneous contacts means there is less emphasis on emotion and sentiment and more on utility. The overall effect of these changes is the rapid undermining of traditional social support networks, leaving little time for new institutions to emerge to replace these supportive functions. The cost to mental health could be enormous. The disruptive effect of rapid urbanization on mental health was evident in Europe during the industrial revolution of the early 19th century (Lewis, 1962) when changes were much slower than in Tanzania and other African countries today (Flanagan, 1977).

In traditional Tanzanian society, the extended family, often including several extended families within a larger family group, is the main social institution. This family group provides spiritual and emotional relief, social support, security, and education, and it defines the moral and ethical system within which the community is intricately bound together. The elders and grandparents bestow their knowledge, skills, wisdom, attitudes, and values on their grandchildren through years of tutelage and close inter-generational contact. A disruption of this system may have a negative effect, due to loss of purpose, direction, and social support, on mental health. Hughes (1962) has suggested that social disintegration may be accompanied by an increase in the prevalence of mental disorders. In his study among the Egba of Nigeria, twice as many individuals were mentally disturbed within the socially disintegrated as compared with those who were socially integrated. The difference was even more dramatic among women than among men. Only 6% of women in the disintegrated population were completely free of symptoms of mental disorder as compared with 60% among the socially integrated population. Asuni (1962) and Cooper and Sartorius (1977) have also observed that social disintegration, which ensues as a result of rapid socio-technological change, is associated with increased mental disturbance and suicide rates mainly among young men.

Historical Development of Mental Health Services in Tanzania

Traditional System

In traditional Tanzanian societies, the process of healing is intimately related to the traditional religious experience. This religion also implies the state of being healthy, and the healing process has been described elegantly by Mbiti (1969) as an ontological phenomenon:

> The individual is immersed in a religious participation which starts before birth and continues after his death...to live is to be caught up in a religious drama ... man lives in a religious universe. Both that world and practically all his activities in it are seen and experienced through a religious understanding and meaning.

To be healthy is to be whole in the intricately intertwined spiritual, mental, social, and physical realms. There is a sacred continuity of purpose and communication between the living, the ancestors, and the gods who inhabit both the spirit world and the physical environment in which the community lives. Various animals, forests, and celestial bodies are consecrated shrines where the ancestors and the gods dwell. The state of being healthy, therefore, not only entails harmony among individuals in the community, but a harmonious relationship between the community and the physical environment as well as the spiritual world of the ancestors and the gods who sustain them. Disturbance in any area of this complex relationship can lead to mental and emotional disharmony (Simmons, 1991). The healer and the healing process, therefore, must address this whole system. Even the empirical herbalist who provides a remedy for parasitic infestation requests that the patient seek harmony within the social and spiritual realms as a prerequisite to the healing process. The whole community is involved in the healing process, which taps into the huge wealth of emotional, familial, and social resources.

This traditional healing system has developed over generations in Tanzanian societies and similar communities in the region as a response to the needs of the people. When new diseases like smallpox and tuberculosis were introduced, healers had a very difficult time responding to them, resulting in epidemics. The slave trade, the European conquest, the partition of Africa, and the rapid transformation of social and economic life not only led to the introduction of new diseases, but upset the delicate balance between the communities and their healing systems, leaving epidemics in their wake (Good, 1987).

The increased human mobility brought about by industrialization and urbanization further compromised the ability of the healers. Since the healing process is intricately woven into the environment from which they obtain their healing powers, healers are most effective when operating within this traditional system. Traditional healers may, therefore, be less effective in urban areas where there is a more heterogeneous definition of the universe (Swantz, 1990).

The introduction of Western medicine to Tanzania came at a time when the healing system was already in a state of flux and was, therefore, susceptible to misinterpretation. Colonialists and Western missionaries failed to recognize the value of the traditional healing system (Good, 1987; Swantz, 1990) and even discouraged it. The system, however, has endured. Today it serves a large proportion of the population in East Africa as well as in the rest of Africa. This is apparent from the overlapping use of both traditional and western healthcare systems. More than half the patients attending health clinics in western Kenya have also consulted traditional healers (Acuda, 1983). In Tanzania, 25.5% of patients with psychiatric complaints in a primary healthcare setting had already consulted a traditional healer (Schulsinger and Jablensky, 1991). The traditional healing system is more accessible to these people and will remain so for quite some time. In rural Tanzania, for example, the ratio of western-trained doctors to the population is 1:20000 while that of the traditional doctors is 1:25 (Swantz. 1990). The traditional and modern systems exist side-by-side. There is the possibility for a reconciliation and synthesis of the two systems (Neki et al., 1986); for example, the traditional system can provide another way of treating and rehabilitating mental patients (Harding, 1975). The appreciation of traditional African beliefs in the healing system can open up new avenues in a therapeutic relationship where the western-trained therapist understands the world view of the client. Lambo (t964) in Aro Abeokuta has demonstrated how the integration of the two systems can lead to a marked improvement in care. Here, mental patients, together with their families, move to a village where they have daily interactions with tolerant, healthy individuals. In this setting, the traditional healing system with its emphasis on group healing reinforcement accompanies western healing practices.

Western Mental Health Services

The documented history of western mental health services in Tanzania begins with the activities of the Church Missionary Society in the wake of Livingstone's journey of "discovery." In 1877, the Church Missionary Society opened the first hospital at Mamboia. This and other health facilities set up by the German administration between 1888 and the turn of the century had little impact on mental health services for native peoples. This was because the few existing hospitals had been established for Europeans. The German government did not make any financial resources available for healthcare facilities for indigenous Africans. A dispensary was established for natives, Arabs, and Indians in 1893 by an Indian magnate, Sewa Haji. This dispensary was upgraded to a hospital in 1897. However, no separate mental health services existed until 1905, when Lutheran missionaries converted an asylum for freed slaves at Lutindi in the Korogwe district into a "lunatic asylum." This asylum, like most other asylums in the world at that time, provided mainly custodial care for long-term patients. The German defeat led to the establishment of the British administration in 1918, which led to some expansion of health services. By 1919, the country had 1,200 hospital beds, of which 86 were for mental patients (Titmuss *et. al.*, 1963). In 1927, Mirembe, a national mental hospital, was opened in Dodoma in central Tanzania. Although Mirembe had approximately 1,000 beds, there were often more than 1,500 in-patients (Titmuss *et. al.*, 1963; Margetts, 1958). Many patients had traveled hundreds of miles on very poor roads to be treated at Mirembe. In 1951, the Broadmoor

Institution for "the criminally insane" was opened next to Mirembe, but under the administration of the prison system. It had a capacity of 600 beds. The growing need to put mental patients in institutional care led to the opening of Irente Mental Hospital at Irente, Lushoto District, by the Lutheran missionaries in 1962. This hospital had a capacity of 200 patients. The overall approach to the management of mental patients up to this period can be characterized as institutional (Kilama *et. al.*, 1974).

This was the situation that existed in the country in the early 60s when Tanganyika obtained independence from the British Trusteeship. An evaluation report (Titmuss *et. al.*, 1963) noted with dismay the overcrowded conditions in the existing institutions and the absence of facilities for the mentally ill in outlying hospitals other than 11 holding beds in Dar es Salaam which were "barred cells ... not suitable for modern psychiatric treatment." It was also reported that although there were plans for the establishment of regional psychiatric units, there were no funds to implement them. Furthermore, in a country of ten million people, there was only one psychiatrist who worked as a government psychiatrist in the Dar es Salaam clinics. He was also employed as a forensic psychiatrist for patients at Mirembe and the Isanga forensic psychiatric hospital in Dodoma. The report further noted:

> All hospitals in Tanganyika suffer in varying degrees from lack of funds, but the financial position of Mirembe Hospital is particularly strained. The patients are housed, fed, clothed and treated for an average cost of only four shillings a day, of which one shilling goes on food. These figures are in line with other government long-stay hospitals but not with those giving acute, short-stay treatment. About half the patients at Mirembe stay for less than one year and the length of stay ranges upwards from a few weeks.

The report also criticized the practice of keeping mental patients in police cells and sending them to prison while awaiting certification. With admirable foresight uncharacteristic of the times, the report went on to recommended the decentralization of mental health services and the training of medical and supporting personnel to this end:

> ... [I]nstruction in mental health and disease must be an important item in the training of the Tanganyikan medical practitioner both before and after he qualifies, so that the health center can become the first place of reference for mental cases [and] will spare the mental hospital the admission of many patients who would be successfully treated near their own homes... It is important that one mental

> hospital at least in Tanganyika should be brought up to the standard required to offer postgraduate training at house officer and registrar level.

The same difficulties regarding facilities and staffing existed in neighboring countries like Kenya. For instance, Margetts (1958) reports that Mathare, the main psychiatric hospital established in 1910 in Kenya, had only one psychiatrist, one junior medical officer, seven European nurses, and some indigenous nurse-assistants by 1958. This meager staff ran the 500-bed mental hospital which overflowed with 700 patients since it was the only mental hospital serving the 6 million people of Kenya.

The decentralization of services in Tanzania began in the mid-60s with the opening of a psychiatric unit at Muhimbili Medical Center in 1965. Other regional psychiatric units and wards followed in Moshi, Tabora, Mwanza, Mbeya, and Songea. The establishment of district mental health services, however, had to wait for 20 years until primary mental healthcare was instituted throughout the country. A postgraduate training program for the psychiatrists who were to oversee the district psychiatric services is yet to be realized. Peripheral services, therefore, continue to rely on district medical officers, mental health nurses, and auxiliaries.

The Burden of Mental Disorders in Tanzania

Psychiatric Disorders

Evidence points to psychiatric morbidity in Africa that approaches the level in industrial countries (German, 1987). Evidence also suggests that, in general, recognized categories of mental disorders in the West are also found in Africa (Woeber, 1975; Odejide, 1979: Ben-Tovim, 1985; Westermeyer, 1985).

In a study of four developing countries, Harding *et. al.* (1980) found that out of 1,624 patients in primary healthcare facilities, 225 or 13.9% had mental disorders. In a community-based survey in Ethiopia, Giel and van Luijk (1969) found that 9.1% of the population had mental disorders, of which 0.3% could be diagnosed as psychotic. In Uganda, Egdell (1984) found that 5 to 20% of patients attending health facilities had some form of mental disorder. In Dar es Salaam, Holmes and Speight (1975) examined patients who had been referred to a medical clinic and found that, of these referrals, the main complaint was mental disorders in 48% of cases. Schulsinger and Jablensky (1991) estimated the point prevalence of major mental disorders among adults in Tanzania to be 1% and severe disorders among children to be 0.5%. This translates into

148, 500 adults and 60, 750 children with major and severe mental disorders requiring attention from the national healthcare delivery system.

Substance Abuse

As already indicated, rapid socio-technical change, migration to the cities, and increased contact with cultural groups from other countries have lead to a profound transformation of the social fabric and cultural values of Tanzanians. Through film and video, there is more exposure, for example, to western behavior, hairstyles, and fashion. These new styles are equated with the "modernization" to which younger Tanzanians aspire and are quickly adopted by them. As a result, the extended family, traditionally the most important social institution in Africa, is gradually losing its grip on the values and attitudes of emerging generations (Kilonzo, 1989). It appears that substance abuse is the unwelcome guest in this confluence of cultural influences.

The pattern of production and consumption of alcohol, for example, has shifted from ceremonial to commercial and recreational use (Nikander *et. al.*, 1991; Kilonzo and Pitkanen, 1992). Traditional home-brewed alcoholic beverages which make up 89% of available alcohol in absolute terms (Kilonzo, 1989) are being commercialized and adulterated with fusel alcohols (isopropyl alcohol, isobutyl alcohol, methyl alcohol, etc.) and aflatoxins (Nikander *et. al.*, 1991). Since only 49% of urban dwellers and 35% of rural dwellers are teetotal (Kilonzo, 1992a), physical damage resulting from home-brewed beverages is likely to be considerable. The pattern of drinking in East Africa tends to be binging (Partanen, 1991), and alcohol-related problems, such as violence and accidents, have become major contributors to morbidity and mortality (Kilonzo, 1989; Nikander *et. al.*, 1992).

Other substances abused in the country include tobacco, cannabis, khat, and inhalants. Tobacco is likely to be a growing contributor to morbidity and mortality in the country since Tanzania is a major producer of both tobacco leaf and cigarettes. Cannabis grows wild and is available in most areas of the country. Its use is a contributing factor to the admission at Muhimbili psychiatric services of about 150 patients each year. Information culled from student surveys (Kaaya *et. al.*, 1992) indicates that about 7% of students in Dar es Salaam abuse at least one substance on a regular basis, especially alcohol and tobacco. Active use of alcohol was reported among 34.1% of the students. This was despite the fact that 60.7% of the students who participated in the surveys were aware of some of the health-related hazards. Regular cannabis use was reported by 1% of the students.

Substance abuse is very high among certain vulnerable groups such as street children. A study conducted in Mwanza, Tanzania found that 52% of the street children use cannabis, 22% on a daily basis. Furthermore, 17% use inhalants, 5% several times a day (WHO, 1994).

Development of Mental Health Services in Tanzania

Khat has been widely used, especially by truck drivers and other individuals who need to keep awake at night. However, in recent years, this drug is being utilized by an increasing number of people for recreational purposes. The effect of khat and inhalant use on morbidity and mortality is not yet known.

Another disturbing trend is the shift of heroin-trafficking routes from the Asia-Europe corridor to staging points in East Africa (Jablensky and Hauli, 1983; African Concord, 1987). Some of the heroin is spilling onto the streets of Dar es Salaam. About 30 heroin addicts arrive at the emergency psychiatric services at the Muhimbili Medical Center every year. Substance abuse, therefore, represents a growing burden on a healthcare delivery system which is already overworked because of conditions resulting from infections and malnutrition.

Since 1987, preventative aspects of substance abuse have been incorporated into a family life education program that is in place at schools in several regions in Tanzania. Since 1989, the government of Finland, through UNDCP, has provided assistance in the control of drug abuse in Tanzania. The family life education program has been extended to various training institutions such as teacher training colleges, nurses training colleges, and schools of journalism (Kilonzo, 1996). Other aspects of the program include community mobilization through discussions with community leaders, teachers, parents, and youths.

Suicide

There is not much documentation on suicide in Tanzania. A study carried out at the Muhimbili Medical Center in Dar es Salaam (Kilonzo and Kassam, 1986) found that between 1971 and 1975, there were 34 recorded cases of suicide, with a male: female sex ratio of 2:1. Between 1981 and 1985, the figure increased to 60 cases, with a male: female sex ratio of 1:1. 58.3% of suicides were among adolescents and young adults.

In the 70s, the most common method used was hanging, and in the 80's, this changed to drug overdoses, with chloroquine and barbiturates being the most frequently used drugs. Where there was information, psychosocial problems, especially conflicts involving dyadic relationships, seemed to be the main factors leading up to the suicides and attempted suicides. There is a clear need for further study on suicide, the contributing factors, and preventative methods.

In a study of 300 parasuicides at the Muhimbili Medical Center in Dar es Salaam during 1991, 1992, and the first half of 1993, Ndosi and Waziri (1996) observed that parasuicides were common among young adults with a male to female ratio of 1:2.2. The most common method employed was drug overdose. Social conflict was the most common precipitating factor.

Tanzanian National Mental Health Programme

Despite successful decentralization of mental healthcare to regional psychiatric units and wards between 1965 and 1979, the care provided was mostly custodial in nature and could, at best, only reach 20% of those in urgent need (Schulsinger and Jablensky, 1991). The challenge was to provide the needed service with scanty resources, including manpower. In 1979, there were only two psychiatrists in the whole country. There were 5 assistant medical officers with some training in clinical psychiatry and some 40 mental health nurses (Jablensky and Hauli, 1983). None of the 2,000 medical assistants and rural medical aids, who formed the backbone of Tanzania's primary health care system, had any training in mental health. Of the 1,862 beds in psychiatric institutions in the country, only 1,000 were available for short-stay acute cases. In other words, the system was only able to meet the needs of 17% of those suffering from mental disorders (Jablensky and Hauli, 1983).

To meet the challenge of providing basic mental healthcare to all in need, a better and more efficient system had to be devised. This system had to be accessible, affordable, and available at all times with a minimal input of additional resources. As conceived, the system also had to encourage and strengthen community participation in providing social support to individuals with mental health problems (Simmons, 1991). In order to do this, mental health services were to be provided through the existing system of primary healthcare. The training of assistant medical officers, medical assistants, rural medical aids, and nurses became a priority. This training had to be limited to a few of the most prevalent psychiatric illnesses for which care would be provided from the village level up to the regional hospitals level (Jablensky and Hauli, 1983). Using key informants and case vignettes, it was possible to determine the most important target conditions in the community and train primary healthcare workers in recognizing these conditions (Climent *et. al.*, 1980) while providing them with the basic skills for their management. These target conditions included acute and chronic psychosis, drug and alcohol abuse, depression, and epilepsy.

Between 1980 and 1983, with financial assistance from Denmark and three WHO consultants, the above system was implemented in two pilot regions of the country, Morogoro and Kilimanjaro (Schulsinger and Jablensky, 1991). At the end of a three-year implementation period in the pilot regions, an external evaluation report could conclude that:

1) The estimated number of people in need gained access to the service.
2) The program was cost effective.
3) The program was operational in both pilot regions and a plan to implement the same program in other regions of Tanzania had been put into operation (Schulsinger and Jablensky, 1991).

The efficacy of the program in the two pilot regions can be illustrated by the dramatic drop in the number of patients admitted at both psychiatric units at Mawenzi, Moshi, and Morogoro. In both cases, bed occupancy rates dropped to less than half at the height of the implementation of the program in 1983.

A primary mental healthcare program provides the opportunity to meet the needs of mental patients when human and financial resources are scarce. Giel and Harding (1976) maintain that the expansion of mental health services in developing countries will only take place if:

1) The task is undertaken by primary healthcare workers.
2) Services are directed at the few priority target conditions which contribute greatly to morbidity in the community.

Community Mental Healthcare Teams in Dar es Salaam

Development of Community Mental Healthcare Teams in Dar es Salaam

The development of community mental healthcare teams in Dar es Salaam illustrates the extension phase of the programme.

The psychiatric unit at the Muhimbili Medical Center, which serves the city of Dar es Salaam, was opened in 1965 to serve a population that was only a tenth of the population in 1983. It also served as a teaching and referral center for the whole country. The exploding population as well as an increasing reliance on hospital mental health services led to the overcrowding of clinics and in-patient facilities. This resulted in inadequate consultation time allocated to each patient, since two or three doctors had to attend to upwards of 200 patients in one clinic. Poor compliance of treatment with frequent defaulting and re-admissions were common. Patients came from all over the city and the surrounding areas, experiencing transportation difficulties, some traveling more than 50 km to get to the clinic. The situation was altogether unsatisfactory.

In 1983, plans were made to develop community care teams for 12 catchment areas of Dar es Salaam and its suburbs. The teams consisted of community mental health nurses, medical social workers, and medical officers of the Dar es Salaam City Council under the supervision of two senior community mental health nurses and a psychiatrist from the teaching hospital. This modest team was all that was available at this time, and there were only two trained community mental health nurses.

The main objective of this plan was to provide care and follow-up services for patients as close to their homes as possible for the purpose of involving families in order to improve compliance, reduce relapses, and decrease the out-patient load at Muhimbili to manageable levels and thereby improve the quality of care.

A training program for community mental health nurses was started at the Department of Psychiatry (Kilonzo, 1992b), and in July 1984, the first six community mental health care team nurses completed their training and started working in three peripheral clinics. Twenty-six such community mental healthcare team nurses have since been trained and deployed in the Dar es Salaam catchment areas. An integrated healthcare system of community-based care with the support of psychiatric services at Muhimbili has thus been effectively developed (Kilonzo, 1992a,b).

The efficiency of these measures became apparent within a year of the establishment of community care teams. The number of out-patients at the Muhimbili Medical Center decreased to a manageable level of 20 to 30 patients (Kilonzo, 1992b).

Management of Vagrant Psychotic Patients

The emergence of homeless or vagrant psychotic patients in Dar es Salaam paralleled the growth of the city. This may be related to the social disintegration associated with the transforming social landscape due to rapid socio-technical changes. By the early 80s, homeless vagrant psychotic patients were visible throughout the city. The management of these patients is one of the most challenging tasks for mental health workers and the community. These patients often go through the "revolving door" pattern of repeated re-admissions and discharges.

Between August and December 1987, a census of the population of homeless psychotic patients was carried out in Dar es Salaam for the purpose of planning for their care. Two hundred such patients were identified. Relatives of 81% of these patients were found and contacted. 44% of the homeless psychotic patients had already had some contact with mental health services in the country (Kilonzo, 1992b). Due to financial constraints, only 90 patients have so far been provided with adequate treatment and rehabilitation services. Relatives are usually willing to take the patients in if they are assured of clinical support. Murray (1962) has similarly observed that communities in Uganda take in mental patients willingly due to the apparent absence of stigma associated with mental disorders. Patients without relatives willing or able to take them in after discharge remain long-stay patients in psychiatric agricultural rehabilitation villages.

Psychiatric Agricultural Rehabilitation Villages in Tanzania

Justification for the Villages

Chronic mental patients are a special challenge to countries with scarce financial and trained human resources. Yet, it is a challenge that cannot and should not be avoided, if the community is to maintain its self-esteem. Lamb (1982) has noted that the top priority for the mental health profession is to care for the severely disabled chronic patients. In caring for these patients, it is important to involve them actively in the process of restoring or acquiring the skills and attitudes needed for a meaningful social existence. The patients must feel they can master and cope with the demands of the environment, their internal drives, and those of their symptoms (Lamb. 1982). Confidence, high self-esteem, and a feeling of control over one's life are essential ingredients for success. The careful assessment of patients, the setting of realistic goals, and rewarding work, set the stage for measured achievements which can restore feelings of being able to cope and high self-esteem (Kilonzo, 1992a,b). Adhering to these principles is often costly in terms of time constraints and human and financial resources. The challenge in Tanzania has been to develop services that can operate with meager resources with the realization, perhaps, that the one resource that still exists in adequate supply is the family and social support networks.

Historical Perspective

Despite all efforts, residual disability in some patients serious enough to require continued care is unavoidable. For these patients, a shelter facility would enable them to take gradual steps towards recovering lost functions and increasing control of their own lives at their own pace. A kind of half-way home which offers a variety of activities including work may be the answer. Although such a home would be cheaper than hospital care, it still costs a considerable amount of money. In Tanzania, where the government spends only US$ 1.3 per capita per annum on health, such a facility must be self-reliant to some extent. Agricultural psychiatric rehabilitation villages offer an opportunity for this in a primarily agricultural country.

Agricultural psychiatric rehabilitation villages are creative African contributions to rehabilitative psychiatry. The Tanzanian villages draw their inspiration from the pioneering Aro Village in Abeokuta, Nigeria founded by Professor T. A. Lambo in 1954 (Lambo, 1964).

The Aro village in Abeokuta provided a culturally-conducive traditional environment in which patients and their relatives lived within an existing village population comprising farmers, fishermen, and local craftsmen. Patients were treated by both traditional healers and Western-trained doctors while at this village.

Development of the Villages

The Tanzanian Hombolo village in Dodoma and Mwera in Dar-es-Salaam were built in the late 60s to provide a natural and socially stimulating environment for patients who needed longer periods of supervised treatment or who were in need of restoring lost social skills after an acute psychiatric illness. They were designed to be microcosms of rural villages in terms of social milieu, productive activities, and economic self-reliance. To varying degrees, these villages were also expected to:

1) Provide a sheltered living facility for chronic patients without relatives.
2) Provide long-term treatment of patients who needed continued work training, as well as education in interpersonal relationships with the participation of relatives.
3) A sheltered working place.

The weighing of the above objectives would depend on local circumstances and needs.

The first village built was Hombolo in Dodoma. It was built in 1969 by the patients themselves with the help of the Mirembe psychiatric hospital staff. In the same year, Mwera village in Dar es Salaam was built by patients transferred from Mirembe with the assistance of staff from the Psychiatric Unit of the Muhimbili Medical Center. A generous grant from the citizens of Calgary, Canada, channeled through Canadian Universities Services Overseas (CUSO) and amounting to 10,000 Tanzanian shillings (at that time equivalent to about US$ 1,400), covered the cost of building materials.

During the 70s and 80s, eleven psychiatric rehabilitation villages were developed in Tanzania to meet the growing demand for this kind of rehabilitation, and 3 more villages are in various stages of construction (Kilonzo, 1992a,b). There are about 450 patients in the care of these villages at any given time. The villages vary in terms of services provided and the kind of patients admitted. They all provide a less restrictive environment than the hospital. These villages also discourage regression and dependency by providing agricultural plots where patients can be engaged according to their abilities and stages of motivation. They all provide work that is rewarding in various forms.

Agricultural rehabilitation villages are gaining popularity in Tanzania not only among the medical professionals but also within the community. This, perhaps, indicates that they are meeting a need that is felt in the communities.

Vikuruti Psychiatric Rehabilitation Village

Vikuruti village provides an illustrative case. It is situated 18 km south of the center of Dar es Salaam and stands on 74.7 ha of land. The bulk of this land is used for farming and gardening. It was opened in 1986. The village is situated within an existing agricultural village called Chamazi. The government of Chamazi village provided the land and welcomed the establishment of the rehabilitation village for mental patients. The village was constructed with assistance from the Danish International Development Agency and is non-profit-making. In addition to coconut and citrus, the farm produces poultry products, pigs, dairy products, and vegetables. Over a 6-month period, the turnover is approximately 2 million shillings, about one-third of this representing profit. The patient population includes schizophrenics, alcoholics, epileptics, psychotics as well as those suffering from affective disorders. The farm is run by agriculturalists for the purpose of providing gainful employment and vocational training facilities for patients. There is an increased scope for self-reliance and possible support for such patient welfare activities as sports and other recreational and cultural projects. The success of this village can be attributed to the presence of qualified agricultural and animal experts at the farm.

Therapeutic activities at the village are supervised by a mental health nurse, a nursing assistant, and three artisans (carpenter, bamboo craftsman, and seamstress) who have some training in working with chronic mental patients. With the assistance of a psychiatrist and a medical social worker who visit once weekly, the team provides counseling and fosters a therapeutic milieu in the village. The patients take part in the village government and in the management of community life. The length of stay varies between 3 months and 2 years, with most patients staying for 6 months. Depending on the need of the individual, the management of the patients and length of stay are individualized as much as possible.

Patients freely interact with people of the Chamazi village, and they occasionally conduct cultural activities together. The involvement of traditional healers depends entirely on the individually expressed wishes of the patients or relatives. Relatives are encouraged to visit, especially during weekends, for social activities as well as to observe and take part in other therapeutic activities. Work forms the most important part of the therapeutic milieu.

Value of Work

Work fosters confidence, high self-esteem, feelings of control, mastery over one's own life and experience of success, and provides meaning and satisfaction in one's social existence (Wing and Morris, 1981). It helps in discarding the sick role. It is, therefore, an important part of psychiatric rehabilitation. Regarding long-stay schizophrenics, Wing and Morris (1981) have observed that:

> The most important single factor associated with improvement of primary handicaps was a reduction in the amount of time spent doing nothing. When work is done in an agricultural setting, it is rewarding not only financially, but carries prestige because the patient is contributing a commodity of equal value to that produced by anyone else. An egg or tomato produced by a mental patient has the same intrinsic value as that produced by a king.

Willson (1987) has observed that when work involves gardening or animal husbandry, "each places miracles within the reach of otherwise incapacitated mortals." It provides an opportunity for the experience of success. Working with animals might also have a special meaning for patients. Willson (1987) has again made the following observation:

> Relationships with animals are different from relationships with people. Animals are essentially honest, offer devotion without unjustified criticisms and do not answer back. They also respect one's confidence and respond through behavior rather than through additions to medical records.

It is possible that animals may form a non-threatening bridge to re-establishing healthy relationships with people.

Experience with this therapeutic environment indicates that patients appear to make swifter recoveries with regard to social responsiveness and normalization of behavior than in the hospital environment. One important reason for this may be the close involvement of the family and relatives in the rehabilitation process. Stable social networks are believed to contribute towards a positive outcome (Jilek and Jilek-Aall, 1970; Westermeyer, 1985).

Prospects for the Future

To make the best use of community-based care and rehabilitation within a village setting, training should be extended to a wider variety of professionals such as psychiatric social workers, occupational therapists, psychiatric rehabilitation assistants, community mental health nurses, and psychiatrists. More work needs to be done to involve the community in mental health promotion. The successful implementation of community mental health programs leads to an increase in the demand for services. It is important that adequate resources such as medicines and facilities for training and supervision are made available.

At present, although there is easier access to medication than in previous years, there are still shortages in the public health facilities. Although medication may be available in private facilities, most patients are unable to afford them. In the past, mental health was not awarded the same importance as other fields of medicine. 10 to 20% of patients in primary healthcare settings have mental disorders, and another 20% of hospital beds would be occupied by mental patients if community mental health care was not available. It thus follows that more than 20% of the total health budget should be devoted to the promotion of mental health. This should also be true of training.

With only 4 to 7% of the national budget dedicated to health, there is no other choice but to rely on the community-based care of chronic mental patients. It is fortunate that this choice happens to provide the best opportunity for improving the status and welfare of mental patients.

Collaboration between traditional healers and mental health professionals has existed on an informal basis. The development of more formal relationships, especially with those healers who are based within their traditional communities, with a cross-fertilization of ideas, information, and skills, may improve the care of the vast majority of mental patients with such minor conditions as anxiety and adjustment disorders.

An important challenge for mental health services is to work out strategies to better integrate traditional healing systems into the Western service. The family system, for example, could shoulder most of the burden of social and emotional support. Authentic traditional healers can play an increased role in the management and prevention of stress-related disorders in the community. This could begin with opening up communication channels between Western-trained mental health professionals and traditional healers. In Tanzania, traditional healers have demonstrated a willingness to participate in our training program, showing special interest in our approach to community mental health work and a willingness to share their knowledge and skills in the management of the mentally ill.

In 1995, the traditional healers formed an association called *"Chama cha Waganga na Wakunga wa Tiba Asilia Tanzania"* (Tanzania Traditional Health Practitioners Association). One of their objectives, as laid down in their constitution, is that of encouraging collaboration between Western-trained doctors and traditional healers and of increasing communication between these two sectors through meetings and seminars.

Preliminary results of an ongoing study in Dar es Salaam (Simmons, 1996) indicate a willingness on the part of Western-trained mental health professionals to collaborate with traditional healers.

It is hoped that such collaboration, together with the establishment of more agricultural psychiatric rehabilitation villages and an improvement in the quality and quantity of community involvement in mental health promotion, will all lead to the provision of more efficient and productive mental health services for Tanzanians.

N.B.: This paper was originally published in *Social Science and Medicine* Vol. 47(4) 419-428

Chapter Eleven

The Nature of Parasuicide in Dar es Salaam

Noah K. Ndosi and *M.C. Waziri*

Abstract

In a two-year period, 300 parasuicides were admitted at Muhimbili Hospital. Socio-demographic, clinical characteristics, trigger factors, and employed methods were analyzed and discussed with reference to other studies. Parasuicides were found to be young adults of mean age 23.7 years. The ratio of females to males was 2.2. The majority had seven years of education and were unemployed or under-employed. Four-fifths of attempts were triggered by acute social conflicts, psychiatric and physical illnesses, and socio-economic deprivations partly aggravated by alcohol intake. Two-thirds of parasuicides ingested overdoses of medicaments of which chloroquine constituted 65% of all drugs. Nearly a third of all the attempters had neuropsychiatric illnesses, while 4.3% had physical disorders. Nearly one-fifth or 18.3% of the parasuicides had a history of mental illness in their families, and 12% had an individual or family history of previous suicidal attempts. Forty percent of the attempts were categorized as demonstrative, 31% as genuine, 10.3% were equivocal, and 18.3% were not clarified.

Introduction

Attempted suicide, commonly referred to as parasuicide or deliberate self-harm, is defined as a non-fatal act in which an individual deliberately initiates a non-habitual behavior that, without intervention from others, will cause self-harm or deliberately ingests a substance in excess of the prescribed or generally recognized therapeutic dosage and which is aimed at realizing changes which the subject desires via the actual or expected physical consequences (Kerkhof *et. al.*, 1994). According to Tanzanian law, attempted suicide is a punishable offense. Parasuicide is a complex social behavior with rich meanings and interactions that are deeply rooted in culturally patterned forms of thought and emotional behavior (Hollan, 1990). Suicide attempts help to evaluate the capacity of various social systems to procure happiness and security for their members (Bhugra, 1989). The behavior may begin in adolescence and may persist for decades and result in great personal and social morbidity. Although in a few cases it has been underrated as a distinct syndrome of low lethality and repetitive, direct, self-destructive behavior (Wasserman, 1989), parasuicide is one of the strongest predictors of suicide and should be treated seriously (Diekstra, 1993). It is one of the commonest emergencies in hospital practice (Mengech and Dhadphale, 1984), and it is thought to be 10-20 times higher than rates for suicide (Platt, 1992; Weissman, 1976).

Many traditional African cultures consider life as sacred, and suicidal behavior is not only frowned upon, but also morally condemned. However, rapid social changes in these societies, especially in urban populations, are leading to moral instability and the loss of familiar norms which inhibit suicidal behavior. Although cross-cultural comparisons of parasuicide between countries are difficult, circumstances under which the attempt was made and the choice of means can give some clue as to the seriousness of the risk. It is important to understand the way people explain it so as to enable clinical and community programs to increase awareness of the social contexts in which they occur and to provide relevant and effective interventions.

From biological studies, DSH-serotonergic dysfunction has widely been implicated in suicide, an act of aggression toward oneself, acts of impulsiveness, and aggression toward others—especially in personality disordered individuals. It is unclear whether abnormally low cerebral serotonin levels relate directly to suicidal behavior, aggressiveness, or severity of depression (Fyer, 1988; Stanley and Mann, 1983). Identified common precipitant factors of vulnerability include a past psychiatric history; past parasuicide; drug and alcohol abuse; past criminal and violent behavior; low self-esteem; unstable family atmosphere characterized by poor relationships, violence, and frequent quarrels; lack of social support; and child abuse (Platt, 1992; Kebede and Ketsela, 1993).

Economic problems of Tanzania associated with rapid urbanization continue to cause higher stress rates among the youth and the unemployed. Population mobility due to socio-economic shifts, the breakdown of traditional family structures, alcohol and drug abuse, famine, and other deprivations are among frequent predisposing factors to parasuicide (Swift, 1977). The extent and severity of suicidal behaviour can be studied by investigating antecedents of suicidal ideation, plans, threats, and deliberate self-harm (Pearce and Martin, 1994). From clinical observations, suicide attempts in Dar es Salaam appear to be on the rise. This descriptive study aims at finding out the nature of suicide attempts in Dar es Salaam, the contributory risk factors, and the psycho-social circumstances surrounding the acts.

Patients and Methods

This study was conducted in the city of Dar es Salaam, the commercial capital of Tanzania with an estimated population of 2.5 million people. From 1 January 1991 to 30 June 1993, all consecutive suicide attempters identified by doctors working at casualty in the Department of Emergency Medicine of Muhimbili Medical Center, the largest referral hospital in Tanzania, as well as the main university teaching hospital, were reported to the authors within 24 hours after admission.

Three-hundred-and-twenty-eight identified subjects were referred to the Muhimbili hospital from the three districts of the city of Dar es Salaam. Of these, 304 subjects suffered less severe physical injuries and were admitted and treated in the medical ward, 13 cases with lacerations and sprains were admitted to the surgical ward, eight critically ill subjects were admitted to the intensive care unit, and three patients suffering from acute mental symptoms were admitted to the psychiatric unit.

When the patients had recovered from the adverse effects of parasuicide and had attained full consciousness, the purpose of the study was explained to patients, close relatives, and friends. Informed consent to participate in the study was sought from the patients and/or caregivers for those patients who exhibited mental symptoms with diminished insight and judgment at the time of admission. Initially, 328 patients consented to participate in the study, but in due course, 28 absconded or did not report in the follow-up as expected. The study cohort was thus reduced to 300.

A semi-structured interview technique was used to collect the individual socio-demographic data; the means employed to attempt suicide; and the number of previous attempts by the patients, their parents, siblings, and second-degree relatives. The attempters and their close relatives were also interviewed in depth about people who had committed suicide in their families. The kinds and amounts of alcohol taken by each parasuicide six hours prior to the attempt were also enquired from the patients and attendant relatives or friends. Indepth interviews focusing on the psycho-social circumstances surrounding parasuicide were conducted on each subject and key informants by the investigators to elicit the motives and risk factors underlying suicidal attempts. The key informants were people who knew about the events leading to deliberate self-harm relatively well and were present at the time of the act. A thorough physical examination was then conducted on each patient. Consultation with the attending physicians was also sought where necessary to delineate the clinical findings on admission.

All the patients who had significant mental symptoms had an indepth psychiatric history taken and a formal mental state examination by each investigator to establish working psychiatric diagnoses before treatment. These patients were followed in the out-patient psychiatric clinic at intervals of one week and four weeks after discharge. A few psychotic patients whose compliance was irregular with slow treatment response were followed up to six months to ensure recovery from suicidal ideation. The clinical symptoms of the mental patients were compared and discussed by the investigators so as to determine one most likely diagnosis. The psychiatric diagnoses were confirmed using guidelines in ICD 10 (WHO, 1992). Except for the mental patients and the severely injured attempters, the majority of patients were admitted for an average duration of three days. The results are tabled below.

Results

Socio-demographic Characteristics of Suicide Attempters

The average age of all the parasuicides who comprised 57 ethnic groups was 23.7 years (range 13-60 years). The average age for the 94 males was 25.7 years, while that of 206 females was 22.8 years. The proportion of females to males was 2.2. As shown in Table 1 below, 62 of 189 singles were students, 104 subjects were married, and seven divorced; 55.7% of the patients were Christians, of whom Catholics were the majority; Moslems comprised 43.3% of parasuicides, and three attempters belonged to other religions; 47.6% of the respondents were simple skilled workers and petty businessmen. The unemployed, who were predominantly women, comprised 31.7% of the study cohort. Nearly three-quarters of the suicide attempters had primary school education and the rest secondary school education and higher.

Triggers of Attempted Suicide

Social conflicts were found to trigger or to contribute to attempted suicides in about four-fifths of cases, as shown in Table 2.

Table 1: *Socio-demographic Characteristics of Parasuicides*

Sex

	No	*%*
Females	206	68.7
Males	94	31.3
Total	300	100.0

Marital Status

Singles	189	63.0
Married	104	34.7
Divorced	7	2.3
Total	300	100.0

Religion

Christians	167	55.7
Moslems	130	43.3
Others	3	1.0
Total	300	100.00

Employment Status

Employed	143	47.6
Unemployed	95	31.7
Students	62	20.7
Total	300	100.0

Educational Level

0-4	32	10.7
5-7	188	62.7
10-14	76	25.3
University	4	1.3
Total	300	100.0

Source: *Computed from Research Findings*

The conflicts were comprised of interpersonal strains between parents and children (17.3%), infidelity largely committed by male partners (17%), other marital misunderstandings (17%), quarrels among siblings (16%), conflicts with other people (8.3%), and unwanted pregnancies (5%). Other contributory factors included severe poverty and acute financial problems (8.3%), recurrent mental illnesses (5%), chronic physical illnesses (4.3%), and bereavement (1.6%).

Table 2: *Reported Triggers of Attempted Suicide*

Trigger	*No*	*%*
Social conflicts	242	80.7
Financial problems	25	8.3
Chronic mental illness	15	5.0
Chronic physical illness	13	4.3
Bereavement	5	1.7
Total	300	100.0

Source: *Computed from Research Findings*

Means Employed by Suicide Attempters

Of the 272 parasuicides who swallowed overdoses of medicaments and poisons, 198 were females. Of medicinal drugs employed, 65% were chloroquine tablets (average dose 1.5 gm), as shown in Table 3. Antibiotics, aspirin, Panadol, and psychotropic drugs were the other types of drugs employed. Rat poisons, dilute sulfuric acid, kerosene, antiseptic solutions, and glass were ingested by 74 patients (24.7%). Twenty patients employed hanging, stabs with knives, jumping from heights, head-banging, and shooting. Of these patients, 17 were males.

Table 3: *Means Employed by Suicide Attempters*

Means	*N*	*%*
Medicaments	206	68.7
Poisons	66	22.0
Ingestion of glass	8	2.7
Hanging	8	2.7
Stabs with knives	4	1.3
Jumps from knives	4	1.3
Head-banging	3	1.0
Shooting	1	0.3
Total	**300**	**100.0**

Source: *Computed from Research Findings*

Table 4: *Mental and Physical Disorders in Parasuicides*

Disorders	*N*	%
Psychosis	37	12.3
Major depression	27	9.0
Neurotic disorder	23	7.7
Drug abuse	12	4.0
AIDS	12	4.0
Epilepsy	5	1.7
P.T.B.	1	0.3
Total	117	39.0

Source: *Computed from Research Findings*

Mental and Physical Disorders

As shown in Table 4, 104 suicide attempters had significant neuropsychiatric disorders. These consisted of acute episodes of recurrent schizophrenic psychoses (12.3%); major depression (9.0%); neurotic disorders (7.7%); alcohol, cannabis, and heroin abuse (4%); and epilepsy (1.7%). Twelve patients (4%) who had advanced AIDS with scanty means of living and poor social support had attempted suicide to end their suffering, and one grossly emaciated patient with pulmonary tuberculosis lost hope of recovery and swallowed an overdose of anti-TB drugs.

History of Mental Illnesses, Parasuicide and Suicide in Patients and Family

A total of 18.3% of all cases had a history of family mental illness. In 3% of cases, parents had suffered from major mental illnesses, while in 4.3%, siblings had been afflicted, and in 11%, second-degree relatives had suffered from mental disorders.

Eleven subjects had previously attempted suicide once, four had made two attempts, and one patient had attempted thrice. In four cases, parents had attempted suicide once, and in 12 subjects, second-degree relatives had attempted suicide once. Two suicide attempters had lost parents through suicide, while three had each lost a sibling through suicide.

Intentions of Suicide Attempters

Analysis of the interviews regarding the suicidal intent yielded the categories in Table 5. Forty percent of respondents made their attempts to solicit help and social sympathy during acute social problems, while 31.3% of them claimed to have had the intention to take their lives. Thirty-one patients (10.3%) could not clearly specify their motives. They claimed both to have been overwhelmed by acute emotional pain and to have acted impulsively.

Table 5: *Intentions of Suicide Attempters*

Intentions	*N*	*%*
Demonstrative	120	40.0
Death wish	94	31.3
No response	55	18.3
Uncertain motive	31	10.3
Total	**300**	**100.0**

Source: *Computed from Research Findings*

The remaining subjects refused to render any information regarding their motives of attempted suicide.

Finally, 73 patients had drunk various amounts of alcohol (industrial beer, local brews, cognac, illicit brew) about six hours prior to attempting suicide, and most of them smelled of alcohol on admission

Discussion

Socio-demographic Characteristics

To understand the nature of parasuicide, it is necessary to identify various underlying factors which enhance and precipitate it. In this study, suicide attempters were found to be young people of an average 23.7 years. The ratio of females to males was 2.2. Females were slightly younger than men. In the majority of African cultures, females are usually expected to bear greater family responsibilities which expose them to greater psychological distress particularly in poor, overcrowded, and challenging city environments. The majority of the unemployed and underemployed subjects were women with lower education. Their young age is likely to have strained their adaptive capacities of coping with the overwhelming psychological stresses they experienced. Studies from Singapore, Western Europe, North America,

Nigeria, and South Africa (Tsoi, 1982; Weissman, 1976; WHO, 1974; Odejide et al., 1986; Naidoo and Pillary, 1993) found the age of parasuicides to be between 20 and 30 years. The prevalence of depression as a symptom or clinical disorder among young women is known to be high and consistently more common in women than men (Retterstol et al., 1993; Klerman, 1986; Miles, 1977; Morano, Cisler and Lemerond, 1993). Two-thirds of the 27 depressed parasuicides were females.

Unemployment featured in 31.7% of adult parasuicides. The urban population in Tanzania has increased from 7% to 34% of the total population in the last 30 years, and over half the increase of this population has occurred in the city of Dar es Salaam which, together with a deteriorating national economy has severely limited the procurement of basic amenities of life (World Bank, 1993). Forty percent of the city population is currently either unemployed or under-employed. Unemployment creates feelings of hopelessness, which adds further stress to the economically and psychologically vulnerable individuals (Pritchard, 1992). Unemployed men have been found to be at a 3.4 times greater risk of suicide than the employed. A strongly significant association has been found between unemployment and self-poisoning (Jones, Forster and Hassanyh, 1991). However, it is unclear to what extent unemployment itself contributes to suicide risk. The effects of unemployment on mental health could increase suicidal risk, but it is also true that people with poor mental health are at an increased risk of becoming unemployed (Smith, 1985). Even though the impact of religion on parasuicide has not yielded consistent results (Stack and Lester, 1991), among the attempters in this study, 167 were Christians, of which two-thirds were Catholics, while their proportion among Christians in Dar es Salaam city is less than half.

Psycho-social Risk Factors

Over 80% of suicide attempters were found to have high stress emanating from severe social conflicts. Quarrels between parents and children characterized by a lack of parental warmth, authoritarian parenting, firmly enforced rules, control of autonomy, and harsh punishments were found in 17.3% of the attempters. Sixteen percent of parasuicides occurred when elder siblings assumed parental roles of punishing their younger ones for deviant behavior. Three percent of these cases had received severe beatings. The lack of family support and feelings of hopelessness, coupled with low self-esteem and acute emotional pain, are among risk factors which enhance suicidal behavior (Horwitz and White, 1991). Infidelity, particularly among male partners, and other marital misunderstandings led to hostility, and intolerable emotional outbursts gave way to parasuicidal acts. Some wives became jealous of their husbands' other sexual partners and dreaded contracting sexually transmitted diseases and severe social hardships brought by separation or divorce. Living in poverty and congestion as squatters enhanced risks to emotional crisis, especially among the 73 attempters who had taken alcohol prior to the acts. Alcohol has the effect of altering the mood of the consumer, increasing paranoid ideation, panic, suicidal thoughts, and impulses to self-mutilation (Lewinsohn, Rohde and Seeley, 1994; Murphy et al., 1992). Fourteen pregnant girls attempted suicide after their boyfriends refused to marry them. A study from Singapore (1982) found the main reason for attempted suicide to be relationship problems involving threats of separation from boyfriends (Tsoi, 1982). Unwanted pregnancies lead to acute stress reactions with loss of self-esteem, anxiety, feelings of guilt, hostility, and hopelessness which sometimes culminate in self-mutilation.

Eight percent of suicide attempters in severe financial deprivation claimed that life was not worth living. Seventeen subjects lived in hardcore poverty and were unwell, while eight had unexpectedly experienced dramatic losses in petty business. Poor people and those in debt report more psychiatric symptoms, harbor feelings of hopelessness, are less in control of events around them, and receive more psychiatric diagnoses. They tend to have greater suicidal intent (Hatcher, 1994). Bereavement following the loss of parents in two instances and loss of a sibling in three others provoked feelings towards self-mutilation. Loss traumas, especially in African cultures, tend to increase the risk of suicide, particularly in females. This risk is particularly high in individuals with a history of psychiatric disorder and/or suicidal behavior before bereavement and who are lacking family support following the loss (Mehlum, 1992; Buch, 1972).

Clinical Factors

The incidence of parasuicides and suicides has been found to be highest among individuals suffering from mental and physical illnesses. Psychiatric illness is one of the most powerful indicators of suicide and probably the most relevant one in the clinical context (Buck, 1982; Alleck and Allgulander, 1990). At least a third of all parasuicides suffered from significant neuropsychiatric disorders. Of these patients, 35.6% had psychotic disorders of which 16 cases had chronic recurrent schizophrenia. These patients suffered from poor therapeutic compliance and could not afford to buy the needed medicaments. The lack of enduring social support made them feel lonely, and they were tired of taking dugs with unpleasant side effects. Six patients had florid psychotic symptoms. They claimed to have obeyed voices instructing them to take their lives. A third of the psychotic patients had taken alcohol several hours before the attempts. About 10% of patients with schizophrenia commit suicide, and that stigmatization, in addition to relapses, remissions, and consumption of alcohol, especially among young schizophrenics, heightens the risk of suicidal behavior (Landmark, Cernovsky and Merkey, 1987; Wilkinson, 1982). Twenty-seven depressed patients suffered from severe distress and decided to end their suffering. Depression has previously been found to be a strong correlate of suicidal behavior, with prevalence among self-harm patients ranging from 30% to 66% (Naidoo and Pillary, 1993; Retterstol et al., 1993). Moreover, suicide risk among affective disorders has been estimated to be 30 times higher than that of the general population, and this risk is highest relatively early on the course of the disorder (Bartels, Drake and McHugo, 1992; Guze and Robins, 1970; Hawton, 1987).

Twelve-and-a-half percent of the psychiatric patients had acute organic brain syndromes whose main etiology comprised infections, substance abuse, and metabolic disorders. Of the 12 who abused drugs, eight drank over two liters of beer with considerable amounts of illicit brew *(gongo)* per day. Three parasuicides abused heroin, and one abused cannabis. These patients accumulated financial debts from their abuse and had provoked severe interpersonal conflicts which heightened their emotional outbursts, leading to autoaggression. The risk of suicide among male heroin addicts has been estimated to be approximately 20 times that of the general population (James, 1967). Slightly over 7% of the attempters suffered from neurotic disorders. They exhibited lower emotional tolerance and had frequent, acute, emotionally charged conflicts within their families. Patients suffering from depressive neurosis or panic have been reported to have increased risk of suicidal behavior (Sims and Prior, 1978). Chronic seizures for about six years featured in five parasuicides. These patients who exhibited inter-ictal personality changes expressed hopelessness and disappointment about regularly taking anticonvulsant medication without sustained relief. Risk of suicide in epilepsy has been estimated to be fivefold, and this risk may be very much higher in people with temporal lobe epilepsy (Barraclough, 1981). Twelve patients suffered from clinically and serologically proven acquired immunodeficiency syndrome, and one suffered from tuberculosis. They claimed worsening, unendurable suffering combined with inadequate socio-economic support. Previous studies have shown the risk of patients with HIV infections to be 35-40 times higher than that of HIV-negative persons. The risk in this group is particularly high if the stage of HIV infection is advanced and accompanied by disabling intercurrent illnesses in poor socio-economic conditions (McKegney and O'Dowd, 1992; Rajs and Fugelstad, 1992).

Genetic and Repeated Parasuicide Factors

Members of a family tend to suffer from similar illnesses because of common genetic predispositions. Although the causal mechanisms are complex, they significantly involve socio-environmental factors. Polygenic inheritance of suicidal behavior in depressed patients with a history of attempted suicide has previously been reported (Papadimitriou *et. al.*, 1991). In this study, parental history of major mental illnesses was found in 3% of cases, while in siblings the history was positive in 4.3% subjects and 11% in second-degree relatives. This finding is lower than that found in Budapest (1988) in which a positive family history of mental disorders was found in 27% of male and 29% in female suicide attempters (Arato *et. al.*, 1988). This difference is likely to be due to under-reporting because of fears of stigmatization of psychiatric disorders in African cultures. Deliberate self-harm is thought to be learned socially, and those who repeat the act are thought to have had significantly more prior contacts. Several studies have also shown that 10-60% of suicide attempters had previously inflicted deliberate self-injuries (Wang and Brille-Brahe, 1972; Kienhorst *et. al.*, 1990; Mishara, Baker and Mishara, 1976; Myers, 1988; Platt, 1993). Five percent of cases had a history of one previous attempt, 3.7% had attempted once, 1% had repeated twice, and one case had made three attempts. Parents of four parasuicides had a positive history of attempted suicides, while second-degree relatives of these parasuicides had attempted suicide. In two cases, parents had completed suicide, while in three cases, siblings had committed suicide. These findings should be taken cautiously as parasuicide and suicides are culturally seen as taboos in Tanzania. People do not volunteer information readily on intimate family matters because they fear social sanctions and marginalization.

Means Employed

Over two-thirds of parasuicides in this study employed overdoses of easily obtainable medicinal drugs; 65% used chloroquine tablets (average dose 1.5 gm). The number of females who employed chloroquine, antibiotics, aspirin, psychotropics, de-worming medicaments, and other unknown drugs was at least three times that of men. Panadol was, however, about equally used in both sexes. In San Diego (1993), women were found to be more than four times as likely as men to employ drugs, particularly Panadol, in suicide (Mendelson, 1993). The motivation to take an overdose of medicament is often complex, frequently involving a simultaneous interplay of different psychological motives in an individual (Farmer, 1987). A study from South Africa found that the majority of parasuicides who employed self-poisoning were single and had experienced early parental loss (Naidoo and Pillary, 1993). In continental Europe, benzodiazepines remain the drug of choice for suicide attempters (Neeleman, 1994), although overdoses of paracetamol are also rampant there and in Nigeria (Eferakeya, 1970; Asuni, 1967). More females than males also ingested various types of poisons. Poisoning was found in a third of all admissions into the intensive care unit at Kenyatta National Hospital in Nairobi (Kauho, 1980). Eight parasuicides were males who employed more aggressive means, such as hanging, jumping from heights, banging heads against walls, and shooting. It has been reported that when males attempt suicide, they often use more lethal and violent methods than females (Spirito *et. al.*, 1993).

The evaluation of the in-depth interviews of the extent of the death wish in the parasuicides was not clear cut in all cases. However, 31.3% of the attempters were serious ideators who indicated a premeditated death wish and an intention to take their lives. Two-fifths of attempters, the majority of which were women, had carried out the acts of deliberate self-injury demonstratively to solicit public sympathy and help in their miseries. Ten percent expressed equivocal deliberations, and 18.3% did not volunteer any intentions. Some of the latter requested exemption from explaining their motives, while the others remained silent. Many parasuicides developed guilt feelings associated with their suicidal behavior as they learned that they transgressed the law. It is, therefore, not surprising that only about a third of the study cohort volunteered their intent in the affirmative.

Conclusion

Although suicidal behavior is difficult to predict even in high-risk groups of suicide attempts, parasuicide was found to be at least twice as common in young women as in young men. The attempts were found to be embedded within socio-economic deprivations and recent acute interpersonal conflicts often aggravated by ill health and the mood-altering effect of alcohol. A previous history of mental illness in the family and a positive history of parasuicide in the patient and relatives, including suicides in the family, were other risk factors. The majority of deliberate self-injuries by women employed overdoses of readily available medicinal drugs, particularly chloroquine. A third of the subjects expressed a genuine death-wish, two-fifths attempted suicide as a means of crying for help, and the rest remained silent or were equivocal about their suicidal intention. Closer surveillance of suicidal mental patients at home would facilitate a timely referral to the hospital. Furthermore, the availability of medicinal drugs calls for greater control to limit misuse. Further studies on parasuicide and suicide rates are needed to determine the seriousness of this psychological suffering so that appropriate interventions can be sought.

N.B.: This chapter was originally published in Social Science and Medicine, 44:55, 1997.

PART FOUR

POVERTY AND THE POLITICAL ECONOMY OF HEALTH

Chapter Twelve

The Impact of Structural Adjustment Policies on Women's and Children's Health in Tanzania

Joe L.P. Lugalla

Abstract

Since 1981, in an attempt to deal withTanzania's present social and economic crisis which dates back to the late 1970s, the government has adopted a variety of policy measures including The National Economic Survival Plan (NESP), Structural Adjustment Programme (SAP), Economic Recovery Programme (ERP) I(1986) and II (1989), the Economic and Social Action Plan (ESAP), and Priority Social Action Plan (PSAP) (1989). The principal objective of these adjustment measures has been to attain macroeconomic balance by bringing national expenditure into line with national income to reduce inflation and to increase exports. Other objectives have been to maintain egalitarian income distribution and the provision of basic social services to the majority of the population. In order to realise these objectives, the government has been controlling credit and has removed subsidies on certain food items and agricultural inputs, introduced a system of progressive devaluation, liberalised trade and has been trying to reduce government expenditure by introducing cost-sharing measures in the education and health sector.

The erosion of real incomes and increased poverty has had a devastating effect on women and children. Rural women have yet heavier workloads as males migrate to the urban areas to look for work, there is increased maternal mortality, and chronic malnutrition and poverty are rendering the implementation of HIV/AIDS intervention strategies difficult. But most of all, the danger lies in the lack of care for future generations.

Introduction

In 1981, the World Bank published the Berg Report on the social and economic crisis in sub-Saharan Africa which engendered a major paradigmatic shift in development assistance to the region. The report focused on issues related to the mismanagement of both the economy and natural resources by state bureaucrats who were corrupt and unaccountable. Implicitly, the report seemed to suggest that it was these internal factors which were solely responsible for the crisis. The crisis of sub-Saharan Africa was seen to be characterized by negative trends in the growth of the economy leading to falling GDP per capita; the declining performance of the agricultural sector, and more particularly, the export sector, leading to shortage of foreign exchange; deteriorating internal and external accounts; and increasing internal and external borrowing. Due to these tendencies, development defined in terms of social economic progress came to a halt in some countries, reversed in others, and the number of people living under conditions of abject poverty and squalor increased in all countries. The magnitude of the crisis in sub-Saharan Africa necessitated, in the language of international monetary institutions, 'Structural Reforms.' What does this mean?

In brief, structural reforms mean adjusting structurally the economy in order to manage properly the balance of payments, reduce the fiscal deficits, increase economic 'efficiency,' and encourage private sector investments and export- oriented production. The major measures include the control of money supply; the devaluation of local currency; the reduction of public borrowing and government expenditure, particularly in the social sectors and introduction of cost-sharing (user-charges in education and health). Other measures include trade liberalization, reduction of tariff rates, and the institution of other measures in order to encourage foreign investors, such as the abolition of price controls, the privatization of public parastatals, the reduction or withdrawal of subsidies, the retrenchment of workers, wage freezes, and the deregulation of laws protecting job security. Most of the countries in sub-Saharan Africa have been forced to adopt these measures as a conditionality for aid and loans from international monetary institutions and other donor agencies.

Since SAPs have now been operating in sub-Saharan Africa for more than a decade, what is at issue is not what will happen as a result of SAPs, but rather what has happened/is happening and how this is going to affect the future of these countries. And if development is to be seen in terms of social progress, we need to know what SAPs mean to different social groups; who suffers most and with what results? The objective of this chapter is to perform a general assessment of the impact of SAPs in the Health Sector in Tanzania. The chapter will go on to look at what these changes mean for the health conditions of vulnerable social groups, i.e. children and women.

Tanzania, SAPs and the Health Sector

The health sector has been severely affected by the economic crisis and its accompanying SAP measures. The share of health in the national budget declined from 7.23 per cent in 1977/78 to 4.62 per cent in 1989/90. As the crisis has deepened, government commitment to the health sector has diminished, creating many problems in terms of intersectoral allocations of resources. For example, it has been difficult for the government to maintain its priority on rural healthcare and the preventive approach to healthcare which started in the early 1970s. More money kept going to recurrent rather than to development expenditure. Per capita spending on health declined by over a third between 1980 and 1986 (World Bank, 1990; Afro-Aid, 1991), and the devaluation of the Tanzanian Shilling in 1986 meant the prices for drugs went up by 300-400 per cent in 1988.

The scarcity of financial resources for health has affected the sector in several ways. First and foremost is that the government has been unable to establish more health facilities and to recruit more health personnel in order to cater for the rapidly rising population. As a result, population per health facility has been increasing year after year. A World Bank study in 1993 shows that population per doctor increased from 19,053 in 1981 to 24,880 in 1990, while population per nurse rose from 3,310 people in 1970 to 5,470 people in 1990. Lack of resources and personnel has led to overcrowding in health institutions, and this has diminished the quality of service provided. Deterioration of medical infrastructure has led to a decline in the delivery of both curative and preventive services (Vuorella, 1992). To date, the availability of medical equipment and essential drugs continues to be a serious problem. An Essential Drugs Programmes (EDP) monitoring study in December of 1987 revealed that the availability of anti-malarial drugs in rural areas was only 51 per cent. An Economic Research Bureau (ERB) survey in October of 1988 of households in Dar-es-Salaam showed that 20 per cent of the 1,000-person sample reported the availability of drugs in hospitals as good, while 70 per cent said it had declined seriously, and 52 per cent of the sample said that the drugs in dispensaries were sold illegally by staff (Ibid). The last response requires some qualification.

SAPs have not only affected the health sector, they have fuelled inflation. Prices of commodities have gone up at a time when salary increases have remained stagnant. Cutbacks in government expenditure have squeezed salaries, and the high cost of living has reduced the real earnings of health workers. The monthly wages offered to health personnel do not correspond with the monthly household cost of living. This has bred corruption in the medical sector. Drugs are sold illegally while prescriptions and medical attention are mostly available to those who can pay or have influence. Kickbacks have become the medium of exchange for medical attention. The majority of health personnel are increasingly involved in private income-generating activities. Some medical personnel invest more effort and time in either officially recognised private practices or in illegal medical units operating behind the doors of their household units using public resources (including official working hours). Others are busy in income-generating activities such as rearing chickens, urban dairy farming, owning piggeries, and operating pirate taxis *(teksi bubu)*. Some health personnel have left the public service and joined the private sector either within or outside the country. This demonstrates the inability of the government to retain physicians.

In the context of the decline in public health infrastructure, unrealistic wages, and worsening conditions of work, demoralised health workers are now reacting bitterly against the state. Doctors' strikes and nurse go-slows, events which never characterized the Tanzanian health sector before, became common in the 1990s. Since the state is unable to meet most of the demands for increased wages and improved conditions, it has sometimes resorted to draconian measures in order to silence opposition. In 1991, the state used the well-trained Field Force Police Unit to end a doctors' strike at Muhimbili Medical Centre (which is the biggest referral and consultant hospital in the country). The Police Unit harassed, beat them and their families, and removed them by force from hospital-owned housing. Growing hostility between the state and health personnel has worsened the delivery of health services even further with a deleterious effect on people's health.

Notwithstanding the declining trend of the Tanzanian people's income, the government has introduced a cost-sharing principle in social services on the basis of user charges. The costs calculated for a variety of medical problems are beyond the reach of the majority of the poor and will lower their access to medical services. In the past, low income earners avoided private hospitals and those owned by Non-Governmental Organisations (NGOs) because they charged fees. But in the 1980s and 1990s, the poor quality of services in the public hospitals and increased official and unofficial costs (e.g. bribes) have made public services very expensive for the poor. The Tanzania Gender Networking Programme (TGNP, 1993) has noted that medical care for a simple case of malaria (an endemic disease among children, women, and men) in low-cost private hospitals and pharmacies consumes as much as half the monthly wage.

There are consistent, broad features of change in health policy due to SAPs . These include a replacement of pro-active health policies by health sector measures which accommodate the interests of SAPs . This has led to a widening gap between the affected communities and policy makers, leading to alienation and social tension with social response ranging from individual coping mechanisms to social resistance. And health, which was regarded as a basic right in the Tanzanian context, has now become a commodity for those who can pay, while the have-nots must rely on charity. In sub-Saharan Africa, the policy debate in the health sector has shifted markedly from demand-oriented questions on what the population needs and what would be feasible and effective to meet those needs, toward supply-oriented questions of what is affordable and cost effective (Loewensen, 1993:724).

It is also important to acknowledge the fact that good health is not only a function of good healthcare facilities. There are other variables, like people's income, which are also important in influencing health conditions and which have not been spared by SAPs. Closely related to the issue of good health and wellbeing is water supply, housing, and sanitation facilities. Water supply is one of the most important services in terms of the health of the people, and it is a necessity for day-to-day life. As the crisis has intensified, water has been one of the most difficult and expensive services to provide, especially in urban areas. The rapid population growth and extensive urban growth have further complicated the situation. Improved water supplies were built to serve some 50 to 70 per cent of the population in urban areas and about 45 per cent in the rural areas, but in both cases, problems of inadequate maintenance have reduced the number of people actually served to about 25 per cent (Kulaba, 1989). The 1991/92 Household Budget Survey (HBS, 1991/92) revealed that 67 per cent of rural households use water from unsafe sources.

Related to the question of water supply is the problem of housing and sanitation facilities. The housing situation is deplorable in urban areas where 70 per cent of the population live in squatter settlements without facilities like drainage and sewerage systems or garbage collection. Urban councils have not been able to improve these services due to restrained budgets. While the urban population has been expanding over the past decade at an annual growth rate of almost 12 per cent, the capacity of urban authorities to collect and dispose of an increasing amount of refuse and solid waste has been declining.

Indeed it is at the level of sanitation, drainage, and urban transport facilities that the impact of the crises in urban areas can be openly seen.

Dar es Salaam's central sewage and drainage system was designed and built during colonialism. This system serves only 10 per cent of the houses of Dar es Salaam. Of the 20 regional headquarters (towns), only eight have central sewerage systems which serve less than 10 per cent of the population of each town. In 1990, Dar es Salaam, a city of over 2 million people, had only 15 public toilets, none of which was functional (Lugalla, 1990). The situation of the collection of garbage, foul water, and refuse is also alarming; in 1985/86, the city generated 1,200 tons of solid waste daily. The city needed 120 vehicles to remove all this garbage, but had only 12. In order to be able to remove all waste water, the city needed 150 emptiers, but by March 1988, the city had only 20 cesspit emptiers (Lugalla, 1990). A survey carried out in Dar es Salaam in 1987/88 shows that despite additional new refuse collection vehicles and cesspit emptying vehicles given by Japan to Dar es Salaam, the City Council was able to collect only a small percentage of solid and liquid waste generated from January 1987 to June 1988. Recent data on households show that 5 per cent of households in Tanzania have no toilets, and 87 per cent have pit latrines although their use by all members of the family is questionable because of cultural beliefs and taboos. Only 7 per cent use flush toilets while 65.6 per cent have garbage pits outside their compound, and only 6 per cent have rubbish bins (HBS, 1991/92). Lack of sufficient refuse collector trucks as well as cesspit emptier trucks means that a lot of garbage is left uncollected, and streets often overflow with sewage. SAP measures are exacerbating the crisis by further restricting government investment in social service infrastructure. If the situation is appalling in affluent areas of Dar es Salaam, one may imagine the conditions of life in the forgotten, unplanned squatter settlements of Buguruni and Manzese where houses are floating in their own sewage and streets are stinking due to decayed, uncollected garbage. There is no doubt that this appalling environment has a far-reaching impact upon the health of the urban population. A recent study by TGNP confirms that common health problems for women and children in Tanzania are associated with contaminated water and food from unhygienic and unsanitary facilities.

SAPs do not mean the same thing to everybody. It is therefore important to understand how SAPs are affecting different social groups, particularly the vulnerable ones like women and children.

IMPACT OF SAPs ON WOMEN'S AND CHILDREN'S HEALTH

On 5 June 1988, the *Daily* Newspaper of the Tanzanian government reported that during the first thirteen weeks of the year, 71 mothers died during labour in the Muhimbili Medical Centre; this number was four times the death rate of previous years. The increase appeared to be due to a shortage of blood and essential obstetric drugs such as lasix, diazepam, ergometrine, pitocin, and hydralazine. The shortage of blood was attributed to a lack of transport from donor to recipients (Vuorella, 1992).

The Berg Report's gender blindness did not render SAPs gender neutral. Poor women and children have been negatively affected (Gladwin, 1991; Schoepf, 1991; TGNP, 1993). The impact of SAPs on women's and children's health is multi-dimensional and is direct as well as indirect. Throughout Africa, the repercussions of SAPs have been exacerbated by women's subordination within the household, by continuing constraints on peasant productivity, and also by mass unemployment (Schoepf, 1991).

In Tanzania, SAPs are negatively affecting the health of women and children in a variety of ways. The rising cost of living, increased production costs in the rural agricultural economy where most of the resources are generated by women, and stiff competition with minimal returns in the urban informal sector have increased women's responsibility in the domestic household economy. The workload of women has increased with concomitant increasing rates of pauperisation, poverty, and misery. The woman's working day is much longer than the man's. On average, women work more than 16 hours per day. They wake up at 4.30 or 5.00 a.m. in many places and don't rest until 9.30 p.m. or later. Data produced by the Danish International Development Agency (DANIDA) in four villages of the Iringa Region show that 25 per cent of women's working hours (totalling 14 hours) was devoted to farm work, 28 per cent to food preparation, 8 per cent to washing and cleaning, 8 per cent to collecting water and firewood, 2 per cent to child care, 15 per cent to other activities, and only 14 per cent to resting (TGNP 1993:66). Women have remained responsible for domestic work and maintaining their household while expansion in school enrolment has increased their workload as access to the labour of older children became seasonal. However, due to SAPs, children in some families are dropping out of school in order to assist in the household domestic economy (girls) or in petty trading activities (boys) (TGNP 1993).

Erosion of real incomes and increasing poverty has intensified gender inequality and the power of men over women in almost every sphere of social life. This has increased gender exploitation since the majority of women—particularly in urban areas—depend on their husband's incomes. Even in situations where women operate their own income-generating projects, at the end of the day, it is the husbands who normally determine how the money is going to be used. Since women are the mainstay of the household economy, decisions unfavourable to them have become detrimental to the population as a whole. This situation is also making women more vulnerable to poor conditions of work and social life with deleterious effects on their health. The majority of urban women are being forced to secure their means of livelihood via marginal informal economic activities which lack safety and job security. Others have joined the 'entertainment industry' where they earn their living through commercial sex. Others, married or unmarried, entertain multiple sex partners in order to ensure their own and family survival. To some women, commercial sex has become necessary for them to support themselves and their dependants. The presence of the deadly HIV virus has turned prostitution from a 'survival strategy' into a 'death strategy' (Schoepf, 1991). On the other hand, erosion of women's economic power, particularly for those who are married, means increasing dependence on the husband's income potential. This situation is exacerbating further the existing culturally sanctioned unequal sexual relations within the household. This jeopardises the opportunities women currently have to determine the mode of their emotional and sexual relations with their husbands.

Due to poverty, women are forced to maintain marriage relations not only because they fear the negative stigma of divorce inherent in Tanzanian society, but because, under such circumstances, marriage becomes a survival strategy. The use of condoms in such relations becomes a taboo, sexual pleasure becomes meaningless, and such women continue to remain objects of men's sexual pleasure and desires. This is reflected in the following comment of one married woman in Dar es Salaam:

> *Sisi wanawake tuna shida. Tunawategemea sana waume zetu siku hizi kwa sababu maisha ni magumu. Hata kama mumeo ni malaya, ni lazima uvumilie. Ukimuacha utakwenda wapi? Utakula nini? Nani mwingine atakuoa mtu uliye na watoto tayari? Basi, inabidi uvumilie. Nina uhakika kuwa kuna baadhi ya wanawake wanaopata ukimwi kwenye vyumba vyao vya kulala.*

(We women have problems. We nowadays depend much on our husbands because life is difficult. Even if your husband is promiscuous, you have to tolerate it. If you desert him, where will you go? How are you going to survive? Who else will marry somebody with children already? Anyway, you have to tolerate it. I am sure some women get HIV/AIDS in their own bedrooms (author's translation from a 1993 interview).

In brief, lack of access to and control of resources at the household level and a lack of decision-making power in issues related to sexual relationships are important factors which make women vulnerable to HIV transmission.

Women's issues are also children's issues. Busy families do not have time to care for their children, who are, thus, left unsupervised. Economic and matrimonial hardships at home have a tendency to push children to search for other life alternatives. In Tanzania, this is leading to rapidly increasing numbers of unsupervised children in urban areas. The number of street children has increased tremendously during the last decade, and this is now an issue of public concem. The majority have no proper or healthy living places and survive by eating food collected from garbage which is a health hazard. The girls engage in commercial sex at a very tender age and risk unwanted pregnancies, clandestine abortions, and contamination by sexually transmitted diseases; some are beaten and go unpaid for the services they have provided. The boys join urban gangs and call themselves *Watoto ma Maskani, Watemi,* and *Magangwe* which basically means those who are tough, used to problems, and carefree. Some smoke *Widi, Bangi* (marijuana); others sniff glue and petrol in order to make themselves high. Most of them survive by robbery and pick-pocketing in the urban-based, congested *Daladala* buses and risk severe beatings or death at the hands of mob justice. Some practice homosexuality in exchange for money.

Due to poverty and increasing economic hardships, women are increasingly being subjected to sexual harassment. A poor, desperate woman may be forced to entertain the sexual desires of a would-be employer or her immediate boss in order to obtain employment, promotion, fringe benefits, or to maintain job security in the face of SAP retrenchment programs. A study by Shaidi (1991) on sexual harassment of women in four different formal work places in Tanzania revealed that some 95 per cent of women interviewed had experienced some kind of sexual harassment. Urban school girls are also at risk. With increasing difficulties in the urban transport system, such girls find it difficult to escape the sexual trap of car lift offers by 'sugar daddies.' It is also important to note that in an education system characterized by corruption, some school girls may be forced to grant sexual favours to their male teachers in order to get examination papers, better grades, and other advantages.

Interviews which I conducted with female and male students at the University of Dar es Salaam in 1994 reveal that this kind of behaviour is becoming increasingly common.

The majority of workers in the urban-based entertainment industry (i.e. bars, pubs, hotels, and restaurants) are females who experience very poor working conditions. Most of them receive minimal pay and are expected to hustle for tips from customers. In reality, many waitresses in pubs and bars are disguised prostitutes and are therefore expected to provide sexual services as part of their job (TGNP, 1993:67). What does this mean as far as HIV/AIDS is concerned?

The statistics for HIV/AIDS in Tanzania are alarming for women. The number of HIV infected persons in Tanzania is about 800,000, or 3 per cent of the total population. The 1992 estimates of HIV sero-prevalence in the adult male population was 5.8 per cent and 7.1 per cent in adult female women. Some 400,000 women were expected to be infected by the mid-1990s according to the National Aids Control Programme NACP (quoted by TGNP, 1993); these are underestimates as only one out of every four cases is reported (TGNP, 1993). According to a NACP analysis of new AIDS cases reported during 1983-1991, women were affected at an earlier age than men, probably a reflection, in part, of gender differences in sexual behaviour (Ibid). There is no doubt that women are more susceptible to HIV infection than men. A study by the World Bank (1991:21) estimated that the probability of heterosexual transmission was 0.03 (3 out of 100) during any one contact between an infected male and an uninfected female and 0.01 (1 out of 100) during any one contact between an infected female and an uninfected male.

Furthermore, the increasing economic hardships of life make women more vulnerable to sexual harassment and violence and lowers their ability to negotiate for safer sex. Poverty is again rendering the implementation of HIV/AIDS intervention strategies difficult. Condoms, if available, are unaffordable to the majority of the poor in rural as well as in urban areas. Health centres for blood screening and voluntary HIV/AIDS testing are almost non-existent in the countryside. This adds to the problem. In the case of HIV infection, poverty restricts nutrition, resulting in low body immunity and causing early death due to AIDS.

Good nutrition is an equally important issue and is the foundation of good health. Culturally, women tend to sacrifice their food intake in favour of other members of the family, particularly husbands and children, and are thereby nutritionally deprived. Recent statistics show that of the 7 million women in Tanzania, 1 million suffer from chronic undernutrition while 4 million or 57 per cent live in absolute poverty. Since access to health services and nutritious food depends on the ability to pay, the majority of women are being forced to survive without such services, making them vulnerable to ill-health. Unhealthy mothers cannot bear healthy children and are more likely to experience maternal problems. In Tanzania, data on the maternal mortality rate has been estimated at 200 to 400 per 100,000 births; two to four thousand out of 7 million adult women die from pregnancy-related causes each year (TGNP, 1993). There are also studies which show that more than 40 per cent of children's deaths recorded in hospitals are due to low birth weight (LBW). About 50 per cent of children suffer from malnutrition while more than 2 million are moderately undernourished (under 80 per cent standard weight for age), and nearly 300,000 or 7 per cent of mainland children are malnourished (under 60 per cent of standard weight for age) (UNICEF, 1990).

The Tanzania Demographic Health Survey observed that almost half of the children (47 per cent) were found to be stunted and 20 per cent severely stunted. This indicates that chronic malnutrition is a major public health problem in Tanzania. These studies also confirm the fact that there is a close relationship between socio-economic status, child mortality, and poor health. Maternal and child mortality are further intensified by the fact that poor women in both urban and rural areas have to be attended by Traditional Birth Attendants (TBAs), most of whom lack experience, equipment, and often work in unsanitary and unsafe conditions. Poor communication infrastructure in rural areas aggravates the problem.. Despite the tremendous achievement of the Child Survival Protection and Development Programme (CSPD) carried out by the government in collaboration with UNICEF, some 200,000 children under five years of age die every year - about 547 per day. This is a national calamity which should receive far more attention (TGNP, 1993:98).

Since SAPs have increased women's workload, they now have less time for food preparation and child care and are resorting to early weaning or not breast-feeding at all. Some leave their infants in the care of young children or inexperienced housegirls who are unable to prepare food properly. Some are forced to dilute and divide the milk supply among many infants so that it lasts longer, and others who can afford to have become vulnerable to accepting cheap breast milk substitutes advertised in the media by multinationals like 'Lactogen,' 'Nespray,' and others.

There is a close relationship between the crisis in women's and children's health and the crisis in women's education. Reduced budgets in the education sector and the introduction of cost-sharing policies in education is again negatively affecting more women than men. Parents are likely to invest more in the education of male children rather than females. Some parents argue that they would not dare to invest much in the education of their daughters because most of them are expelled from school due to pregnancies, and that means suffering double losses (Cooksey, Malekela and Lugalla, 1993). Others would rather let their daughters get married earlier in order to enjoy the bride price. These, and of course those who exploit the labour of their daughters at the expense of their daughters' education, are using their female children as a source of capital accumulation as well as a survival strategy. Since knowledge of health and hygiene is closely related to the level of education, less educated women are bound to experience difficulties in understanding health education and campaigns. The data derived from the 1991/92 Tanzania Demographic Health Survey (TDHS, 1993) confirms this. The study noted that women with a secondary education had a fertility rate of 4.2 children per woman, those who completed primary education had a total of 6.0, and those with incomplete primary education or with no formal education at all had total fertility rates of 6.4 and 6.5 respectively. Health education assists women in avoiding high-risk fertility behaviour. Educated women have the highest median age at first marriage (23 years), compared with women with complete primary education (20 years) and incomplete or without education whose median is 17 years. The timing of births has implications for both fertility and mortality. A woman who births spaced close together will most likely complete her childbearing years with more children than the one who spaces her births further apart. Children who are born within short intervals are vulnerable to poor health which also puts the mother at risk. The TDHS shows that among most educated women (women with the least nutritional risk), there is an increase in age at first birth and that birth spacing is long.

The level and type of education determines the type of employment one gets and, of course, the salary. Lack of education and employment opportunities for women is central to HIV transmission. Those who cannot find jobs often use sex as a means of support (Schoepf, 1991). Education also has a strong influence on family planning issues. The TDHS observed that the percentage rates of those who have never heard family planning messages on radio or television were 86.7 per cent for those without education, 77.8 per cent for those with incomplete primary education, 70.3 per cent with complete primary education, and only 46.4 per cent for those with secondary or higher education. The percentage rates of women who believe that it is acceptable to have messages about family planning on radio and television were 57 per cent for those without education, 70.8 per cent for those with some form of primary education, 79.3 per cent with complete primary education, and 88.5 per cent for those with secondary or higher education. There is no doubt that this influences the acceptability and use of contraceptives. It was also noted that 42.4 per cent of women with secondary and higher education used some method of contraception as opposed to 3.7 per cent, 12.9 per cent, and 14.6 per cent for those with no education, incomplete primary education, and complete primary education respectively. This indicates that a better educated woman has a higher chance of experiencing good health since she is more likely to understand the relationship between family planning and physical wellbeing.

Conclusion

It is now evident in Tanzania that SAPs have done and continue to do more harm than good to the general population. As far as the health sector is concerned, the basic right to good health has been curtailed, and women and children are suffering most as a result. By affecting women negatively, SAPs are basically threatening the whole system of human reproduction in Tanzania. The role of women is dual – producers and reproducers. Yet in Tanzania, they are producing and reproducing by sheer luck. At the same time, due to the difficult conditions of life in rural areas, men are migrating to urban areas in search of waged employment, mostly without their families. Hence, women who remain in the rural areas suffer from increased poverty, lack of companionship, and risk of HIV infection from HIV-positive returning husbands. Schoepf (1991) argues that multiple partner relationships appear to be increasing in both rural and urban areas as a result of the economic crisis. However, this is not to say that SAPs have been instrumental in causing all these problems. Some of these problems are long-standing. SAPs have just intensified the nature of these problems and made the government less able to finance strategies that might have solved some of them.

The SAP prescription of 'market forces' is failing to produce good results in the health sector. The liberalisation of health and medical services in Tanzania constitutes a health hazard. Quality control of both drugs and services becomes problematic in a situation where services are scarce and people are desperate. Cases of expired drugs being sold after faking labels seems to be the order of the day. The number of private clinics being opened, some of which are housed in unhealthy environments, continues to increase. The medical and health personnel working in these clinics leave much to be desired. Some cleaners and nurses pose as competent doctors and prescribe medicine. The activities of these fake personnel flourish because of widespread ignorance on the part of patients, the elitism that characterizes the structure of health care services, the cheapness of services offered by quacks and their make-shift dispensaries, and the problems of access to genuine personnel given the present economic crisis (Falola and Ityavyar, 1992:12-13).

Self-medication and non-compliance with medical instructions are also widespread. The reasons are many: ignorance, the high cost of consulting a doctor, lack of access to medical facilities, the time lost in hospitals by those who have no 'connections' with staff, very easy access to drug stores and hawkers, and reliance on 'cure all' capsules. These are the after-effects of the liberalization of health services in an underdeveloped, dependent economy like Tanzania's. Women and children are among the vulnerable social groups that are being negatively affected by SAPs, but their voices are hardly being heard. They indeed constitute a 'social periphery,' or as Ramphele (1991), Heggenhougen (1993), and others are calling it, 'The Underside of the Underside.'

In the meantime, the government is thinking about the proper procedure of introducing user charges in the health sector. Since it is clear that people are already suffering, going ahead with such policies adds insult to injury. SAP policies have been a bitter pill in Tanzania. They have brought real suffering, increased health risks, and have reduced much access to health care for the poor in general— particularly for women and children.

Although people have found their own coping mechanisms, these policies are alienating them from the state and as a result, Tanzania is now witnessing the growth of social resistance with severe political implications. Policies aimed at improving the health conditions of women can only be effective if they are accompanied by strategies empowering women socially, economically, politically, and culturally. However, the empowerment of women is hampered by the fact that Tanzanian policies do not strive to question the existing unequal gender relations, some of which are culturally and politically sanctioned.

N.B.: This chapter was originally published by the *Review of African Political Economy* No. 63 of 1995.

Chapter Thirteen

Women, Poverty and HIV/AIDS in Africa: The Fate of Young Women working as Maids in Tanzania

Peter A. Kopoka

Introduction

Poverty and AIDS are without a doubt the major challenges facing the African continent in the twenty-first century. This chapter focuses on these inter linked problems facing Africa and how they impact the lives of those most vulnerable in society. There is little doubt that the impact of poverty and AIDS on the entirety of African society has been devastating. This is particularly so on the lives of women and children. Being the most vulnerable, young women have been the most affected. Amongst this group are those young girls and women who work as housemaids and barmaids.

In this chapter, we seek to examine the link between poverty and HIV and the impact of this linkage on the lives of poor women working as barmaids and housemaids. We draw on the experiences and viewpoints of these poor women working as housemaids and barmaids in the city of Dar es Salaam in Tanzania. The chapter is divided into four parts. The first part discusses the need for a better understanding of the relationship and root causes of poverty and HIV/AIDS in the African context. This part provides an overview of the poverty situation and the AIDS pandemic in Africa, drawing on the experience of Tanzania. There is little doubt that women are more exposed to poverty and AIDS. This is particularly so for the poor women of Africa who are the poorest of the poor. It is for this reason that the central focus of this paper is on the plight of young girls working as maids in Dar es Salaam.

The second part of the chapter reflects on the experiences and testimonies of poor women expressed in in-depth interviews and narratives from young women working as housemaids and bar maids in Dar es Salaam. Here, we seek to examine the working and socio-economic environment in which these women work and the extent to which this environment puts these women at risk of HIV infection. We shall attempt to show that as these young women seek to escape from a life of poverty in rural areas, their likely reward or destination appears to be the inevitable embrace of HIV/AIDS. Our focus on poverty does not mean that it is the only dominant factor which facilitates HIV/AIDS transmission in Africa or elsewhere. We acknowledge the influence of other factors. Other factors besides poverty that put women at risk of contracting AIDS include drug abuse and traditional norms and customs which perpetuate gender inequalities. There are also the devastating impacts of the free market economies in African countries, which are leading to increased marginalization, poverty, and HIV infection. We are also aware of the devastating impact of poverty and HIV/AIDS on other sections of African society. Therefore, it goes without saying that suggestions for overcoming these twin problems are also applicable to other segments of society.

The third part of this chapter focuses on existing and planned attempts to address the twin problems of poverty and AIDS in Tanzania. Here we note that there are no joint efforts to address the problems of poverty and HIV/AIDS. There is clearly much more that is still required in the battle against poverty and HIV/AIDS. Finally, the fourth section is a look at the way forward and examines what needs to be done if Africa and Tanzania in particular are to find lasting solutions to the twin problems of poverty and HIV/AIDS.

The chapter is based on a study carried out in 2001 in Dar es Salaam in the district of Kinondoni. The study is based on a study of 50 barmaids, aged between 15 to 33 years, working in the district. In-depth interviews, narratives of maids and observations are the major instruments used to collect data for this study.

The Socio-Economic Context of HIV/AIDS and Poverty in Africa

In the public discussion of HIV/AIDS in Africa, we constantly hear about the numbers – infection rates, prevalence rates, and mortality rates of HIV/AIDS. However, seldom do we hear of the circumstances that these people are living in and which situations put them more at risk of HIV infection. For instance, we do not hear of the extreme poverty, disease, human degradation, and destitution and their linkage to HIV/AIDS. In other words, what about the people behind those numbers? What about the men, women, and children living with HIV, struggling to make it through each day? What about the life and experiences of those people who are vulnerable and most at risk of contracting this terrible disease? Answers to such questions are seldom reflected in studies on HIV/AIDS in Africa. In an attempt to remedy this situation, this paper examines the link between women,

AIDS, and poverty in Africa. The paper attempts to reflect on the experiences and compelling circumstances that led young girls to work as house girls and barmaids and the circumstances that put them at more risk than any other section among women in Tanzania.

Many studies of HIV/AIDS associate the disease with specific risky factors/behaviors, risky social groups, and risky areas. These studies explain the reasons for the magnitude of the epidemic in terms of high prevalence of STDs, population movements, high-risk sexual practices, blood transfusion, limited access to health services, and "harmful" traditional practices. The suggested or implemented interventions tend to follow the same logic: abstinence, zero-grazing, faithfulness, avoid prostitutes, safe sex, emphasis on condom use, blood screening, treatment of STDs and other opportunistic infections. In terms of target groups, they tend to focus on prostitutes, long-distance truck drivers, pregnant women, drug addicts, and homosexuals (Lugalla, 1999).

In order to understand the prevailing poverty situation in African countries such as Tanzania, it is our contention that one needs to examine the ways in which national economies, shaped by a century or more of colonial rule, have given rise to an increasingly marginalized peasant labor force. One also needs to examine the social disintegration of the rural society, massive migration to cities in search of work, and the unprecedented growth of rural poverty with attendant unemployment and prostitution.

Looking at the AIDS pandemic, Lugalla (1999) argues that HIV/AIDS in Africa is facilitated by socio-economic, cultural, and political conditions. In Africa, Simonsen and colleagues (1990) were among the first biomedical researchers to examine social factors in relation to HIV transmission. While calling for the "reduction of the social circumstances which create the necessity for women to resort to prostitution," they did not actually focus on poverty and inequality as causal factors in the pandemic itself. This paper seeks to make a modest attempt to address this limitation. Our starting point is to provide a general overview of poverty and the HIV/AIDS pandemic in Africa.

Overview of Poverty in Africa

The World Health Report of 1995 correctly notes that the world's biggest killer and the greatest cause of ill health and suffering across the globe is listed almost at the end of the International Classification of Diseases. It is given the code Z59.5 – extreme poverty. The report points out that poverty is the main reason behind many of the world's health problems. One cannot but agree with this observation made by the WHO. If one is to move this argument further, one cannot fail to conclude that poverty –extreme poverty—is a major cause of the spread of HIV/AIDS infection in poor countries in the world. As Africa moves further into the 21st century, poverty and AIDS continue to reap death and despair on a vast scale in Africa.

When one takes a look at the African continent, chief features of the African socio-economic landscape are increasing mass poverty, destitution, and human degradation. Poverty continues to be widespread in almost all parts of the African continent and threatens the very fabric of human existence in this region. Indeed, as Adedeji (1995) points out, human deprivation and pervasive poverty have become the plight of the broad masses of Africans with a devastating impact on the lives of millions of Africans.

Poverty as a dynamic force requires individuals to reprioritize their lives based on survival, often at the expense of wellbeing. Poverty destabilizes lives, crushes self-esteem, and creates despair leading to actions that often tend to lead to risky sexual behavior. Poverty marginalizes, stigmatizes, and erodes human agency and leads to dependence and powerlessness. Poverty effectively prevents individuals from reconceptualizing problems, imagining different alternatives, and creating new solutions. This is clearly indicated in our study of poor working women employed as maids in Tanzania.

NEPAD (2001) indicates that in Africa, 340 million people or half the population live on less than US $1 per day. The mortality rate of children under five years of age is 140 per 1000, and the life expectancy at birth is only 54 years. Only 58 per cent of the population have access to safe water. The rate of illiteracy for people over 15 is 41 percent. There are only 18 mainline telephones per 1000 people in Africa, compared with 146 for the world as a whole, and 567 for high-income countries. The above statistics go some way in highlighting the extreme poverty situation facing most of the African population.

However, they are neither able to fully portray the misery, human suffering, destitution, and degradation of millions of Africans living in extreme poverty nor the things that they are forced to do in order to survive. The statistics are unable to reflect the intractable pain, despair, and hopelessness of those living in extreme poverty. It is our contention that it is only by fully comprehending the situation of those living in poverty that we can fully understand the factors involved in the increase of the AIDS pandemic in Africa.

The Magnitude of HIV/AIDS in Africa

Nearly 24 million people in Africa currently live with HIV/AIDS, and the epidemic continues to ravage the development prospects for millions of Africans throughout the continent. In 1999, about 3.8 million Africans were infected with AIDS, and a total of 10.7 million children were estimated to be orphaned by it. At the national level, the 21 countries with the highest HIV prevalence are in Africa. In South Africa, Botswana, and Zimbabwe, one in four adults are infected. A child born in Zambia or Zimbabwe today is more likely than not to die. In many other African countries, the lifetime risk of dying of AIDS is greater than one in three (World Bank, 2002).

South Africa, where 20 percent or five million people are living with HIV/AIDS, is the worst affected country in the world. According to UNAIDS and WHO, by the end of 1999, women comprised 55 percent of the 23.3 million people in sub-Saharan Africa who have been infected with HIV (UNAIDS, 1999). Since the beginning of the epidemic, a total of 4.7 million have died from AIDS (Briggs, 1999). According to these sources, every day more than 5,000 women become infected with HIV, and 500 women die of related illnesses. In every five women living with the HIV virus in the world, four of them live in Africa. The main mode of the spread of HIV infection in sub-Saharan Africa is heterosexual contact, accounting for more than 4/5 of the transmission routes. In Africa, the women to men ratio is now 6:5.

Poverty in Tanzania

Tanzania is one of the poorest countries in the world. Poverty in Tanzania, as in other African countries, is not a story or dream, but a grim reality. With each passing day, an increasing number of people are falling into poverty. Between 15 and 18 million Tanzanians live below a poverty line of 65 cents per day. Nearly 12.5 million live in abject poverty, spending less than 50 US cents per day on consumption. This is according to a year 2000 country study by the World Bank. According to the UNDP's latest report (2001), Tanzania has some people living on even less than a half-dollar (US$ 0.50) per day. A number of reasons have bee5n put forward to explain this situation. Tanzania's economy is heavily dependent on agriculture, which accounts for 57% of GDP, provides 85% of exports, and employs 90% of the work force. Despite its paramount position in socio-economic development, the traditional stronghold of poverty has always been the rural sector. As Bagachwa (1994) observes, poverty in Tanzania is overwhelmingly pervasive in rural areas.

While agriculture is the mainstay of the economy, the rural sector remains neglected and backward. At only 3.5 percent, the real value-added growth of agriculture in 2000 was lower than expected, reflecting the impact of adverse weather and underlying structural problems in the sector (URT, 2001:12). The relatively weak growth performance of the agricultural sector coupled with the collapse of export prices for cashew nuts, coffee, and cotton pose not only a major challenge for the poverty reduction strategy, but is also forcing increasing numbers of young people to flee from rural areas.

The liberalization of the agricultural sector has not led to the improvement of the sector. Indeed, the situation appears to be worse. What we see is the removal of subsidies, shortage of credit, declining productivity leading to food shortages and food insecurity, as well the decline in the quality of cash crops. The government has continued with its efforts to attract foreign investors, but foreign investors continue to evade investing in the agricultural sector. The sector is avoided like a very infectious disease.

The unfavorable condition of the rural sector in Tanzania is without doubt a major factor in the massive exodus of young people from rural to urban areas in search of better living conditions. The result has on the whole been disappointing for the vast majority, with thousands of young women being forced to work as maids in conditions akin to modern-day slavery!

In their efforts to survive the harsh economic and social conditions in rural areas, young girls with little or nothing to lose are flocking into urban areas for work, and the only form of employment that they can secure is that of housemaids and barmaids.

It is not only the abandonment of the rural sector that is fuelling poverty and human destitution in Tanzania and other African countries. The growth of mass poverty in these countries has external links. The introduction of structural adjustment programs (SAPs) in Africa by the international financial institutions has undoubtedly contributed to the impoverishment of the continent. There is increasing evidence that SAPs and the ongoing process of globalization are linked to the increasing state of mass poverty in the developing world, particularly in Africa. Poverty has become a breeding ground for an increased risk of HIV infection.

Messkoub (1996) points out that what is at stake with adjustment policies is not only the immediate effect of, for example, a cut in food subsidies on the nutritional intake of children in poor households, but also changing *opportunities for different groups and classes in the society*. The validity of this observation is becoming increasingly clear when we see a large segment of the traditional "middle" class in Tanzania, including professionals, being thrown into poverty. The educated elite from collages and universities who were previously assured employment are now being thrown into absolute poverty with their prospects of acquiring employment relevant to their skills diminishing.

Other leading economic researchers and planners are also in agreement that ten years of SAPs in Tanzania have not alleviated the problem of poverty and unemployment in Tanzania. Rather, they have accelerated them. For instance, Musoke (1992) argues that the various SAP recommendations have had a very adverse economic and social impact on various social categories in Tanzanian society, with the poor and vulnerable social classes bearing the brunt. Shao (1996) also points out that the current IMF/WB sponsored structural adjustment programs have had an adverse impact on the poor and particularly on women and children in the rural sector.

Contributing to the debate, Simmons *et. al.* (1996) argue that as "Economic Recovery" and Structural Adjustment Policies shifted national burdens to the poor, many families' incomes were outpaced by hyperinflation in the costs of basic necessities. Those who were just scraping by in the 1980s have since fallen into extreme poverty. In cities, where people had been accustomed to eating two and three meals per day, now eat a single meal or skip food for days; malnutrition is widespread. Ever more desperate economic conditions have reduced poor and formerly middle-class families to "zones of non-existence." School attendance has declined, especially among girls.

A study by Lugalla (1997) shows how SAPs have created classes of "new poor" and "chronic poor." The majority of these new classes of the poor are women who have become the poorest of the poor. The poor in Africa continue to be marginalized by powerful forces beyond their control. The introduction of the free market economy and the ongoing process of globalization are ushering in a new era of mass impoverization in most African countries with the hardest hit being women and children. It can thus be concluded that, today, the majority of Tanzanians have become poorer as a result of SAPs. The consequence has been to force women, particularly those most vulnerable, to work under conditions that put them at great risk of HIV infection.

Living in Poverty – The Fate of Women in Tanzania

A disregard for the rural sector has gone hand in hand with the marginalization of Tanzania's key resource – women. Women in Tanzania are not only the majority population, but are at the forefront of economic and social development in the country. Today, women in most parts of Tanzania play a leading role in both economic development and in the home. Women, in addition to their domestic role of looking after the family, do most of the agricultural work. Women are not only the major producers in rural areas, producing up to 80% of household food requirements, but are also important bread earners in most urban households. Despite the significant input of women in the development process, women still remain at the bottom of the ladder in terms of equality and access to economic and social opportunities. To date, three overriding features characterize women's position in the country. They have little or no control over resources such as land; they have little or no autonomy or decision-making voice; and they have little or no freedom of movement, that is, they tend to be both physically and socially secluded. One consequence of this unfortunate situation has been the rapid spread of HIV/AIDS among women.

Women's Poverty and HIV/AIDS in Tanzania

Tanzania, like most African countries, is in the throes of an ever-deepening economic crisis. In these times, poor women bear the brunt of an increased work load, declining incomes, and increased sickness. Poor women are also more at risk of infectious diseases including sexually transmitted diseases (STDs) and HIV/AIDS. They are more at risk because many are unemployed, and the fortunate few who are employed are low paid. Women, particularly the young and uneducated, are concentrated in the lowest-paid and often unlicensed activities. These include petty trade, food preparation, sewing, hairdressing, domestic work, smuggling, and prostitution. Most of the occupations done by women yield very low and often erratic incomes, and at the same time render their practitioners vulnerable to extortion, violence, and disease.

In their attempts to make ends meet, they engage in risky sexual behavior with multiple sex partners. Prevention is also made more difficult by women's lack of access to effective treatment for STDs. STDs increase the risk of acquiring HIV from an infected partner. While only a small portion of urban women with disposable income can consult private practitioners and pay for a full course of antibiotic treatment, this is extremely difficult, if not impossible, for women living in poverty. Poor women's access to treatment is further limited when user-fees are charged, a policy mandated as part of the structural adjustment programs imposed by the World Bank.

In Tanzania, according to the NACP, there were approximately 1.4 million adults living with HIV by the year 1998. Roughly 7 percent of all women were infected, compared with 5.4 percent of all adult men. Among sex workers, from 49.5 up to 60 percent were found to be HIV positive. In Dar es Salaam City, 50 percent of all bar workers were infected with the HIV virus. In the Mbeya and Moshi Municipalities, 52 percent and 32 percent of barmaids respectively were infected with HIV (NACP, 1997).

According to recent estimates in Tanzania, an estimated 1.2 million people are suspected of being infected with the HIV virus (President Mkapa, 2002). President Mkapa further pointed out that research carried out in the city of Dar es Salaam and the districts of Morogoro Rural and Hai in the Kilimanjaro region showed that AIDS has been responsible for the deaths of hundreds of people. AIDS was responsible for 42 percent of deaths amongst men and 45 percent amongst women in the city of Dar es Salaam. In Morogoro, AIDS was linked to 51 percent of deaths amongst men and 43 percent amongst women. In Hai district, AIDS was responsible for 37 percent of deaths amongst men and 26 percent amongst women. The World Bank estimates that by the year 2020, Tanzania will have lost 27,000 teachers whose replacement will cost the nation 35 bn Tshs. (The Tanzanian Guardian Newspaper, July 15, 2002).

"It is Tough Being Poor and a Woman" The Lives and Times of Maids in Dar es Salaam

The Plight of Young Girls Working as Housemaids

The most common form of employment among younger women of rural origin is that of servants commonly known as house girls: "in the cities, the {economically} active 10-14 year old girls are essentially all domestic…These 'restaveks' find themselves at the very bottom of the social hierarchy." (Neptune-Anglade, 1986:209). It is this social position that will later determine, to a large extent, their increased risk of HIV infection. It is important to underscore that these young girls are at the very bottom of the social hierarchy because they come from poor and economically marginalized groups in rural and urban areas. They are unable to sustain themselves and their families. Poverty leads to powerlessness, making these girls the lowest of the low. Mistreatment of girl domestic servants through overworking, sexual harassment, and low pay is still rampant in Dar es Salaam and other urban centers. An investigation conducted by the Guardian Newspaper (August, 02 2002) in the Manzese and Tabata suburbs has established that many school- age children employed as housemaids have either been raped, sexually abused, or discriminated against by the employer's family members.

According to our findings, children are forced into labor because of poverty, harassment, and abuse from parents, among other reasons. Many of these children drop out of school due to their parent's inability to meet school requirements including school fees, uniforms, and other numerous contributions that are required by schools. Others drop out of school to take up family responsibilities. These are the ones who are found selling groundnuts, ice cream, and other foods from one place to another. Our study indicates that the average age of house girls is 15. They receive an average "salary" of around Tshs.10, 000 - 15,000/= per month and work for over 12 hours a day. These girls are constant victims of sexual abuse and rape and have no recourse to legal assistance, as is indicated in the cases of Farida and Paulina.

The Story of Farida

Farida Bakari, a standard three dropout from Same District in Kilimanjaro, started work as a housemaid at the tender age of twelve. Working as a housemaid, Farida had to carry 20 jerry cans of water every night from 8.00 p.m. to 12.00 a.m. (midnight). "I used to clean the house, utensils, and wash clothes, and I would not be allowed to eat or go to bed before I completed all the household chores," said Farida. After two years, she could bear it no longer, and in consultation with a neighboring housemaid, she decided to leave her employment and try her luck at becoming a barmaid at a local bar in Manzese. The bar had one small room where all the barmaids slept on a mattress on the floor. Working as a barmaid, she was at least free to move about, and the boss did not require them to sleep in their room. Farida was soon spotted by a number of men who "requested" her to have sexual relations with them. She was in no position to refuse their request, because in the course of the night, these men would buy her drinks and food and provide her with some money for her upkeep. She soon had three regular guys, and since all three did not come each night, she could manage them easily. Of course, there was also the odd customer with whom she would go out if any of the three regulars were not around. When asked why she continued with such behavior in the midst of HIV/AIDS, her quick answer was "Brother, I have to survive in this town or do you want me to eat at the police station?"

The Case of Paulina, A Housemaid From Arusha

The plight of housemaids is well illustrated by the case of a ten-year old house girl who, in June 1999, was admitted to the Mount Meru Hospital, Arusha in a critical condition after her employer severely burnt her on the buttocks for failing to cleanse kitchenware to the satisfaction of the employer. Narrating the ordeal, little Paulina Anthony said her employer, Joyce Baraka, 27, beat her on the head using a piece of wood before using glowing splinters to burn her on both buttocks. So excruciating was the experience that the child fainted. The burns will leave life long scars unless she gets plastic surgery treatment, medics said, adding that the psychological trauma was enormous (Daily Mail, 1999).

Paulina's case is not an isolated incident, but is a reflection of the growing state of violence against and abuse of house girls. The lure of a better life makes these girls leave one difficult and demanding environment for another equally demanding and exploitative employment situation: barmaid. Before graduating to becoming a barmaid, there is usually a husband or lover who soon abandons her after shedding her youth and innocence. It is at this juncture that these girls become survivors depending on their only asset – their womanhood. While working as barmaids, these women experience numerous problems from society pointing fingers at them for their immoral behavior.

Barmaids and the Struggle to Survive

Women often find themselves in situations where they must weigh the risk of becoming infected against other risks including homelessness, starvation, and loss of essential income. We have to gather an understanding of the social forces that make HIV infection more likely to become embodied as personal risk. Examining the lives of poor women will help make sense of the circumstances in which many poor women are forced to choose between the risk of HIV and other dangers.

"For poor women," notes anthropologist Martha Ward, "AIDS is just another problem they are blamed for and have to take responsibility for. They ask, 'How am I going to take care of my family? I have to put food on the table now. You think AIDS is a problem! Let me tell you –I got real problems.'" (Cited from Farmer, P., 1996). The narratives of the following young women working as barmaids seem to bear out the validity of Ward's observation. These are Ashura, Mwanahawa, Eliza, and Agnes (not their real names), who are working as maids in Dar es Salaam.

The Story of Ashura

Ashura was born just outside of Dar es Salaam in the district of Kibaha in 1973. She is one of six children born to peasant parents. Hers was not a happy childhood as she often had to go to school without any breakfast and would return home not certain of a meal. Their parents were often fighting over the little income that came in as a result of selling coconuts and a petty business that was run by the mother. Ashura remembers her parents having terrible fights in which her father hit her mother, confiscating the little money available for his daily alcohol. Sometimes the children would return from school to find no food for the evening, and Ashura would be forced to visit their small shamba to find whatever she could to cook for her younger siblings. The diet consisted mainly of cassava and maize and greens from the small shamba (farm) owned by the family. Ashura slept in small mud house in a room which she shared with her four other siblings.

Like other rural children, Ashura was born into poverty, and early childhood only strengthened the foundations of increasing poverty and human destitution for the young girl. After completing her primary education (standard seven) at the age of sixteen, Ashura left for Dar es Salaam with an aunt who promised to find her a job as housemaid. She got a job working for a businesswoman in the city. The businesswoman reared about one thousand chickens which Ashura had to look after in addition to her daily duties as a housemaid. Her day started at five in the morning and ended at around midnight. Her salary was 8,000/= a month. Whenever she was sick, her employer did not bother to take her to hospital, and soon her hands were infected by fungus. Ashura could bear the situation no longer, and she soon left her employment to work as a barmaid in Manzese. She has a bit more freedom with her personal time, although the financial rewards for a barmaid are not that much. She receives 12,000 Tshs. After work, she now has the opportunity of supplementing her income through sexual liaisons with her male clients. Ashura admits that she now has three regular boyfriends who help support her financially. She is now able to send some money to support her younger siblings and mother from time to time as well being able to spend money on herself.

Asked about the dangers of HIV/AIDS, Ashura explained that she was indeed in danger of the disease as two of her boyfriends resisted any attempts to use a condom—and anyway, they were often too drunk to bother about any protection. "Circumstances have forced me to work here, and I do as best as I can. Perhaps if I had better education, I would be able to get a better job," so says Ashura whose future remains very much in doubt due to increased exposure to HIV/AIDS through multiple sex partners.

The Story of Mwanahawa

Mwanahawa was born in a rural district in the southern part of Tanzania. Like other families in her village, her parents fed their children by working on a small plot of land and selling produce along the main highway that passed near their village. Mwanahawa's family was poor to the extent that she recalls often going to bed hungry, as there was nothing to cook. She also had to miss school constantly in order to look after her younger brothers and sisters. Rural life become too unbearable for Mwanahawa, and she soon escaped to the district headquarters where she struck up a relationship with a young man who was working on one of the transport buses traveling to Dar es Salaam. They lived together in a single room. Life in town was still difficult as the young man soon started to mistreat her with constant beatings and by leaving her at home with no money. Mwanahawa soon found herself pregnant, and she had no recourse except to return home to her parents. Mwanahawa, soon after the delivery of her baby into a poverty-riddled world at her parent's house, again left home to find means not only of supporting herself and her young siblings, but also of supporting her young child. She ended up in Dar es Salaam, where she shortly gained employment as a housemaid for a middle class family in Mwenge. Getting little pay, she soon became employed as a barmaid in Sinza. She now gets a monthly salary of 15,000/= , and she sends some of this money back home to support her baby son and family.

Her salary as a barmaid is obviously not enough, and Mwanahawa admits to having a boyfriend that helps support her financially. She is also available to other customers for sex in the absence of her regular friend. Mwanahawa has hopes of renting her own room and being able to bring her son to stay with her. She freely acknowledges that she stopped using a condom after knowing her boyfriend for two months. She also admits to having had two abortions unknown to her boyfriend. Once again, Mwanahawa's future is very much clouded by the increased risk of HIV/AIDS.

What immediate advise/assistance do we offer Mwanahawa and other young women in similar situations? Do we simply tell her the obvious - that

AIDS is a terrible disease and that she will get it if she does not change her behavior? Or do we advise/supply her with a condom? Or should we provide her with more education and awareness of HIV/AIDS?

These are burning questions that require urgent answers if there is to be any hope of rescuing Mwanahawa. We are of the strong opinion that the starting point in rescuing the life of this woman and many others is addressing the acute poverty situation that this woman finds herself in. This includes improving her working conditions. Since the government has a statutory minimum wage of 30,000/=, it should ensure that maids are not paid below this amount. There should also be some legal protection for maids and for other women in low-income employment. But over and above that, the underlying causes for the predicament in which these women find themselves must be critically examined and understood. This viewpoint is supported by Schoepf (1993: 70) who argues that "Unless the underlying struggles of millions who survive in the midst of poverty, powerlessness, and hopelessness are addressed, and the meanings of AIDS understood in the context of gender relations, HIV will continue to spread."

Eliza's Story

Eliza is twenty-five years old and hails from the central part of Tanzania. She arrived in Dar es Salaam after failing to continue with her studies following primary school in 1999. Eliza's father had passed away the previous year, and her mother was no longer able to effectively look after the family. With family responsibilities being put on her young shoulders, the young Eliza set of for Dar es Salaam to seek salvation from poverty. In Dar es Salaam, while staying at a relative's house, Eliza became sexually engaged with a married male neighbor. The neighbor was able to spend a good amount of time and money on Eliza, and it did not take long for her to become pregnant. Soon after the birth of her child, the sexual relationship came to an abrupt end. Left on her own with no financial support, Eliza found work as a barmaid in a nearby bar. The manager of the bar soon developed a sexual relationship with Eliza. This was partly a result of Eliza's need for financial security and also security for her employment. Needless to say, Eliza soon found herself in search of new employment after the bar manager got tired of her. The fact that Eliza became pregnant and gave birth to two children within a short period illustrates her vulnerability in terms of negotiating for safe sex. Eliza is now working in another bar and has decided not to stick to only one man for her economic survival.

As Eliza's case illustrates, sexual patron-client relations and multiple partner strategies that supplement poor women's incomes have become increasingly important for survival. "What do you expect me to do- let my children starve or eat at the police station?" replied an angry and frustrated Eliza in response to why she had to go out with several men who wanted her.

As to the question of whether she was afraid of HIV/AIDS, she responds despairingly that *"Ukimwi ni ajali kazini"* ("AIDS is an accident at work"). In her struggle for survival, Eliza has without a doubt put herself at the forefront of risk in terms of getting the disease (if she is not already infected!).

In her struggle against poverty, Eliza and other vulnerable girls in similar situations are, as Lugalla & Mbwambo (1996) point out, forced to accept sexual behavior that is harmful to their health. Since they are already vulnerable, negotiating condom usage or practicing safe sax becomes a near impossibility. Given these circumstances, contracting the deadly HIV virus becomes inevitable.

The Story of Agnes

Agnes is a young girl from Iringa who found her way to Dar es Salaam at the age of seventeen after finishing her primary education in her local village in the northern part of Tanzania. She joined a group of three other girls to come to Dar es Salaam in search of work. An older "sister" hailing from the same village took Agnes and her friends in and was able to find them jobs as maids in the neighborhood.

Agnes is the second born from a family of seven other siblings. Her parents were very poor and could not afford the costs of her continued education. Indeed, soon after the completion of her primary education, the parents soon placed much of the family burden on the shoulders of young Agnes. Agnes's younger siblings were also in need of money to keep them in school. It is under these circumstances that Agnes found herself working as a housemaid in Dar es Salaam. Work as a housemaid was not easy, and with a monthly salary of 8,000/=, she could not take care of the family responsibilities at home. Agnes is now working in a bar in Mwenge after quitting her job as a housemaid. She lives with three other girls in a rented room. Her main source of income is through men who go out with her for sex. She gets an average of around 5,000/= each night she sleeps with one of her numerous boyfriends.

"I have since given up on having a regular/steady boyfriend because they are not to be trusted," so says Agnes, *"Mie bwana ni dei waka"* (Casual day worker) in regard to sexual relationships. Sex, to Agnes, is a casual/ business arrangement with no formal ties. The business starts with cash negotiation with the potential male partner and ends in the morning after payment of an agreed amount. This response indicates the extent of the despair of this woman. To her, being able to put food on the table for herself, being able to pay the rent, and being able to have some money to send home to her family is more important than her own personal safety. "Getting sick and dying are some of the hazards that people like myself must face up to - we are all in the hands of God."

There is little doubt that this young girl, like the others, is on the fast track to getting infected by the HIV virus.

Lessons from Ashura and Her Friends

The above life experiences of young girls and women such as Ashura are multiplying daily. We could tell these stories as hundreds and hundreds of individual accounts of suffering, each with its own unique configuration of personalities and circumstances. In other words, the stories of Ashura and many others may be individual life stories, yet tales like these are similar for most young girls and women in urban settings working in low paid employment. They are stories about women and poverty, about extreme exploitation, deprivation, and human destitution. From the individual narratives of the young women above, we learn that most of the young women working as maids have been born into and are still living in poverty. Their attempts to escape poverty by working as maids are long bets that are doomed to fail –with AIDS as their likely form of failure. The saying "out of the frying pan into the fire" cannot be a better description of the fate of these young women.

The stories of Ashura and others have been recounted in detail in order to bring into sharp focus the unique circumstances leading to their current situation. Thus, the increased risk of HIV/AIDS is placed on a most vulnerable section of the population. We are of the opinion that, embroiled in increasing poverty, their chances of avoiding HIV are slim. As young women, they have all been driven to the glittering lights of Dar es Salaam by the lure of an escape from the harshest of poverty in rural areas. However, their chances of escaping from poverty are very slim. This becomes very clear when one looks with scrutiny at the work of a barmaid.

Having heard the narratives of the young girls and women working as maids, we now move on to take a closer look at the socio-economic conditions these women are working in and how these conditions more or less determine the destiny of these girls.

The Socio-Economic Context of Barmaidship in Dar es Salaam

Working as a barmaid has become a major form of employment for many young girls and women in Dar es Salaam. Even though work as a barmaid is hard and exploitative, it is seen as a better and higher stage of employment than that of a housemaid. When asked why they prefer this form of employment, the response from barmaids is that the only qualification required is a beer opener and a nice smile! The usual salary of barmaids in Dar es Salaam ranges from Tshs. 5,000 to 20,000/=. For the lucky few who work behind the counter and as matrons, the salary can be as much as 40,000/=. A study by Mbaga (2001) also reports monthly salaries of barmaids in Dar es Salaam as being between Tshs.10, 000/= and 19,000/=.

It is unheard of that any of the barmaids get their salary in full (few of the girls receive their full salary). This is because they have to pay for any glasses or furniture breakage, and often customers run off without paying. Their salary is also deducted if one arrives late for work. The average take-home pay is therefore between 8,000 and 10,000/=.

According to our study, many barmaids interviewed complained of late payment- as late as near the end of the following month. Others also complained of being paid in small installments of 2,000 to 4,000 shillings. Most of the girls are afraid to complain very much in case they get the sack. Others, upon getting employment in another bar, just quit, leaving behind their salaries. One can indeed say that these are deliberate attempts by bar owners to refuse payment to barmaids for work being done. It is in these circumstances that these women resort to having multiple sex partners.

The average working day is from 6.00 a.m. to 9.00 a.m., at which time all the girls are required to clean the business premises. They start again in the afternoon from 4.00 p.m. to past midnight. The job of a barmaid carries no job security, and it is difficult to find a girl/woman who has worked in the same bar for five years.

Simple arithmetic indicates that no individual can live on a monthly income of 10,000/= in a city such as Dar es Salaam. It is therefore inevitable that these young girls find extra income from somewhere. The quickest and easiest way is having multiple sex partners. This puts these young women at an increased risk of contracting the deadly HIV virus. The bar, therefore, becomes a place of getting access to men who can support their daily existence. They are also unable to negotiate safer sex. Having multiple sexual relations is clearly seen as a survival strategy among barmaids. Such working conditions put these women at risk of HIV infection, STDs, and unwanted pregnancies.

Women working as barmaids are generally perceived as a risk group for HIV infection. Mhalu (1989) notes that female barmaids, prostitutes, as well as hoteliers are people who, due to the unpredictable economic status of their jobs, have to supplement their inadequate income by selling sexual favors for money. This aspect is also noted by Simmons, *et. al.* (1996), who argue that poverty plays a large role in restructuring dependent relationships with a male partner, whether that relationship be marriage or any other type of union. It is, however, worth noting that from the narratives of Ashura and her friends, these poor women do not usually enter into multiple relationships with men on their own accord, but are more or less victims of circumstances. None of the women indicated that they went out with multiple sex partners just for the love of sexual pleasure. Indeed, the terms used to describe their male companions are derogatory and show a lack of love and respect for these men. The relationships are more or less an economic necessity.

The deepening economic crisis propels most of the barmaids to seek financial godfathers (popularly referred to as *"mabuzi," "bingo," "tenda,"* etc.) to make ends meet. The literal translation of these names indicates that these godfathers are nothing else to these girls except men for "skinning" or "exploiting" as a means of survival and escaping from poverty. The reality is, while they are able to extract some financial gains from the men, these young women are putting themselves at risk of HIV infection, making them the losers at the end of this deadly game. One can argue that these young women are putting themselves at risk due to unbearable poverty and dire circumstances. It can therefore be argued that the major risk factor of these young women is being poor. Being poor places these women in settings in which they cannot safely demand that their partners use condoms, thus putting them at risk of HIV infection. Table 3 below shows the distribution of respondents according to age structure, income, marital status, level of education, income, and religion in the Kinondoni District in Dar es Salaam.

Table 1: *Socio-economic Characteristics of Barmaids in Dar es Salaam*

Socio-Demographic Characteristics	*Respondents*
1. Number of dependents	**Total (%)**
1- 2	12 (24%)
3- 4	32 (64%)
5+	6 (12%)
Total	50 (100%)
2. Age structure (years)	
15- 17	4 (8%)
18- 24	27 (54%)
25- 29	15 (30%)
30+	4 (8%)
Total	50 (100%)
3. Income	
0- 9,000	7 (14%)
10,000 - 15,000	33 (66%)
Above 20,000	10 (20%)
Total	50 (100%)
4. Marital Status	
Single	26 (52%)
Married	3 (6%)
Living with a partner	5 (10%)
Did not reveal Status	16 (32%)
Total	50 (100%)
5. Religion	
Catholic	16 (32%)
Moslem	25 (50%)
Protestants	7 (14%)
Traditional	-
None	2 (4%)
Total	50 (100%)
6. Level of Education	
No Education	2 (4%)
Primary Education Incomplete	10 (20%)
Primary Education	33 (66%)
Secondary Education	5 (10%)
Total	50 (100%)

Source: *Research Findings, Dar es Salaam, 2001*

The above information indicates that most of the respondents—62 percent—were aged between 17 and 24 years. 52 percent were single, and another 32 percent were unwilling to reveal their marital status. It can be assumed that these respondents do not have any permanent attachments and are in many regards, still single. Most of the respondents – 66 percent—had only completed primary education. Lack of education placed these women at a disadvantage in terms of securing better employment, and they were thus condemned to life as a barmaid. Many respondents - 64 percent—had more than two dependents. This put heavy burdens on the shoulders of these women, forcing them to work under very harsh and difficult circumstances. Multiple sexual relationships were noted from our interviews. The types of partners ranged from regular sexual partners to casual sexual relationships to boyfriends. Almost all of the sexual relationships were purely for cash payment.

The overall situation of barmaids was one of hardships due to low income and the limited opportunities of earning a living through alternative means. There is little doubt that urgent steps need to be taken by all stakeholders, especially the government which has been taking center stage in the battle against poverty and HIV/AIDS. In the next part, we examine some of the initiatives being taken to eradicate poverty and to counter the threat of HIV/AIDS in Tanzania.

Eradication of Poverty and HIV/AIDS

Most African governments, with the assistance of international organizations, are spending massive amounts of money on trying to create awareness of the dangers of HIV/AIDS. There appears to be a growing belief/conviction that once people become aware of the devastating impact of AIDS and are knowledgeable on the best ways to protect themselves—practicing safe sex; using a condom; having only a single partner; or, as the religious institutions would suggest, abstaining from sex before marriage—then the spread of the disease would be contained.

We argue on the contrary. There is almost no way a desperate young woman with two young children to look after will abstain from sex or avoid having multiple sex partners as a means of survival. It is unrealistic to suggest that a barmaid who receives a monthly salary of Tshs.15, 000/- (less than 20 US$) with no job protection will take seriously the dangers of contracting HIV. This is where you get responses such as *"ajali Kazini."* Much more focus must be put on addressing the root causes of poverty, particularly among the most vulnerable in society. Unfortunately, this has yet to be given due emphasis by Tanzania and other African countries.

Outlining the progress made in implementing Tanzania's poverty reduction strategy during the financial year 2000/01 the government indicates that during 2000/01, the implementation of the poverty reduction program focused on initiatives to strengthen growth prospects, especially in the pro-poor sectors. The initiatives included an increase in material and other forms of support for the priority areas, the development of an effective framework for monitoring poverty, and elaborate strategies and cost interventions for the key sectors (URT, 2001).

The government is convinced that the continuing consolidation of the macroeconomic situation lays a good foundation for an effective struggle against poverty. We are not so convinced as the prevailing reality for millions of Tanzanians is increased poverty. Without disputing the necessity of the economic reforms being introduced by the Tanzanian government, it is clear that not enough is being done to address the problems of specific groups of people in society. Women living in absolute poverty and the likely consequences of this situation—including increased risk of HIV/AIDS—need to be addressed. Without identifying specific requirements for different groups in society, the benefits of economic growth are unlikely in the struggle against poverty and HIV/AIDS.

During FY2000/01, Tanzania's struggle against the pandemic focused mainly on "awareness" campaigns by political, religious, and civic leaders at all levels. Public media (notably newspapers, radio, and television) were used intensively; school curricula were modified to include coverage of HIV/AIDS; and theoretical presentations encompassed skits on AIDS. The government, assisted by domestic and international partners, encouraged and supported (financially) the general use of condoms. Special efforts were also made to discourage traditional and cultural practices that compound the problem of HIV/AIDS (URT, 2001). On the institutional side, the Government established TACAIDS as a quasi-autonomous agency to coordinate all interventions related to AIDS, including the mobilization of resources from domestic and external sources. More specifically, the responsibilities of TACAIDS will also cover policy formulation, strategic planning, advocacy, monitoring and evaluation, and the public dissemination of information on HIV/AIDS. While we applaud these initiatives, we are of the opinion that they are not sufficient and that they are not being directed towards addressing the root causes of poverty and HIV/AIDS.

The struggle against AIDS, in our view, must center on eradicating poverty, particularly for poor women. Endeavors focused on AIDS, though critical, must be linked to efforts to empower poor women and society in general. It is of little use to preach on the danger of HIV to a destitute young woman who has not had a decent meal for two days or whose children are starving not to go out with a man who is likely to offer her some cash. Unfortunately, the risks of HIV infection are also greater. We are of the view that if you improve the general living standards of the general population, particularly of women, you significantly improve the environment of tackling HIV and AIDS.

The Road Ahead

We have attempted to show that poverty is putting young women working as maids at increased risk of HIV/AIDS and have therefore suggested that efforts to combat the AIDS pandemic go hand in hand with efforts to eradicate poverty. This can be largely achieved by putting the interests of young people at the top of Africa's development agenda. Africa's greatest asset in the midst of growing mass poverty and the AIDS pandemic is their youth who are the most dynamic elements. However, Africa's youth population are not only being denied the opportunity to play an effective role in the development process, particularly in poverty eradication, they are increasingly being put at risk of HIV infection. Indeed, it can be argued that a major tragedy of Africa is her inability to promote, invest, and utilize the youth population. The observed conditions indicated in our study of young women working as maids are testimonies to this observation. It is little wonder that the major victims of poverty and HIV/AIDS are the youths of Africa. This situation can slowly be addressed by empowering the youth population to take control of their own destiny.

Progress towards attacking the twin problems of poverty and HIV/AIDS is also being obstructed by the lack of political will. It is the responsibility of African governments not only to undertake measures to increase antiretroviral therapy to all sections of society, but to ensure that the root causes of the disease are addressed.

Regarding the HIV/AIDS pandemic, our findings clearly indicate that the time has come to abandon the false belief that individual behaviors and cultural norms, once they are "corrected," will prevent the further spread of HIV. It is our contention that individual behaviors are largely dependent on prevailing socio-economic circumstances. There is an increasing need to introduce multiple approaches to addressing the economic and social deprivation of women and young girls/women working as house girls and barmaids. The socio-economic and political conditions that put these women in a vicious cycle of poverty and AIDS must not only be understood, but meaningful steps must be taken to break down this vicious cycle. It is only then that we can find lasting solutions to the AIDS pandemic that threatens the lives of these young girls and many others.

Conclusion

We have noted that the AIDS pandemic is advancing most rapidly among women living in poverty. This is particularly the case for young girls and women who are employed as house girls and barmaids in most urban areas in Africa. This leads to the observation that poverty is an important co-factor in the AIDS pandemic. Therefore, preventing AIDS will also require recognition and redressing of the global and local forces that perpetuate poverty. This means that we have to re-examine Africa's position in the ongoing process of globalization. We have to look at the forces which are contributing to Africa's marginalization and the possibilities for addressing this situation.

It is becoming more and more apparent that the prevention of HIV transmission to women will require a serious consideration of the means by which poverty enhances transmission of HIV. More powerful explanatory frameworks are therefore required to address the problem of HIV transmission. These must be dynamic, systematic, and critical. They must explain the pandemic's rapid change and predict its future course; they must reveal its transnational linkages eluded to in many accounts based on national reporting; they must reveal the ways in which inequalities inevitably play a role in local sub-epidemics and in the larger pandemic.

It is easy to demand that the life conditions of the poor, particularly those of young women, are improved through compassionate and effective medical, social, economic, political, and legal strategies for change. The difficulty will be in finding the means of making these demands heard by those who hold the balance of power—the developed capitalist countries—and the will and determination to persue these demands. In part, this requires joint and concerted action from African leaders and their people.

Chapter Fourteen

A Return to Arusha: Structural Adjustment Indeed! Violence, Globalization, Health and Human Rights

Kris H. Heggenhougen

Development strategies that attempt to make improvements in the lives of the rural poor without addressing the underlying structural causes of poverty serve to deflect attention away from the real needs of impoverished communities (Green, L., 1989).

According to UNICEF "...the total cost of providing basic social services in the developing countries including health, education, family planning, clean water, and all of the other basic social goals outlined at the World Summit for Children would cost about $30-$40 billion annually, less than the world spends annually playing golf" (UNICEF, 1995:59).

Introduction

This century has seen tremendous progress in the field of physical public health: increased childhood immunization and significantly decreased infant mortality rates; increased life expectancy, in places, by decades; and, though still requiring attention, a substantial reduction in the threat of infectious diseases - the eradication of smallpox being an outstanding example. But while we should duly recognize these accomplishments, we must also take note of the re-emergence of old diseases such as TB and the emergence of new ones such as HIV/AIDS which are wrecking havoc on past progress, making the public health situation in most countries far from bright. Similarly, we must be aware of, and attempt to address, powerful socio-economic forces, especially those associated with growing poverty, disparity and marginalization, including human rights abuses of various kinds and their negative effect on public health. It is the public health importance of these social changes which are exacerbating social pathologies and the emphasis on the relevance of the socio-economic and political roots of disease and human welfare to which I attempt to draw your attention in this chapter. Through this, I am calling for a different public health emphasis than usually practiced - a renewal of a public health perspective voiced by those such as Rudolph Virchow in the 19th century. In fact, I am affirming the importance of what has now become known as the 'new public health' which emphasizes interdisciplinarity and a human rights perspective.

The Largest Markets

A discussion of public health on a global scale must begin, I believe, by stating that the sale - the "pushing" - of military hardware and illicit drugs constitutes two of the world's largest markets. Of the major weapons, some of the smallest and cheapest are land-mines - much in the news these days. There are now 110 million land-mines scattered in 68 countries (Brown *et. al.*, 1996; UNDP, 1997). Land-mines and the "... mass production and mass trade of especially small hand weapons and modern explosives, easily available everywhere and their sale actively promoted in a global market, argue in favor of increased violence..." (Kloos, 1993) affecting the health of people throughout the world. These and other enterprises, such as the tobacco industry, are but the most obvious examples of powerful global interests for whom public health consequences pale against the paramount concern for profit - profit derived at the cost of what has become known as "commerciogenic pathology."

The creation of a treaty to ban land-mines, the awarding of the Nobel Peace Prize to the International Committee to Ban Land-Mines, and the inroads made against the tobacco companies in the United States are clearly positive steps against such pathologizing forces and a sign that something can be done. Yet, markets are only shifting from one country to another. The sale and use of tobacco and of illicit drugs is increasing in developing countries. There is also reason for some skepticism regarding the effects of the land-mines ban treaty since the biggest producers - Russia, China, and the U.S.- have refused to sign.

Globalization

We live in a period of increasing globalization. Though many examples can be found to show the benefits of this - in a few instances, even for the poor (China is used as one example, India as another) - much of the evidence points in the opposite direction to the damaging effects, especially on the lives of the poor. According to the 1997 UNDP Report, "the accelerating process of globalization is expanding global opportunities without distributing them equitably. The playing fields of globalization more often than not slope against the interests of people and countries" (UNDP, 1997). The report of a conference, organized by Jesuits in San Salvador in January 1994, came to a similar conclusion but stated it in more forceful language: 'Central America today is experiencing globalization as a more devastating pillage than what its people underwent 500 years ago with the conquest and colonization' (Chomsky, 1994). And, according to a recent North American Committee on Latin America (NACLA) Report, "Globalization has become associated in our minds with corporate profit, growing income concentration, the decline of workers' rights, environmental degradation and increased corporate power" (NACLA, 1996).

"The 350 largest corporations now account for 40% of global trade" (UNDP, 1997). Yet, from 1982 to 1992 "... the world's top five hundred firms...shed 400,000 workers yearly... notwithstanding the upsurge of their combined revenues [or perhaps because of it]." "...[A]bout 30% of the world's labor force was unemployed in January 1994" (Chomsky, 1994). The UNDP (1997) states that in industrialized countries "...unemployment has soared to levels not seen since the 1930s and income inequality to levels not recorded since the last century."

As Russell Baker (1995) recently pointed out in one of his *New York Times* pieces entitled "Those Vital Paupers," "...there must be something wrong with the health of an economic system which depends on a good supply of paupers [another aspect of 'commerciogenic pathology']." If all were employed, wages would rise and profits and stocks would decline.

Mega-corporations make up 50 of the 100 largest economic entities in the world, while countries make up the other half (UNDP, 1997). According to Laxer (1995), "Global citizenship rights for corporations enables them to escape obligations to country. The implicit threat is: Bring in strict anti-pollution regulation... or higher minimum wages and we the corporation will move out. You, the wage-earners and citizens who voted for such policies will be left hurting. Not us: we are mobile and responsible to shareholders, not communities. Global corporate-citizenship rights enhance the trans-nationals' ability to use blackmail to discipline democracies." The UNDP (1997) states the same in more moderate language: "...national governments go out of their way to attract foreign direct investment by offering to relax labor or health standards that will hurt the poor and set off a 'race to the bottom' that will lower standards worldwide."

Cavanaugh & Broad (1996) point to a specific example: "Over the past two decades, Nike closed its... factories [in the U.S.] and increasingly sub-contracted work to factories it did not own in Korea and Taiwan where workers were poorly paid and denied basic rights. As unions spread in both of those countries, Nike shifted its suppliers primarily to Indonesia, China, and Thailand where they could depend on governments to suppress independent union-organizing efforts.... In 1993, Nike paid part-time employee Michael Jordan more than the combined yearly income of the 30,000 young women who toiled under horrendous conditions to piece together Nike sneakers for suppliers in Indonesia." Here is another example: The (US) National Labor Committee (1996) reports that the Walt Disney Corporation paid 11 cents per hour to workers living in the slums of Haiti to sew Mickey Mouse and Pocahontas pajamas while paying CEO Michael Eisner $97,000 per hour (Holtz, 1997).

Noam Chomsky (1994) asks us to compare two recent events: "The 1992 riots in south-central Los Angeles and the Mayan uprising in Chiapas, Mexico on January 1, 1994. In both cases, the uprisings reflected the increasing marginalization of people who do not contribute to profit-making under prevailing institutional arrangements, and therefore, lack human rights or value." NACLA notes that when "The Zapatista [rebels in Chiapas, Mexico] were asked if they were against globalization, they responded in a communique: 'Our struggle is not against the future, but about who shapes that future and who benefits from it'"(NACLA, 1996).

Some Sobering Statistics

For some, it may seem surprising that private finance to developing countries increased five fold between 1990 and 1996 to $234 billion, rising from $44 billion in 1990 (with donor support leveling off at $64 billion in 1995). By 1996, 84% of international capital moving into the developing world was from private sources. In 1993, investment in emerging stock markets increased from 8% to 30% of all private investment world wide (Brown *et. al.*, 1996; French, 1997).

"In 1988, developing countries sent $1.5 billion more to the North in debt payment than they received in private and public finance. In 1995, the net transfer from North to South was $126 billion" (Brown *et. al.*, 1996). But this transfer of funds (in stock market investment and in direct investment) is concentrated in a small number of countries: 50% of foreign investment in (so-called) emerging stock markets were in Brazil, Mexico, and South Korea, and more than 50% of direct investment went to Argentina, China, Malaysia, Mexico, and Thailand (Brown *et. al.*, 1996). "Just 12 countries account for some three-quarters of all private flows to the developing world" (French,

1997). The North-South economic gap is narrowing for a few countries but is still widening for the vast majority (Broad & Cavanaugh, 1995/96).

The external debt of developing countries has grown 22 times over the past 25 years: in 1970, it was $100 billion; in 1980, around $650 billion; and by the end of 1996, it was $2.2 trillion. The ratio of external debt to Gross Domestic Product (GDP) is now 50% higher than in 1982 (UNICEF, 1995).

The difference between rich and poor nations is increasing, as is the difference between the rich and the poor within countries. According to the UNDP (1997), the economic disparity between the top and the bottom 20% of the world's population, which was 30 to 1 in 1960, grew to 61 to 1 by 1991 and had grown to 78 to 1 by 1994.

"In 1992, the richest 20% of the population controlled 83% of total world income, while the poorest 20% had to survive on 1.4%" (UNDP, 1994). Their share is now 1.1% (UNDP, 1997). "The least developed countries, with 10% of the world's people, have 0.3% of world trade - half their share two decades ago" (UNDP, 1997). The Human Development Index - based on a number of social, health, and human welfare indicators - which has been rising for countries since it was first reported in 1990, has now, for the first time, fallen for as many as 30 countries (UNDP, 1997). A growing underclass is being created to the effect that:

- The proportion of the world's population which had an income of $1-a-day or less declined from 34% to 32% from 1987 to 1993, but the number of income-poor people increased from 1.2 to 1.3 billion people (UNDP, 1997).
- In Sub-Saharan Africa and in Latin America, there has also been an increase in the proportion of the poor.
- At least one fifth of the world's population lives in absolute poverty.
- Seventy percent of people living in absolute poverty are women. Indigenous communities suffer poverty at rates far above national poverty rates (Buvenic *et. al.,* 1996:16-18).
- There are an estimated 100 million street children worldwide.

"The number of people in the world with a fortune greater than $1 billion climbed from 145 in 1987 to 358 in 1994. Quite a number were from developing countries. These billionaires accumulated $761.9 billion, equivalent to the annual per-capita income of 45% of the world's population of more or less 2.6 billion people" (Forbes, 1994; see also i.e. Wac, 1997). 358 individuals equated to 2.6 billion people! Something is obviously wrong!

An example from Mexico: "...half of all Mexicans (or 42 million people) lived in poverty in 1990, and 18 million lived in conditions of extreme poverty.... To illustrate the extreme concentration of wealth and income, the wealthiest Mexican... was said by Forbes magazine (18 July 1994) to be worth 6.6 billion dollars. The assets of this one man alone total more than the annual income of the poorest 17 million [Mexicans] combined" (Hayride & Parcel, 1995).

- "In Mexico, between 1980 and 1992, infant deaths due to nutritional deficiencies almost tripled to rates higher than those in the seventies" (Hayride & Parcel, 1995).
- Between 1986 and 1994, the life expectancy dropped in at least 11 African countries, and maternal mortality rates increased in a number of African countries (Epprecht, 1994: 37).
- In Ghana, child mortality was higher after 10 years of so-called economic recovery than it was in the "dark days" following Nkrumah's socialism (Epprecht, 1994: 38).
- "From 1979 – 89, the income of the poorest 20% of all families (in the US) fell 10% while that of the richest 1% of families increased 105%" (Fernandez, 1994).
- "In Brazil, in 1971-89, real GNP per capita grew by 3.3% annually, but the income of the poorest 20% grew by only 0.8%. In 1968-88 in the United Kingdom, GNP per capita grew by 2.2% and the income of the poorest 20% by only 0.3%. Sweden also had 2.2% growth in that period, but the income of the poorest 20% grew by 6.3%" (UNDP, 1997: 73). It is possible.

These statistics are not inevitable. Interventions can be made, and examples of these can be found at local, national and international levels. The solution is obviously not the elimination of large enterprises, but rather the democratic establishment of effective and enforceable national and international laws and safeguards to protect the welfare of labor and that of the general population. Even corporations such as Reebok and Levi Strauss have led the way in constructing codes of conon the danger of HIVduct for their corporations. There are also examples of other large corporations which are environmentally responsible and concerned with workers' rights. But these examples need to be multiplied and strengthened. Significantly strengthened, especially in the face of the powerful countervailing forces.

Some years ago, Structural Adjustment Policies (SAPs) were implemented in many developing countries in an attempt to improve GNP and presumably also the welfare of all their citizens. Previously quite harsh, we are now told these are "structural adjustments with a human face." Maybe! But I am not convinced. I am not convinced that human welfare is served. The evidence I read increasingly convinces me that this human face is not the smiling child's face we see on the cover of certain books, but rather a crying face - the crying face of a child in misery! (e.g., Lugalla, 1995a&b).

The former Executive Secretary of the UN Economic Commission for Africa, Adebayo Adedeji, stated that "to permit orthodox SAPs as we have known them in the 1980s to dominate the 1990s would reduce Africa to an abyss so low that it would be virtually impossible to emerge from it" (Asante, 1991).

In 1992, UNICEF reported that the number of women dying in childbirth in a number of African countries had doubled over the first two years of the Economic Structural Adjustment Program (ESAP). ESAP was dubbed "Extended Suffering for African People" by slum residents in Harare (Ankomah, 1993). *The Economist* noted: "Stabilization and structural adjustment have brought magnificent returns to the rich" (Green, D., 1995). Even the World Bank is beginning to question the wisdom of these SAPs we have come to know so well.

The Epidemiology of Functional Apartheid and Structural Violence

Why These Statistics in This Context?

Those concerned with public health and human welfare must be poignantly aware of the growing pauperization of the world and of the global forces which affect the everyday lives of people in local communities. People's political, economic, social class, and human rights situations, the degree to which they can live with dignity, are directly reflected in epidemiological patterns - in patterns of disease. This holds true throughout the world, in the North as well as in the South. The public health literature has also clearly established that inequity - the degree of economic disparity within a country, more than its overall degree of wealth as measured by GNP per capita - is the significant factor influencing overall health status. This explains not only the positive health indicators for rich countries such as Japan and the Scandinavians, which have modest income differentials, but also why relatively poor but more egalitarian countries have better health indicators than those considerably richer but with greater internal disparity, i.e. Good Health at Low Cost (Halstead *et. al.*, 1985).

On the 24th of April, 1994, we saw the collapse of Apartheid in South Africa. Yet, in countries throughout the world, the structure and practice of a functional apartheid - in the United States (Bourqois, 1996; Brooks *et. al.*, 1991) and in other industrialized countries - persists. While we may share in the celebration of the collapse of Apartheid in South Africa, we should not be blind to the tenacity of apartheid in its various guises and its destructive consequences throughout the world. Groups of people are marginalized, exploited and abused as a result of both their ethnicity and their class (and gender and geography) for being "the other." They are those often considered to be less than human - the "gooks," "trash," "inditos," or "subversives," - the expendable ones - supposedly not true or equal citizens in their own countries. In 1974, Vincente Navarro spoke metaphorically and dramatically but, I believe, not incorrectly, when he stated that the equivalent of twenty nuclear bombs explode every year in Latin America without making a sound. From all accounts, they are more numerous today. And not only in Latin America. There is violence in the world, in all parts of the world. Civil wars, homicide resulting from a whole range of motives, torture (whether state sponsored or not), rape, and a pervasive climate of fear in the lives of all too many (millions and millions too many) have been a part of our recent and current history. We know full well the horrors which occurred next door in Rwanda, in Bosnia, and in Cambodia, and.... Our news media report on such violence every day:

- In the 1970s and 1980s, crimes increased worldwide by 5% a year.
- In the U.S., there are two million victims of violent crime every year.
- It is estimated that a third of married women in developing countries are battered by their husbands (UNDP, 1997:31) (It is not much different in developed countries).
- Of the thirty armed struggles in 1995, none was a war between states, but internal conflicts largely killing and maiming civilians.
- Around two million children died as a result of armed conflict in the past decade.

Navarro's point, however, is that violence is not always direct or overt - it is also covert and silent. It is the violence resulting from the structure of *de-facto* apartheid (of "otherness," "segregation") - and whether such apartheid is official government policy or "only" functional makes little difference to those for whom it is a fact of repetitive assaults and degradations experienced as part of their everyday lives. It is a structural violence that according to the Pan American Health Organization, for example, claims more than one million Latin American lives a year - and millions of lives elsewhere. They may not talk about it in terms of apartheid or violence, but to state that "more than one million children under age five are dying each year, the majority from diseases which are preventable with today's technology" (Knouss, 1992) is not too far apart.

By mentioning this here, I mean to make a direct relationship between inequity, poverty and violence - as well as to suggest that the growing disparity in the world is itself a profound and insidious form of violence. Functional apartheid - the discrimination against or the so-called "setting apart" of "disposable people" - and structural violence - hierarchical and iniquitous social systems which condemn people to poverty - are directly related to the public's health; that is, if we are concerned with improving the health of the more than one billion of the world's most marginalized people (Farmer, 1996; Heggenhougen, 1995a).

It is difficult to speak of social pathologies when discussing health patterns. People's eyes glaze over, and they throw their hands up in despair when "poverty" and inequality are wheeled out as the underlying root causes of disease. The problem, then, becomes too overwhelming, the required tasks too difficult. But, though difficult, the evidence (in the public health literature) for such a connection - for the social and human rights roots of disease - is inescapable. The public health statistics are undeniable! Poverty and inequity are associated with malnutrition, hunger, and with disease, and they are directly responsible for 17 million people dying of starvation each year and for malnutrition affecting 24% of the world's population every day (Desjarlais, *et. al.*, 1995; Heggenhougen, 1995b).

This is nothing new, of course. Our public health predecessors, Rudolf Virchow, Peter Panum, William Farr, and many others clearly pointed to this relationship more than a century ago, and their lessons remain as relevant now as they were then - in fact, even more so.

In 1990, Amnesty International rightly called attention to the brutal killing of (according to their report) 400 street children in Rio de Janeiro which justifiably caused worldwide condemnation. As reported by Dorothy Logie, one Brazilian pediatrician strongly criticized the Amnesty Report, not because of any lack of compassion since he had dedicated his life to working with

Rio's street children, but because of what was not said. "His objection was the lack of any similar campaign or international outrage over the deaths of the 350,000 Brazilian children under the age of five who had died during 1990 from starvation and preventable diseases - deaths not caused by death squads but from unfair social and economic conditions which include the massive financial haemorrhage from Brazil in the form of debt repayment" (Logie, 1993). Former President Mwalimu Nyerere of Tanzania asked "Must we starve our children to pay our debt?" UNICEF estimates that 10,000 children die every week from the effects of the debt crisis (Logie, 1993; see also Nash, 1994; Heggenhougen, 1995b).

Conclusion : A Return to Arusha

Thirty years ago, at the same time the World Federation of Public Health Associations was initiated under the leadership of former President Mwalimu Julius Nyerere in Arusha the Arusha Declaration was formulated and confirmed as government policy. I remember one of my graduate-school professors at the time holding it up as an example for the rest of the world as an attempt to establish an equitable society. (I realize some Tanzanians and others may not have positive memories of the effects of the Arusha Declaration and may even suggest it caused economic disaster.) Mistakes were made, no doubt, and the reality might not always have reflected the ideals put on paper. But I would argue that, as public health professionals, we should work for a "Return to Arusha" - perhaps not as it was formulated in detail, but a return to what Arusha symbolized. A return to a renewed Arusha, to the creation of policies - in the North and in the South, at national and at international levels - which would combat the social and economic disparity so prevalent and so destructive to the health of significant segments of the world's population - for the sake of their health and that of us all.

If we are truly concerned with the public's health and welfare, we must not only narrowly focus on vectors, infectious agents, and harmful environmental and biological risk factors - important as these are - but also on the social roots of disease, on the underlying causes of "Why are people sick?" and particularly on the destructive elements in most societies of structural violence, of functional apartheid, and of inequalities of all kinds - including the harmful effects of globalization and of ethnic strife.

We should, and must, be outraged at the killing of street children in Brazil, Guatemala, Colombia, and of community health workers and ordinary Maya women and children as well as men in Guatemalan villages and in villages elsewhere - of individuals whom we have known, whom I have known: Francisco Curruchiche, Sefarino, Chepe ...they are all too many. But we should be equally outraged at the more widespread, though less immediately personal, violence and breaches of human rights - the insidious forms of structural violence which condemn an increasing number of people to lives of misery.

Combating structural violence and functional apartheid - the growing divides which separate us - is the work of public health and human rights. A health transition of any positive consequence, depends on such a focus - on an examination of the root causes of inequity and the growing pauperization of the world. It depends on a shift in the dominant public health perspective.

Yes, indeed! This does require structural adjustments; it is central to our task to formulate and fight for such adjustment - for the return to a renewed Arusha, if you will; but these are adjustments of quite a different kind than those we have come to know all too well (Heggenhougen, 1995).

Conclusion

How Should Tanzania Improve People's Health?

Kris Heggenhougen and Joe L.P. Lugalla

Introduction

We conclude the book as we began. This book is about "social change and health in Tanzania." We believe the contributors have demonstrated, with concrete evidence, that the forty years of Tanzania's independence have been accompanied by a variety of social, political, economic, and cultural changes which are reflected in new epidemiological patterns for different segments of Tanzania's population. These changes have created positive and negative social and economic contradictions and have ushered in new challenges that have to be addressed in the post-colonial state if the welfare of Tanzanians is to improve.

A critical examination of the processes of social change and development in Tanzania since independence suggests that the optimistic view held by most development planners and politicians - that independence, structural adjustments, and the winds of globalization have enhanced the ability of the majority of Tanzanians to participate in determining their own destiny and that Tanzanians have benefited from overall development processes - must be questioned. The chapters in this volume suggest more pessimism than optimism about the development trends and changes that have characterized Tanzania since independence. It is evident from the chapters that the majority of Tanzanians continue to suffer from the consequences of poverty, and consequently, from unacceptably deleterious health conditions. Poverty is dominant in rural as well as in urban areas. There is ample evidence suggesting that there is a growing divide between the majority of people living in difficult circumstances and the relatively few who have access to wealth, power, and upper-class social status. For most, even making ends meet to maintain their own and their families' livelihood continues to be problematic. As a result, the majority of Tanzanians continue to suffer ill health caused by an inadequate living environment, poor housing, lack of clean water, inadequate nutrition, lack of basic sanitation, and lack of easy access to basic but effective primary health care (including basic immunization services). The chapters in this volume have demonstrated how these problems manifest themselves in people's health. The truth is, for many rural residents of Tanzania, "death" (due to diseases) continues to be a common visitor. Another way of putting it is that it seems easier for people to find a bottle of beer or coca-cola than a glass of clean water. Why is this so? We can understand the failure of Tanzania in achieving equitable growth and improved health for its entire people if we analyze both the internal and external dimensions of the social and economic problems confronting Tanzania.

The Internal Dimension

Tanzania is among the very few countries in Africa that have at least tried to bring basic/primary health care within the reach of all. The political slogans of *"Mtu ni Uhai"* (A Human Being is Life), *"Mtu ni Afya"*(A Human Being is Health), and several other slogans helped a great deal in directing the implementation of equitable health policies that aimed at improving the health condition of all Tanzanians. These policies worked well from the mid 1960s to the early 1980s, particularly because of the will and receptivity of the people and their leaders as well as the policy guidelines of the Arusha Declaration of 1967 which vowed to build a society based on principles of human justice and equality. Besides the specific health policies that were adopted at that time, it is important to note that people's health was considered an integral part of the entire development process. Supplementing a specific policy on health were other policies which, in effect, also improved people's health including policies on education (which, of course is interrelated with health, e.g. the health of educated women and their children is better than that of illiterate women and their children) which aimed at creating a Tanzanian nation of people who would be both literate and healthy. By the early 1980s, Tanzanian schools had achieved a gross enrollment rate of 98 percent for primary education (Kuleana, 1999). As far as health was concerned, by the 1980s, Tanzania had established an extensive network of functioning health facilities which were relatively easily accessible to most people. Emphasis had been on equity and the distribution of health services in both rural and urban areas. The government viewed access to health services as a basic human right for all Tanzanians. The focus was on primary and community healthcare, and the main objectives of primary healthcare were to strengthen district management capacity, to foster multi-sectoral collaboration, and encourage community participation.

Despite these achievements during the first two decades of independence, there has been a subsequent decline in the quality of health services. The poor performance of the health sector is not simply or necessarily a result of the relative weakness of the Ministry of Health or the inadequacies of health planners, but rather it is a result of the apparent inadequacies of the overall planning machinery of the country as a whole. Policy planning in Tanzania is currently sectoral (and decentralized), which tends to limit the importance placed on comprehensive social and development planning. Currently there are national policies aimed at eradicating urban and rural poverty, with a directorate of poverty eradication having been established in the office of the Vice President, and these policies should also lead to improved health outcomes. But it is not clear how the proposed poverty eradication strategies fit in with the country's overall socio-economic development plans. The strategies seem to neither clearly identify nor to include the interested stakeholders in this key process or who is to do what, where and when.

Successful planning requires people's participation. The poverty eradication initiatives being proposed do not specifically state how the voices of the poor will be heard or how they will actively participate in improving their own welfare. An examination must be made of the extent of the truth of the claim that due to poor governance, corruption, lack of accountability, and the absence of democratic participation in development planning and implementation, there seems to be a wide gap between policy announcements and practices in Tanzania. We have no doubt that government policies can succeed if they incorporate people's ideas, from the bottom up, in a democratic, integrated, and well coordinated manner.

We stated in the introduction that Tanzania has been through four main ideological and developmental phases since independence in 1961. During each of these phases, Tanzania underwent significant social and economic transformations which had both positive and negative health and social welfare implications. The negative consequences seem to predominate in the present period.

The fundamentals of primary healthcare and the emphasis on community health that was advocated during the period of the Arusha Declaration are now less evident, if evident all. The health infrastructure is in a state of disrepair, with many hospitals, rural health centers, and dispensaries lacking basic medical equipment and medicines. Poor wages for health personnel have produced demoralized workers, and some have resorted to corruption in order to bridge the deficit in income. A few of them have opted out from public service and have opened their own private clinics, and some have left the country for employment in Botswana, South Africa, and elsewhere. Others continue to work in the public health facilities but spend much of their time moonlighting in private clinics. All this has led to the sub-optimal management of public health facilities and lack of accountability. How can this situation be addressed?

Although these problems are increasingly becoming evident, Tanzania is fortunate in that an extensive network of health infrastructure still exists throughout the country, which, if rejuvenated, could be used to improve at least the healthcare services for the majority of Tanzanians. Before the adoption of structural adjustment policies, sixty percent of healthcare services were being provided by the government, and the remaining services were being provided by non-governmental organizations. By the early 1990s, there were four major referral hospitals at the national level, one of which was a teaching hospital. All regions had a regional hospital, and there were a total of 152 hospitals in 106 districts (DHS, 1992). At divisional levels, there were 373 rural health centers, and at the ward level, there were about 3,000 dispensaries. It is estimated that Tanzania had some 5,550 community health workers at the village level. At present, Tanzania has five medical schools. In the area of education, Tanzania currently has a network of more than 11,000 schools and over 100,00 teachers, which, if improved, could also serve as a good source for basic preventive health education as well as regular primary education. While this can happen if there is political will - government commitment and people's participation - there is considerable concern about how this can occur at the same time that the government has embraced policy reform packages advocated by the World Bank and the International Monetary Fund. This leads us to an examination of the external dimensions of Tanzania's social, political, and economic problems.

The External Dimension

Putting aside the legacy of colonialism and the structures of dependency and underdevelopment, Tanzania, at independence, began a development process heavily influenced by policies of equity and improvement in social services. This process was also supported by outside donors, especially the Scandinavians. But, as indicated above, these so-called socialist policies were put aside by the mid 1980s. Since then, Tanzania's development process has continued to be heavily influenced by donors, but also by the policies of the Bretton Woods institutions - the World Bank and the International Monetary Fund (IMF) and the World Trade Organization (WTO). The adoption of structural adjustment policies (SAPs) and the full-scale embracement of the globalization process is an evident result of these recent developments. Due to these policies, Tanzania has been forced to introduce unpopular reforms in the provision of social services as well as in a variety of other areas. The health as well as education policy reforms advocate the introduction of user fees and the participation of private institutions in the provision of health and education services.

The current reform packages have been criticized for a variety of reasons including that they are primarily based on the conceptual work of short-term outside consultants, who, no matter their formal qualifications, are unlikely to be competent and conversant with the dynamics of the problems confronting Tanzania and its people. Further, many have argued that these social or development policies have not been designed to fit the true priorities and needs of the majority of Tanzanians and that they also contradict Tanzanian cultural norms.

For example, the application of structural adjustment policies (SAPs) has had severe negative consequences on people's health. By reducing government expenditure on health and other social services, there have been serious shortages of health supplies, medical equipment and medicines that have led to the deterioration of available government health services. The introduction of user fees in health has made it very difficult for the poor majority to access these services. The externally mandated SAPs have also made it difficult for the government to pay health workers livable wages. This has created an unbearable working environment which has demoralized most health workers who are now reacting bitterly against the state. Doctors have gone on strike, and nurses have staged go-slow actions. These are events which were previously unknown in Tanzania, but which have become common since the 1990s (Green, 2001). For example, in 1991, the state acted swiftly, using the well-trained Field Force Police Unit to end the doctors' strike at the Muhimbili Medical Centre in Dar es Salaam, the country's largest health facility. The police units were reported to have handled the doctors and their families roughly and to have removed them by force from their residences in the hospital owned housing. The growing hostility between the state and health personnel has worsened the delivery of health services even more (Lugalla, 1995; Green, 2001). As Charles Green (2001) has argued, throughout Sub-Saharan Africa, the policy debate on healthcare has shifted from demand-oriented questions on what the population needs and what is feasible and effective, toward supply-oriented questions of what is affordable and cost effective.

The SAPs have had severe consequences on education, too. Due to these policies, some children are dropping out of school in order to assist in the household economy by being involved in either commodity production or in petty trading activities. Those who are less fortunate have been abandoned by their hard pressed families and are ending up as street children, resulting in deteriorating health and other negative consequences.

The policies that advocate free trade and liberalization have forced Tanzania to privatize most of the previously state-owned institutions such as banks, transport, communication infrastructure, and other corporations. Foreign companies have bought many of these corporations at throwaway prices. The sale of the National Bank of Commerce to a banking conglomerate of South Africa (ABSA) in 1997 is but one example of this. Liberalization without control is resulting in a situation where the entire lucrative mining business is currently dominated by foreign multinational companies, and small-scale Tanzanian miners have lost their mining rights on their own soil. The strong influence of liberalization and globalization is reversing Tanzania's previous development agenda. Due to these influences, those whom the Arusha Declaration labeled as "colonialists," "capitalists," and "economic exploiters," are now being invited to participate in developing Tanzania according to a definition of development which equates it with creating conditions attractive to "foreign investors." The newly adopted investment policies tend to favor foreign investors rather than local ones. Tax holidays are being granted, and the state machinery assists by creating labor laws that restrict strikes and the degree to which labor can be organized. Privatization of state-controlled institutions has led to the retrenchment of workers and to increasing rates of unemployment. Free trade and importation of material goods from abroad have jeopardized local industries and severely affected people's incomes. People are also increasingly enticed to sell their land to foreign investors, which may have short-term gains but long-term losses. All these processes are generating a situation of poverty for the majority of the people with catastrophic consequences for their health.

Tanzania can not escape the "winds of globalization." But to therefore assume that Tanzania's problems are rooted solely in its situation of dependency and the politics of donors like the World Bank and the International Monetary Fund is deceptive. It is true that the accelerating process of globalization is expanding global opportunities without distributing them equitably. Globalization is associated with corporate profit, increased corporate power, growing income concentration, decline of workers' rights, environmental destruction, and with poverty. But Tanzania is not a passive playing field for external forces. Yet, we must ask: Is the Tanzanian government willing and capable of dealing with the negative impact of globalization?

In order to deal with increasing corporate power, Tanzania requires a political regime that is powerful, has political will, and is committed to improving the welfare of the majority of its people. The qualities of such a regime are certainly clear. Tanzania needs a regime that is democratic, respects human rights, listens to the voices of the poor, and puts the needs of poor people first in all social and development plans. In any state where the above qualities are lacking, the prospects for meaningful change, real social development, and empowerment of the people will most likely remain unrealized. Tanzania, in comparison with other countries of sub-Saharan Africa, is not in a hopeless situation. There is some ground for optimism when we consider the social, economic, and political culture which the current Tanzanian government seems to be advocating. The country has been relatively stable since independence and has moved through different political and development phases including periods of economic turmoil without bloodshed caused by a civil war which has been the case in so many other countries. The multiparty political system that was adopted in the early 1990s is surviving and growing roots. In general, the majority of people are now beginning to understand the essence of democracy and of participation in political and development affairs. If this climate persists, it can become the basis for a real transformation of the socio-economy of Tanzania for the interest of those who have been deprived of the benefit of development for a long time. Health problems in Tanzania are unlikely to be resolved if the main underlying causes for poor health—poverty and inequity—are not adequately addressed. This is a major challenge for Tanzania and its supporters as far as future development is concerned. What are the best strategies for fighting poverty and inequity? In Tanzania, people's health and social welfare will depend on the outcome of that fight.

Alleviating Poverty and Improving People's Health

In order to successfully combat poverty, one must understand that poverty implies that the condition of people's lives is inadequate for obtaining the minimal necessities for daily living such as food (nutrition), housing, safe water, good health, and adequate education (Lugalla, 1995). Poverty is a material condition, but that material condition is derived from an inequitable social power relationship. Poverty and inequality have been examined by a variety of social scientists. While economists may prefer to use concepts of "income" and "income distribution" in denoting various aspects of the problem, sociologists and anthropologists prefer to use concepts of "class," "stratification," "marginality," and "social inequality." These are, in turn, not only analyzed in terms of how they allude to income, wealth, prestige, and power, but also to accessibility of basic necessities of life and to social services such as education, health, good housing and security. These variables are also analyzed in terms of hierarchical social structures which influence the accessibility of various social groups to the major means of livelihood such as land and tools of production in the rural areas and employment opportunities in the urban areas. This way of understanding poverty can be helpful in identifying who the poor are, where they are, and what they currently do in order to survive. This may also influence the design of policies that target and listen to the voices of the poor. Poverty reduction policies and programs need to be based on an understanding of how the poor respond in times of economic crisis. Otherwise, however well intentioned, programs may undermine rather than complement and support the actions taken by the poor themselves to improve their situations. Poverty alleviation policies vary from one country to the other, and they also vary within countries. For example, policies aimed at addressing rural and urban poverty in Tanzania tend to vary considerably. However, for poverty alleviation strategies to succeed, it is important to understand that the real experts on poverty are the poor themselves. In most cases, the poor have long been the victims of development plans designed for their benefit, though typically without their consultation, by national governments, international agencies, and non-governmental organizations (Watkins 1996). And some are beginning to wonder why they are poor despite these plans, while others are noting that they may, in fact, remain poor, precisely because of some of those plans. Poverty eradication requires the input of the poor and creation of an enabling environment at national as well as international levels which will assist the poor in becoming their own liberators.

As Watkins (1996) has argued, there are five building blocks upon which any successful poverty eradication strategy should be built. We refer to Watkins' (1996) writings here at some length: The first of these building blocks is *increased equity*. "High levels of inequality and widespread poverty are a source of economic inefficiency." It is important to have wider distribution of productive assets and secure and equitable forms of employment. Policies that discriminate against the majority and benefit only a small wealthy minority of elites must be discouraged. Second, Watkins highlights the importance of *enhanced opportunity.* People's accessibility to productive assets, which are important to maintain sustainable livelihood, is important in alleviating poverty. People need the opportunity to develop greater autonomy (agency/power) through education, health care, and provision of clean water and sanitation. People themselves ought to be in control of the common resources on which their survival depends. Third, Watkins emphasizes *peace and security.* "Without peace and security, genuine human development will remain an elusive goal." In all situations where instability prevails, the poorest women and children who are most vulnerable tend to be those who suffer much more than others. Fourth, *People's participation* can only become effective if there is open and accountable governing of political structures that are run democratically at village, district, national, and international levels. It is important to note that the concern of what we presumptuously call "true development," which is akin to the UNDP's definition of development, is to enhance people's capacity to become masters and drivers of the engine of their own social change. Fifth, according to Watkins, creating *sustainable development* has to be the focus of any strategy aimed at eradicating poverty. The vulnerability of the poor and the impoverishment of their lives can only be reduced if they have a secure livelihood. And one way by which this can be achieved is to spend much more effort in considering both the sustainable and the equitable use of currently available, but limited, resources.

Looking at the social, political, economic, and cultural structure of urban and rural Tanzania, the following weaknesses are evident. In rural Tanzania, land is the primary means of income. In the urban areas, the majority of people have nothing except their labor power. Therefore, selling their labor and the availability of employment opportunities are the major factors influencing their survival. In both rural and urban areas, the old hierarchical structures of colonialism, which had abated somewhat in the 1960s and 1970s, have started to reappear, albeit in a different form. History is beginning to repeat itself through the influence of globalization and the liberalization of trade. People in the rural areas are losing their means of livelihood due to the diminishment of land, forests, and water (due to damning of rivers for the creation of hydro-electric power) and environmental destruction. The climate is further compounded by the inadequate provision of social services such as water, electricity, sanitation, preventive health, education, and other public utilities like roads and phone systems.

Having seen the kind of intervening policies and strategies that may assist Tanzania in her attempt to alleviate poverty, it is important to make clear that these policies are not independent variables but dependent ones. The success of alleviating poverty will depend on whether the government is willing to do so and on whether it is capable in the sense of having the required personnel which have both the motivation and the will.

The government of Tanzania will have to look into these issues seriously if the country wants to have a healthy population in the near future. It is important to note that improved health services are critical for both poverty alleviation and improved productivity. The development of the nation will not take place if the people are unhealthy.

Bibliography

Introduction

Daily News Paper 25-3-1999.

Green, C. (2001): *Manufacturing Powerlessness in the Black Diaspora: Inner-City Youth and the New Global Frontier*. New York: Altamira Press.

Heggenhougen, K., P., Vaughan, E. Muhondwa, & J. Rutabanzibwa-Ngaiza. (1987): *Community Health Workers—The Tanzanian Experience*. Oxford: Oxford University Press.

Lugalla, J.L.P. & Kibassa, C.G. (Eds.) (2002): *Poverty, AIDS and Street Children in East Africa*. The Edwin Mellen Press, New York, USA.

Majira News Paper 21-3-1999.

United Nations Development Program (UNDP), (1997): *Human Development Report*. Oxford: Oxford University Press.

United Republic of Tanzania, (2001): *The Community Health Fund Act* (Acts Supplement).

United Republic of Tanzania, (1999): *The National Health Insurance Fund.*

Chapter 1

AHRTAG (1993): "Promoting Sexual Health." *AIDS Action* 22.

AMMP (1997): *The Policy Implications of Adult Morbidity and Mortality; End of Phase 1 Report.* Dar es Salaam: Adult Morbidity and Mortality Project.

Baldwin J.D. and Baldwin, J.I. (1986): *Behavior Principles in Everyday Life.* Englenwood Cliffs, N.J., University of California Prentice-Hall.

Balmer, DH, Gikundi M.A., Billingsley MC., Kihuno FG., Kimani M., Wang'ondu J., & Njoroge H. (1997): "Adolescent Knowledge, Values and Coping Strategies: Implications for Health in Sub-Saharan Africa." *Journal of Adolescent Health* 21:33-38.

BEST (1990): *Basic Education Statistics in Tanzania, 1987-1988.* Dar es Salaam, Tanzania: Ministry of Education and Culture.

BEST (1994): *Basic Education Statistics in Tanzania, 1989-1993*. Dar es Salaam, Tanzania: Ministry of Education and Culture.

Bledsoe, C.H. and Cohen B. (1993): *Social Dynamics of Adolescent Fertility in Sub-Saharan Africa.* Washington DC: National Academy Press.

Bureau of Statistics (1971): *Population Census Volume 3: Demographic Statistics.* Dar es Salaam: Bureau of Statistics, Planning Commission United Republic of Tanzania.

Bureau of Statistics (1982): *Population Census Volume VII; Basic Demographic and Socio-economic Characteristics.* Dar es Salaam: Bureau of Statistics, Planning Commission United Republic of Tanzania.

Bureau of Statistics (1992): *Population Census Basic Demographic and Socio-economic Characteristics*. Dar es Salaam: Planning Commission United Republic of Tanzania.

Bureau of Statistics (1994): *Statistical Abstract.* Dar es Salaam: Bureau of Statistics, United Republic of Tanzania, Planning Commission United Republic of Tanzania.

Chacha, C.M. (1994): "The Growing Incidence of Youth Unemployment: Strategy and Policy Options." *Journal of Social Work* 2.

Cooksey, B., Malekela, G., and Lugalla, J. (1993): *Parents' Attitude Towards Education in Rural Tanzania.* Dar es Salaam, Tanzania: Tanzania Development Research Group (TADREG) report No. 5.

Fleming A. (1994): "The Next Generation and AIDS." *AIDS* 4.6.

Haub, C. and Yanagishita, M. (1992): *World Population Data Sheet.* Washington D.C.: Population Reference Bureau.

Justesen, A., Kapiga S.H., and Van Asten, H. (1992): "Abortions in a Hospital Setting: Hidden Realities in Dar es Salaam, Tanzania." *Studies in Family Planning* 23.5.

Kaaya, S.F., Kilonzo G.P., Semboja, A., and Matowo, A. (1992): "Prevalence of Substance Abuse Among Secondary School Students in Dar es Salaam." *Tanzania Medical Journal* 7.1.

Kahama, C.G., Maliyamkono, T. L., and Wells, S. (1986): *The Challenge for Tanzania's Economy.* London: James Currey.

Kamm, M. (1977): "The Problem of Youth and School Leavers in the Youth." In *Report of the Child Study in Tanzania - Age 7 to 15.* Dar es Salaam: Tanzania National Scientific Research Council.

Kapiga, S.H., Hunter, D.J., and Nachtigal, G. (1992): "Reproductive Knowledge and Contraceptive Awareness and Practice Among Secondary School Pupils in Bagamoyo and Dar es Salaam, Tanzania." *Central African Journal of Medicine* 38.9.

Kilonzo, G.P. (1992): *The Reduction of Demand for Dependence Producing Drugs - The Tanzanian Experience.* Presented at the International Conference on Drug Abuse Control, Arusha, AICC.

Klepp, K.I., Ndeki, S.S., Thuen, F., and Leshabari, M.T. (1996): "Predictors of Intention to be Sexually Active Among Tanzanian School Children." *East African Medical Journal* 73.4.

Klepp, K.I., Ndeki, S.S., Thuen, F., Leshabari, M.T., and Seha, A.M. (1994): "Predictors of High-risk Sexual Behavior Among Tanzanian School Youth." *AIDS Care* 6.2.

Leshabari, M.T., Mpangile, G.S., Kaaya, S.F. and Kihwele, D.T. (1994): "From Teenage Unwanted Pregnancy to Induced Abortions: Who Facilitates Links." *International Journal of Adolescence and Youth* 4.

Leshabari, M.T. (1988): *Factors Influencing School Adolescent Fertility Behavior in Dar es Salaam, Tanzania.* Unpublished Doctor of Science Thesis, The John Hopkins University, School of Public Health, Baltimore, Maryland, USA.

Leshabari, M.T., Mwanri L.J., Minjas J.N., Yona E.N. (1996b): *Rapid Situational Analysis of the Health Status of School-aged Children in Tanzania.* Report submitted by the Institute of Public Health, Muhimbili University College of Health Sciences, Dar es Salaam.

Leshabari, M.T. and Kaaya, S.F. (1997): "Bridging the Information Gap: Sexual Maturity and Reproductive Health Problems among Youth in Tanzania." *Health Transition Review* 7 Suppl. 3.

Leshabari, M.T.; Kaaya S.K.; Nguma, J.K. and Kapiga, S.H. (1996a): *Household Responses to HIV/AIDS in Kyela District, Tanzania.* A research Report submitted to WHO, Geneva by the Institute of Public Health, Muhimbili University College of Health Sciences, Dar es Salaam.

Liljestrom, R., Masanja, P., Mkai, C.P.B., and Tumbo-Masabo, Z. (1994): The Pubescent Girl - Past and Present, In (Eds.) Tumbo-Masabo Z., Liljestrom R. *Chelewa Chelewa the Dilemma of Teenage Girls.* The Scandinavian Institute of African Studies. Ostersund Sweden.

Liskin, L., Church C.A. Piotrow T., Harris J. AIDS Education; A Beginning. In (Eds.) Rinehart W. *Issues in World Health.* Series L. No: 8.

Lugalla, J.L.P. (1993): Structural Adjustment Policies and Education in Tanzania. In (Ed.) Gibbon P. *Social Change and Economic Reform in Africa.* Nordiska Afrikainstitutet, Uppsala, Sweden.

Lugalla, J.L.P. (1995): *Adjustment and Poverty in Tanzania.* Bremer Afrika-Studien Bd. 12., Lit Verlag, Munster, Germany.

Lugalla, J.L.P. (1997): Where do the Majority Live in Urban Tanzania? In (Ed.) Green C. *Globalization and Survival in the Black Diaspora; the New Urban Challenge.* State University of New York Press, Albany.

Lugalla, J.L.P., Mbwambo, J. (1999): Street Children and Street Life in Urban Tanzania; the Culture of Surviving and its Implications on Children's Health. *International Journal for Urban and Rural Research*, 23 (2).

Lwihula, G., Nyamuryekunge, K., Hamelmann, J.B. (1996): *Baseline Survey of Sexual and Reproductive Health Knowledge, Perceptions and Behavior among School Youth in Kinondoni District, Dar es Salaam.* Report submitted to the African Medical Research Council (AMREF), Dar es Salaam.

Malentlema, T.N. (1977): *Health and Nutrition Report of the Young Child Study in Tanzania Age 7-15 Years*, Tanzania National Scientific Research Council, Dar es Salaam.

Mbunda D. (1991): *Traditional Sex Education in Tanzania; A study of 12 Ethnic Groups.* The Margaret Sanger Center, New York City, NY, USA.

Mbunda, W.M. (1988): *Adolescent Fertility in Tanzania: Knowledge, Perceptions and Practices.* Chama cha Uzazi na Malezi Bora Tanzania (UMATI). Dar es Salaam, Tanzania.

Mhalu, F., Swai, A., Mwakagile D., Sege T. (Eds.) (1992): "Microbial and Sociological Determinants of Acute STD and HIV Infection in Dar es Salaam." In Mpangile G.S., Mbunda W.M. (eds) *Information on Adolescent Sexuality in Dar es Salaam, An Annotated Bibliography.* The Family Planning Association of Tanzania-UMATI/ UNFPA, Dar es Salaam.

Ministry of Health and AMMP Team (1998): *Health Statistics Abstract,* Issue No. 6, July, Ministry of Health and Adult Morbidity and Mortality Project, Dar es Salaam

Mongula, B.S. (1991): " Children Under Especially Difficult Circumstances in Tanzania:

The Case of Street Children." *Population and Development Papers,* 1 (1).

Mosha, H.J. (1988): "Twenty Years After Education for Self-Reliance; A Critical Review." *International Journal of Education Development,* Vol. 10.

Mpangile, G.S. and Mbunda, W.M. (1993): "Introduction." In Mpangile G.S., Mbunda W.M. (eds) *Information on Adolescent Sexuality in Dar es Salaam; An Annotated Bibliography.* The Family Planning Association of Tanzania - UMATI/UNFPA, Dar es Salaam.

Mpangile, G.S., Leshabari, M.T. and Kihwele D.J. (1993): "Factors Associated with Induced Abortions in Public Hospitals in Dar es Salaam, Tanzania." Study Report Submitted to WHO Human Reproduction Unit, Geneva. The Family Planning Association of Tanzania (UMATI), Dar es Salaam, Tanzania.

Msamanga, G.I. (1986): "The Epidemiology and Control of STD in Tanzania. Proceedings of the Symposium on STDs in Dar es Salaam." The Medical Association of Tanzania (MAT), Dar es Salaam.

Mwakagile, D.S., Swai , A.B., Sandstrom E., Urassa E., Biberfeld G., Mhalu, F. (1996): "High Frequency of Sexually Transmitted Diseases Among Pregnant Women: Need for Intervention." *East African Medical Journal,* 73(10).

NACP (1994): "HIV/AIDS/STD Surveillance; Report No. 8." Epidemiology Unit. The National AIDS Control Programme, Ministry of Health, Dar es Salaam.

Nikander P., Honkanen R., Huttunen P., Kilonzo G. P., Pitkanen T. (1992b): "Role of Alcohol in Injuries in the Muhimbili Medical Center Casuality Department, Dar es Salaam Tanzania. In Kilonzo G.P., Pitkanen Y.T. (eds), *Pombe; Report of Alcohol Research Project in Tanzania 1988-90.* University of Helsinki, Institute of Development Studies, Helsinki, Finland.

Nikander P., Kilima, E., Kilonzo G.P. (1992a): "Commercialization of the Traditional Alcoholic Beverages." In Kilonzo G.P., Pitkanen, Y.T. (eds), *Pombe; Report of Alcohol Research Project in Tanzania 1988-90.* University of Helsinki, Institute of Development Studies, Helsinki Finland.

Omari, C.K. (1977): "Family Structure and the Child." In *Report on a Study of the young Child in Tanzania from Age 7 - 15 Years.* Tanzania National Scientific Council, Dar es Salaam.

Population Reference Bureau (1990): *Teenage Parents, Global Patterns.* Population Reference Bureau, Washington DC.

Puja, G.K., Kassimoto T. (1994): "Girls in Education and Pregnancy at School. In Tumbo-Masabo Z., Liljestrom R. (eds) *Chelewa Chelewa: The Dilemma of Teenage Girls.* The Scandinavian Institute of African Studies. Ostersund, Sweden.

Schoepf, B.G. (1992): "Women at a Risk: Case Studies from Zaire." In Hardt G., Lindenbaum (ed) *The Time of AIDS: Social Analysis, Theory and Method.* Sage publication, Newbury Park, California.

Seha, A.M., Klepp, K and Ndeki, S.S. (1994): "Scale Reliability and Construct Validity: A Pilot Study Among Primary School Children in Northern Tanzania." *AIDS Education and Prevention* 6 (6).

Senderowitz, J and Paxman, J. (1985): *Adolescent Fertility: World Concerns.* Population Reference Bureau, Washington DC.

Temu , M., Leshabari, M.T. (1992): "Use of Surrogate Patients in Identifying Dispensing Practices of Urban Drug Stores." Unpublished Report, Faculty of Pharmacy, Dar es Salaam, Tanzania.

UN (1992): *Demographic Year Book.* United Nations Department of Economics and Social Development, Population Division, New York.

WHO (1993): *Women and Substance Abuse; A Gender Analysis and Review of Health and Policy Implications*. Programme on Substance Abuse, World Health Organization, PSA/93.12.

Wilson, M. (1951): *Good Company: A Study of Nyakyusa Age Villages*. Oxford University Press, London.

Chapter 2

Anarfi, J.K. (1993): "Sexuality, Migration and AIDS in Ghana." In *Health Transition Review Supplement* to Vol. 3.

Barnett, T and Blaikie, P. (1992): *AIDS in Africa: Its Present and Future Impact.* The Guilford Press, New York, USA. 1992.

Borgdorff, M. (1994): *Epidemiology of HIV-1 Infection in Mwanza Region - Tanzania.* Royal Tropical Institute. Amsterdam, The Netherlands.

Borgdorff, M., Barongo, L., van Jaarsveld E. *et. al.* (1993): Sentinel Surveillance for HIV-1 Infection: How Representative are Blood Donors, Outpatients With Fever, Anaemia or Sexually Transmitted Diseases, and Antenatl Clinic Attenders in Mwanza Region, Tanzania. In *AIDS* 7.

Bureau of Statistics (1992): *1988 Population Census: Basic Demographic and Socio-economic Characteristics*. Planning Commission, Dar es Salaam.

Cory H. *Ypescript* (1949): Dar es Salaam: University of Dar es Salaam, Library EAF, CORY 104.

Fuglesang, M. (1995): "Red Card or Yellow: Are You Still in Game? Being Young and Reproductive Health in Tanzania. In Fuglesang, M. (ed) *Reports on Sexuality and Reproductive.* Swedish Association for Sex Education, RFSU, Stockholm, Sweden.

Kaaya, S.F., Mbwambo J.K.K., Leshabari S. (1995): *"Report on the Impact of HIV/AIDS on Women and Children: A Case Study of Morogoro Region."* Report Prepared for UNICEF, UNICEF, Dar es Salaam, Tanzania.

Kaijage, F.J. (1992): " The AIDS Crisis in the Kagera Region Tanzania From a Historical Perspective, In Killewo, J.Z.J. and Lwihula G.K. (eds). *Behavioural and Epidemiological Aspects of Research in Tanzania.*" Department of Epidemiology and Biostatistics - Muhimbili University College, Dar es Salaam.

Kessy, A.T. (1995): "Risk Factors of HIV Infection and Other Sexuality Transmitted Disease Among Youths in Moshi Rural District, Kilimanjaro Region." A Dissertation submitted in Partial Fulfilment for the Master of Medicine Degree University of Dar es Salaam.

Killewo J.Z.J. and Lwihula, G.K., *et. al.* (Eds) (1989): *Behavoural and Epidemiological Aspects of AIDS Research in Tanzania.* Proceedings of A Workshop held in Dar es

Salaam from 6th - 8th December 1989. Department of Epidemiology Biostatistics - Muhimbili University College of Health Sciences Dar es Salaam, Tanzania.

Lwihula, G.K., Killewo, J.Z.J., Dablgren, L.A. and Sandstrom, A. (1993): "AIDS Epidemic in Kagera Region, Tanzania -The Experiences of Local People." *AIDS CARE*, 5 (3).

Mpangile, G.S., Leshabari M.T. and Kihwele, D.J. (1993): "Factors Associated with Induced Abortions in Public Hospitals in Dar es Salaam, Tanzania." Family Planning Association of Tanzania (UMATI), UMATl, Dar es Salaam, Tanzania.

NACP (1991): "National AIDS Control Programme AIDS Surveillance Report No. 4," March, Ministry of Health, Dar es Salaam, Tanzania.

NACP (1992): "National AIDS Control Programme Surveillance Report No. 6," Ministry of Health, Dar es Salaam, Tanzania.

NACP (1995): "National AIDS Control Programme HIV/AIDS Surveilance Report No. 9," Ministry of Health, Dar es Salaam, Tanzania.

Ngallaba, S., Kapiga, S.H. Rugobya, I. and Boerma, J.T. (1993): "Tanzania Demographic Health Survey 1991/92," Bureau of Statistics, Planning Commission, Dar es Salaam, Tanzania.

Ngugi, E.N. Simmonsen, J.N. Bosire, M; Ronald A.R. (1988): "Prevention of Transmission of Human Immunodeficiency Virus in Africa: Effectiveness of Condom Promotion and Health Education Among Prostitute." *Lancet*, 2(8616).

Nkya, W.M., Gillespie, S.H., Howlett, W, Elford, J. (1995): "Sexually Transmitted Diseases Among Prostitutes in Moshi and Arusha, Northern Tanzania." *International Journal of STDs and AIDS*, 2 (6).

O'Connor, P., Leshabari, M.T. and Lwihula, G. (1992): "Ethnographic Study of the Truck Stop Environment in Tanzania." Family Health International, Durham, NC, USA.

Obbo, C. (1980): *African Women: Their Struggle for Economic Independence.* Zed Press, London, UK.

Omari, C.K., Shaidi, L.P. (Eds) (1991): *Social Problems in Eastern Africa.* Dar es Salaam, Dar es Salaam University Press.

Rutasitara, W.K. (1980): "Mombasa Bar Girls." Muga, E. (ed) *Studies in Prostitution; East, West and South Africa, Zaire and Nevada,* Kenya Literature Bureau Nairobi, Kenya.

Santhall, A.W. and Gutkind, P.C.W. (1957): *Townsman in the Making: Kampala and Its Suburbs*, East African Institute of Social Research, Kampala, Uganda.

Schoepf, B.G. (1992): "Women at Risk: Case Studies From Zaire." Herdt, G. and Linderbaurn (eds), *Social Analysis in the Time of AIDS*, Sage Publications, Newburry Park California, USA.

Setel, P. (1995): "The Social Context of AIDS Education Among Young Men in Northern Kilimanjaro."Klepp, K; Biswalo, P.1vL and Talle, A. (eds) *Young People at Risk: Fighting AIDS in Northern Tanzania,* Oslo, Finland, Scandinavian University Press.

Swantz, M-L. (1985): *Women in Development: A Creative Role Denied.* Dar es Salaam, Dar es Salaam University Press.

Swai, R.O. (1995): "Patterns of HIV Infection Amongst Youth in Tanzania." Proceedings of a Workshop on Youth Growth and Related Problems in Tanzania, Social Science and Medicine Group (SOSMED), Monogram 3.

Van De Perre, P; Rouvroy, D; Bogaerts, J; and Kestelyn, P. (1984): "Acquired Immunodeficiecy Syndrome in Ruanda." *Lancet* 2.

White, C. (1988): "Domestic Labour in a Colonial City: Prostitution in Nairobi." Strichter, S.B. and Rapport, J.L (Eds) *Patriarchy and class: African women in the Home and the Workplace* Westview Press, London, UK.

White, L. (1983): "Colonial State and African Petty Bourgregeoise: Prostitution Poverty and Class Struggle in Nairobi." Cooper. F. (Ed) *Struggle for the City: Migrant Labour Capital, and the State in Urban Africa,* Sage Publications, Berverly Hills, California, USA.

Wilson G.M. (1980:) "A Study of Prostitutions in Mombasa." Nluga E. (ed) *Studies in Prostitution: East, West and South Africa, Zaire and Nevada.* Kenya Literature Bureau Nairobi, Kenya.

Talle, A., Biswalo, P.M., Scheiner, A.H., Klepp, K. (1995): *Introduction to Young People at Risk: Fighting AIDS in Northern Tanzania.* Scandinavian University Press, Oslo, Finland.

Chapter 3

Adeokun, L.A. (1990): "Research on Human Sexuality in Type II Countries." Chouinard A., Albert J. (eds): *Human Sexuality: Research Perspectives in a World Facing AIDS.* Background Papers and Reports of a Workshop Held at the International Development and Research Centre, IDRC, Ottawa, Canada.

BEST (1994): *Basic Education Statistics in Tanzania (BEST) 1989-1993.* Ministry of Education and Culture Dar es Salaam, Tanzania.

Bledsoe, C.H., Cohen, B. (1993): *Social Dynamics of Adolescent Fertility in Sub-Saharan Africa.* Washington DC: National Academy Press.

Bujra, J.M. (1995): "Women Entrepreneurs of Early Nairobi." *Canadian Journal of African Studies* VI (2).

Caldwell, J.C. (1989): "The Social Context of AIDS in Sub-Saharan Africa." *Population and Development Review* 15(2).

Cherlin A and Riley N.E. (1986): "Adolescent Fertility; Emerging Issues in Sub Saharan Africa." PHN Technical Note 86-23. World Bank, Washington, D.C.

Fundikira, S.R. (1985): "Sexuality, Fertility and Contraception, Knowledge and Attitudes Among Secondary School Girls in Dar es Salaam." Unpublished M.A. dissertation Department of Community Health, Faculty of Medicine, University of Dar es Salaam.

Grunseit, A., Kippax, S. (1993): *Effects of Sex Education on Young People's Sexual Behavior.* World Health Organization. Geneva.

Haram, L. (1995): "Negotiating Sexuality in Times of Economic Wants: The Young and Modern Meru Women." Klepp K., Biswalo P.M. Talle A. (eds): *Young People at Risk; Fighting AIDS in Northern Tanzania.* Scandinavian University Press, Oslo.

Huygens, P., Kajura, E., Seeley, J. and Barton, T. (1996): "Rethinking Methods for the Study of Sexual Behavior." *Social Science and Medicine*, 42(2).

Justesen, A., Kapiga S.H., Van Asten H. (1992): "Abortions in a Hospital Setting: Hidden Realities in Dar es Salaam, Tanzania." *Studies in Family Planning*, 23 (5).

Kessy, A. (1996): "Prevalence and Risk Factors for HIV and Other STDs Among Youth in Moshi Rural District." Unpublished Master of Medicine Dissertation, Institute of Public Health, University of Dar es Salaam, Dar es Salaam.

Leshabari, M.T. and Kaaya, S.F. (1994): "Youth Health and Development in Tanzania." Report prepared for the United Nations Fund for Population Activities (UNFPA),Dar es Salaam.

Leshabari, M.T. (1988): "Factors Influencing School Adolescent Fertility Behavior in Dar es Salaam, Tanzania." Unpublished Doctor of Science Thesis, Johns Hopkins University, School of Public Health, Baltimore Maryland.

Leshabari, M.T., Kaaya, S.F., Nguma, J.K. and Kapiga, S.H. (1996a): "Household Responses to HIV/AIDS in Mbeya Region, Tanzania." Institute of Public Health, University of Dar es Salaam, Dar es Salaam.

Leshabari, M.T., Mwanri, L.J; Minjas, J.N. and Yona E.N. (1996b): "Rapid Situation Analysis of the Health Status of School Aged Children in Tanzania." Institute of Public Health Muhimbili University College of Health Sciences, Dar es Salaam.

Levitt, M.Z., Selman, R.L., Richmond, J.B. (1991): "The Psychosocial Foundations of Early Adolescent High-risk Behavior: Implications for Research and Practice." *Journal of Research on Adolescence,* 1(4).

Lwihula, G., Nymuryekunge, K., Hamelmann, C. (1996): "Baseline Survey of Sexual and Reproductive Health knowledge, Perceptions and Behavior Among School Youths in Kinondoni District." Report submitted to the African Medical Research Foundation (AMREF) Dar es Salaam March.

Maro, P.S. (1975): "Population Growth and Agricultural Change in Kilimanjaro; 1920-1970." University of Dar es Salaam, Bureau of Resource Assessment and Land Use Planning *Research Paper No. 40,* Dar es Salaam, Tanzania.

Mound, W.A. (1988): "Adolescent Fertility in Tanzania: Knowledge, Perceptions and Practices." Family Planning Association of Tanzania (UMATI), Dar es Salaam.

Mpangile, G.S., Leshabari, M.T. and Kihwele, D.J. (1993): *"Factors Associated with Induced Abortion in Public Hospitals in Dar es Salaam, Tanzania."* Family Planning Association of Tanzania (UMATI) Dar es Salaam.

NACP (1994): *HIV/AIDS/STD Surveillance, Report* No. 8 Ministry of Health, Dar es Salaam.

Ntukula, M. (1994): "The Initiation Rite. In Tumbo-Masabo Z., Liljestrom R. (eds) *Chelewa Chelewa the Dilemma of Reenage Girls.* The Scandinavian Institute of African Studies. Ostersund, Sweden.

Sawaya, M. (1995): "School Dropouts and Related Problems." In Proceedings of the Workshop on Youth Growth and Related Problems in Tanzania. Book of abstracts and discussions. Monograph of the Social Science and Medicine Program of the University of Dar es Salaam, No. 1, Dar es Salaam.

Setel , P. (1995): "The Social Context of AIDS Education Among Young Men in

Northern Kilimanjaro." In Klepp K., Biswalo, P.M., Talle, A.(eds) *Young People at Risk; Fighting AIDS in Northern Tanzania.* Scandinavian University Press, Oslo.

TDHS (1993): *Tanzania Demographic and Health Survey 1991/1992*; Bureau of Statistics, Planning Commission, Dar es Salaam, Tanzania.

Van den Bergh, G. (1996): *"Sexual Relations in the Making; The Case of Adolescents in Rombo District, Kilimanjaro, Tanzania."* Unpublished thesis submitted in partial fulfillment of the requirements for the degree Masters of Science in Health Promotion, University of Bergen, Bergen, 1996.

Worthman, C. and Whiting, J. (1987): "Social Change in Adolescent Sexual Behavior, Mate Selection, and Premarital Pregnancy Rates in Kikuyu Community." *Ethos,* 15(2).

Chapter 4

Bassuk, E. and L. Rubin (1987): "Homeless Children: A Neglected Population." *American Journal of Orthopsychiatry* 57(2).

Blanc-Szanton, C. (1994): *Urban Children in Distress: Global Predicaments and Innovative Strategies.* UNICEF Studies, Gordon and Breach, Newark, NJ.

Cohen, E., R. McKenzie and G. Yates (1991): " HEADSS, A Psycho-social Risk Assessment Instrument: Implications for Designing Effective Intervention Programs for Runaway Youth." *Journal of Adolescent Health,* 12.

Knaul, F. (1995a): *Counting the Street Children of Bogota: Defined Away, Missing or Out of Sight.* Working Paper Series no. 95-07, Harvard Center for Population and Development Studies.

Knaul, F. (1995b): "Young Workers, Street Life, and Gender: The Effect of Education and Work Experience on Earnings in Colombia." Ph.D. Dissertation, Department of Economics, Harvard University.

Lugalla, J. (1995): "Crisis, Urbanization and Urban Poverty in Tanzania: A Study of Urban Poverty and Survival Politics." University Press of America, Lanham, MD.

Mutuku, M. and R. Mutiso (1994): "Kenya: The Urban Threat for Women and Children." In C. Blanc-Szanton (ed.), *Urban Children in Distress: Global Predicaments and Innovative Strategies,* UNICEF Studies, Gordon and Breach, Newark, NJ.

Patel, S. (1990): "Street Children, Hotel Boys and Children of Pavement Dwellers and Construction Workers in Bombay - How They Meet Their Daily Needs." *Environment and Urbanization* 2 (2).

Rajani, R. and M. Kudrati (1996): "The Varieties of Sexual Experience of the Street Children of Mwanza, Tanzania." In S. Zeidenstein and K. Moore (eds.), *Learning About Sexuality: A Practical Beginning,* The Population International Women's Health Coalition, New York.

Rizzini, I. Munoz-Vargas, M. & Galeano, L. Brazil (1994): "A New Concept of Childhood." In C. Blanc-Szanton (ed.), *Urban Children in Distress: Global Predicaments and Innovative Strategies,* UNICEF Studies, Gordon and Breach, Newark, NJ.

Sibthorpe, B., J. Drinkwater, K. Gardner and G. Bammer (1995): "Drug Use, Binge Drinking and Attempted Suicide Among Homeless and Potentially Homeless Youths." *Australian and New Zealand Journal of Psychiatry* 29.

UNICEF (1990): *Women and Children in Tanzania: An Overview.* UNICEF and the Government of the United Republic of Tanzania.

Wagner, J. and E. Menek (1990): "The Mental Health of the Homeless Children." Paper presented at the Conference of the American Association of Public Health, New York City.

Chapter 5

Carswell, J.W. (1988): "Impact of AIDS in the Developing World." *British Medical Bulletin,* 44(1):183-202.

Dolmans, W.M., Njelesani, E.K., Van Asten H, Kigadye, F.C., Heessen, F.W., Velema, J.P. *et. al.* (1992): "Prevention of HIV Transmission Through Blood Transfusion in Tanzania." *Tropical Geographical Medicine,* 44:285.

Heydmann , D.L., Edstrom, K. (1991): "Strategies for AIDS Prevention and Control in Sub-Saharan Africa." *AIDS,* 5: 197-208.

Hunter, S.S. (1990): Orphans as a Window on the AIDS Epidemic in Sub-Saharan Africa: Initial Results and Implications of a Study in Uganda. *Social Science and Medicine,* 31 (6):681-690.

Killewo J., Sandstrom A.,Dahlgren L., Wall, S. (1994): "Knowlegde, Attitudes and Perceptions Regarding HIV Infection risk: Communicating With the People on the Basis for Planning Interventions in Epidemiology Towards the Control of HIV Infection. Thesis for Ph.D., Department of Epidemiology and Public Health, Umea University, Sweden.

Killewo J., Dahlgren L., Sandstrom A. (1994): "Socio Geographical Patterns of HIV- I Transmission in Kagera Region, Tanzania." *Social Science and Medicine,* 38(1), 129-134.

Larsson B. (1991): *Conversion to Greater Freedom: Women, Church and Social Change in North Western Tanzania Under Colonial Rule.* Acta Universitatis Upsalienis, Studia Historica Upsaliensia 162, 96.

Lesbordes, J.L., Chassingol, S., Ray, E., *et. al.* (1986): " Malnutrition and HIV Infection in Children in the Central African Republic." *Lancet* (ii), 337-338.

Leshabari, M.T., Kaaya, S.F., Kapiga, S., Nguma, J. (1995): "Community Coping Mechanisms and the HIV/AIDS Epidemic in Mbeya." Conference on The Impact of AIDS on the Family in Tanzania. 20 March. USAID/NACP, Dar es Salaam, Tanzania.

Lwihula, G., Dahlgren, L., Killewo, J., Sandstrom, A. (1993): "AIDS Epidemic in Kagera-the Experience of Local People." *AIDS Care Vol* 5 (3), 347-57.

Mhalu, F. (1993): "Counseling and HIV Testing as an Intervention Strategy in the Control of HIV Infection." *Proceedings of Workshop on AIDS* May 10-11, Bukoba. Kagera AIDS Research Project, Dar es Salaam, Tanzania.

NACP (1995): Review Report No. 10. Ministry of Health Tanzania Mainland and Zanibar, Dar es Salaam, Tanzania.

Mnyika, K.S., Kleep K., Kvale G., Nilseen S., Kissila P., Ole King'ori N. (1994): "Prevalence of HIV Infection in Urban, Semi-urban and Urban Areas in Arusha Region, Tanzania." *AIDS* 8:1477-81.

O'Connor P., Leshabari, M.T., Lwihula G. (1992): "Ethnographic Study of the Truck Stop Environment in Tanzania." AIDSTECH. Family Health International, Durham, NC, U.S.A.

Schuerman L., Seynhaeve V., Bachshmidt I, Tchotch V., Quattara, S.A., De The' G. (1988): "Severe Malnutrition and Paediatric AIDS: A Diagnostic Problem in Rural Africa." *AIDS* 2:232-3.

UNICEF (1990): *Women and Children in Tanzania: A Situational Analysis*, The Government of the United Republic of Tanzania and United Nations Children's Fund Dar es Salaam.

Chapter 6

Adult Mortality and Morbidity Project (2000): "Cause-specific Adult Mortality: Evidence from Community-based Surveillance – Selected Sites, Tanzania, 1992-1998." Morb Mortal Wkly Rep. 49.

Bakari M., Lyamuya E, Mugusi, F., Aris, E., Chale, S., Magao, P., Jossiah, R., Janabi, M., Swai, A., Pallangyo, N., Sandstrom, E., Mhalu, F., Biberfeld, G., Pallangyo, K. (2000): "The Prevalence and Incidence of HIV-1 Infection and Syphilis in a Cohort of Police Officers in Dar es Salaam, Tanzania: A Potential Population for HIV Vaccine Trials." *AIDS* 14.

Barongo, L.R., Borgdorff, M.W., Mosha, F.F., Nicoll, A., Grosskurth, H., Senkoro, K.P., Newell, J.N., Changalucha, J., Klokke, A.H., Killewo, J.Z., Velema, J.P., Hayes, R.J., Dunn, D.T., Muller, L.A.S., Rugemalila, J.B. (1992): "The Epidemiology of HIV-1 Infection in Urban Areas, Roadside Settlements and Rural Villages in Mwanza Region, Tanzania." *AIDS 6.*

Barongo, L.R., Borgdorff, M.W., Newell, J.N., Senkoro, K.P., Klokke, A.H., Changalucha, J., Deville, W., Velema, J.P., Coutinho, R.A., Gabone, R.M. (1994): "Intake of a Cohort Study of Urban Factory Workers in Northwest Tanzania: Risk Factors for HIV-1 Infection." *Trop Geogr Med 46.*

Blackard, J.T., Renjifo, B., Fawzi, W., Hertzmark, E., Msamanga, G., Mwakagile, D., Hunter, D., Spiegelman, D., Sharghi, N., Kagoma, C.(2001): "Essex M. HIV-1 LTR Subtype and Perinatal Transmission." *Virology 287.*

Boerma, J.T., Urassa, M., Senkoro, K., Klokke, A., Ng'weshemi, J.Z.L. (1999): "Spread of HIV Infection in a Rural Area of Tanzania." *AIDS 13.*

Borgdorff, M.W., Barongo, L.R., van Jaarsveld, E., Klokke, A., Senkoro, K., Newell, J., Nicoll, A., Mosha, F., Grosskurth, H., Swai, R., van Asten H., Velema, J., Hayes, R., Muller, L., Rugemalila, J. (1993): "Sentinel Surveillance for HIV-1 Infection: How Representative are Blood Donors, Outpatients With Fever, Anaemia, or Sexually Transmitted Diseases, and Antenatal Clinic Attenders in Mwanza Region, Tanzania." *AIDS 7.*

Bredberg-Raden, U., Urassa, W., Urassa, E., Lyamuya, E., Msemo, G., Kawo, G., Kazimoto, T., Massawe, A., Grankvist, O., Mbena, E., Karlsson, K., Mhalu, F., Biberfeld, G. (1995): "Predictive Markers for Mother-to-Child Transmission of HIV-1 in Dar es Salaam, Tanzania." *J Acquir Immune Defic Syndr 8.*

Bureau of Statistics and Macro International (1993): *Tanzania Demographic and Health*

Survey 1991/1992. Calverton: Macro International Inc. and Bureau of Statistics, Dar es Salaam, Tanzania.

Bureau of Statistics and Macro International (1995): "Tanzania Knowledge, Attitudes and Practices Survey, 1994." Calverton: *Macro International Inc. and Bureau of Statistics,* Dar es Salaam, Tanzania.

Bureau of Statistics and Macro International (1997): "Tanzania Demographic and Health Survey, 1996." Calverton: *Macro International Inc. and Bureau of Statistics*, Dar es Salaam, Tanzania.

Buve, A., Bishikwabo-Nsarhaza, K., Mutangadura, G. (2002): "The Spread and Effect of HIV-1 Infection in Sub-Saharan Africa." *Lancet 359.*

Carael, M., Cleland, J., Deheneffe, J.C., Ferry, B., Ingham, R. (1995): "Sexual Behavior in Developing Countries: Implications for HIV Control." *AIDS 9.*

Carael, M. (1997): "Urban-Rural Differentials in HIV/STDs and Sexual Behavior. In Herdt, G. *(ed): Sexual Cultures and Migration in the Era of AIDS: Anthropological and Demographic Perspectives*." Oxford University Press.

Chum, H.J., O'Brien, R.J., Chonde, T.M., Graf, P., Rieder, H.L. (1996): "An Epidemiological Study of Muberculosis and HIV Infection in Tanzania, 1991-1993." *AIDS* 10.

Fawzi, W.W., Msamanga, G., Hunter, D.J., Urassa, E., Renjifo, B., Mwakagile, D., Hertzmark, E., Coley, J., Garland, M., Kapiga, S., Antelman, G., Essex, M., Spiegelman, D. (2000): "Randomized Trial of Vitamin Supplements in Relation to Vertical Transmission of HIV-1 in Tanzania." *J Acquir Immune Defic Syndr 23.*

Fawzi, W.W., Msamanga, G., Renjifo, B., Spiegelman, D., Urassa, E., Hashemi, L., Antelman, G., Essex, M., Hunter, D. (2001): "Predictors of Intrauterine and Intrapartum Transmission of HIV-1 Among Tanzanian Women." *AIDS 15.*

Fawzi, W.W., Msamanga, G.I., Spiegelman, D., Urassa, E.J., McGrath, N., Mwakagile, D., Antelman, G., Mbise, R., Herrera, G., Kapiga, S., Willett, W., Hunter, D.J. (1998): "Randomized Trial of Effects of Vitamin Supplements on Pregnancy Outcomes and T Cell Counts in HIV-1- Infected Women in Tanzania." *Lancet 351.*

Fothal, D., Mhalu, F.S., Dahoma, A. (1986): "AIDS in Tanzania. Second International Conference on AIDS." Paris, (*Abstract no. S17F*).

Glynn, J.R., Carael, M., Auvert, B., Kahindo, M., Chege, J., Musonda, R., Kaona, F., Buve, A. (2001): "Why Do Young Women Have a Much Higher Prevalence of HIV Than Young Men?" A study in Kisumu, Kenya and Ndola, Zambia. *AIDS 15 (Suppl. 4).*

Gray, R., Wawer, M., Serwadda, D., Sewankambo, N., Li, C., Wabwire-Mangen, F., Paxton, L., Kiwanuka, N., Kigozi, G., Konde-Lule, J., Quinn, T.C., Gaydos, C.A., McNairn, D. (1998): "Population-based Study of Fertility in Women With HIV-1 Infection in Uganda." *Lancet 351.*

Gregson, S., Zaba, B., Garnett, G.P. (1999): "Low Fertility in Women With HIV and the Impact of the Epidemic on Orphanhood and Early Childhood Mortality in Sub-Saharan Africa." *AIDS 13* (Suppl. A).

Grosskurth, H., Mosha, F., Todd, J., Mwijarubi, E., Klokke, A., Senkoro, K., Mayaud, P., Changalucha, J., Nicoll, A., ka-Gina, G., Newell, J., Mugeye, K., Mabey, D., Hayes, R. (1995): "Impact of Improved Treatment of Sexually Transmitted Diseases on HIV Infection in Rural Tanzania: Randomized Controlled Trial." *Lancet 346.*

Grosskurth, H., Mosha, F., Todd, J., Newell, J., Klokke, A., Changalucha, J., West, B., Mayaud, P., Gavyole, A., Gabone, R., Mabey, D., Hayes, R. (1995): "A Community Trial of the Impact of Improved Sexually Transmitted Disease Treatment on the HIV Epidemic in Rural Tanzania: 2. Baseline Survey Results." *AIDS 9.*

Hoelscher, M., Hanker, S., Barin, F., Cheingsong-Popov, R., Dietrich, U., Jordan-Harder, B., Olaleye, D., Nagele, E, Markuzzi, A., Mwakagile, D., Minja, F., Weber, J., Gurtler, L., Von Sonnenburg, F. (1998): "HIV Type 1 V3 Serotyping of Tanzanian Samples: Probable Reasons for Mismatching With Genetic Subtyping." *AIDS Res Hum Retroviruses 14.*

Hoelscher, M., Kim, B., Maboko, L., Mhalu, F., von Sonnenburg, F., Birx, D.L., McCutchan, F.E., and UNAIDS Network for HIV Isolation and Characterization (2001): "High Proportion of Unrelated HIV-1 Intersubtype Recombinants in the Mbeya Region of Southwest Tanzania." *AIDS 15.*

Holm-Hansen, C., Ayehunie, S., Johansson, B., Nkya, W., Shao, J., Haukenes, G. (1996): "HIV-1 Proviral DNA Sequences of env gp41 PCR Amplificates From Tanzania." *APMIS 104.*

Hugonnet, S., Mosha, F., Todd, J., Mugeye, K., Klokke, A., Ndeki, L., Ross, D., Grosskurth, H., Hayes, R. (2002): " Incidence of HIV Infection in Stable Sexual Partnerships: A Retrospective Cohort Study of 1802 Couples in Mwanza Region, Tanzania." *J Aquir Immune Defic Syndr 30.*

Janssens, W., Buve, A., Nkengasong, J.N. (1997): "The Puzzle of HIV-1 Subtypes in Africa." *AIDS 11.*

Kapinga, S.H., Lugalla, J.L.P. "Sexual Behaviour Patterns and Condom Use in Tanzania: Results From the 1996 Demographic and Health Survey." *AIDS Care* (in press).

Kapiga, S.H., Lwihula, G.K., Shao, J.F., Hunter, D.J. (1995): "Predictors of AIDS Knowledge, Condom Use and High-risk Sexual Behavior Among Women in Dar es Salaam, Tanzania." *Int. J. STD AIDS 6.*

Kapiga, S.H., Lyamuya, E.F., Lwihula, G.K., Hunter, D.J. (1998): "The Incidence of HIV Infection Among Women Using Family Planning Methods in Dar es Salaam, Tanzania." *AIDS 12.*

Kapiga, S.H., Lyamuya, E.F., Vuylsteke, B., Spiegelman, D., Larsen, U., Hunter, D.J. (2000): "Risk Factors for HIV-1 Sero-prevalence Among Family Planning Clients in Dar es Salaam, Tanzania. " *Afr. J. Reprod Health 4.*

Kapiga, S.H., Sam, N.E., Shao, J.F., Renjifo, B., Masenga, E.J., Kiwelu, I.E., Manongi, R., Fawzi, W., Essex, M. (2002): "HIV-1 Epidemic Among Female Bar and Hotel Workers in Northern Tanzania: Risk Factors and Opportunities for Prevention." *J. Acquir. Immune Defic. Syndr. 29.*

Kapiga, S.H., Shao, J.F., Lwihula, G.K., Hunter, D.J. (1994): "Risk Factors for HIV Infection

Among Women in Dar es Salaam, Tanzania." *J. Aquir. Immune Defic. Syndr. 7.*
Kapiga, S.H., Vuylsteke, B., Lyamuya, E.F., Dallabetta, G., Laga, M. (1998): "Evaluation of Sexually Transmitted Diseases Diagnostic Algorithms Among Family Planning Clients in Dar es Salaam, Tanzania." *Sex Transm Inf. 74(Suppl. 1).*
Kapiga, S.H. (1996): "Determinants of Multiple Sexual Partners and Condom Use Among Sexually Active Tanzanians." *East Afr. Med. J. 73.*
Kawo, G., Karlsson, K., Lyamuya, E., Kalokola, F., Fataki, M., Kazimoto, T., Kitundu, J., Msaky, H., Munubhi, E., Ostborn, A., Bredberg-Raden, U., Swai, A., Mbise, R., Msengi, A., Mhalu, F., Biberfeld, G. (2000): "Prevalence of HIV Type 1 Infection, Associated Clinical Features and Mortality Among Hospitalized Children in Dar es Salaam, Tanzania." *Scand. J. Infect. Dis. 32.*
Killewo, J., Nyamuryekunge, K., Sandstrom, A., Bredberg-Raden, U., Wall, S., Mhalu, F., Biberfeld, G. (1990): Prevalence of HIV-1 Infection in the Kagera region of Tanzania: A Population-based Study. *AIDS 4.*
Killewo, J.Z., Sandstrom, A., Bredberg Raden, U., Mhalu, F.S., Biberfeld, G., Wall, S. (1994): "Prevalence and Incidence of Syphilis and Its Association with HIV-1 Infection in A Population-based Study in the Kagera Region of Tanzania." *Int. J. STD AIDS 5.*
Killewo, J.Z.J., Sandstrom, A., Bredberg-Raden, U., Mhalu, F.S., Biberfeld, G., Wall, S. (1993): "Incidence of HIV-1 Infection Among Adults in the Kagera Region of Tanzania." *Int. J. Epidemiol. 22.*
Klepp, K-I, Biswalo, P.M., Talle, A. (eds). (1995): *Young People at Risk. Fighting AIDS in Northern Tanzania.* Oslo: Scandinavian University Press.
Klouman, E., Masenga, E.J., Sam, N.E., Klepp, K-I. (2000): "Asymptomatic Gonorrhea and Chlamydial Infection in a Population-based and Work-site Based Sample of Men in Kilimanjaro, Tanzania." *Int. J. STD AIDS 11.*
Klouman, E., Massenga, E.J., Klepp, K-I, Sam, N.E., Nkya, W., Nkya, C. (1997): "HIV and Reproductive Tract Infections in a Total Village Population in Rural Kilimanjaro, Tanzania: Women at Increased Risk." *J. Acquir. Immune Defic. Syndr. 14.*
Konde-Lule, J.K., Tumwesigye, M.N., Lubanga, R.G.N. (1997): "Trends in Attitudes and Behavior Relevant to AIDS in Ugandan Community." *East Afr. Med. J. 74.*
Konings, E., Blattner, W.A., Levin, A., Brubaker, G., Siso, Z., Shao, J., Goedert, J.J., Anderson, R.M. (1994): "Sexual Behavior Survey in A Rural Area of Northwest Tanzania." *AIDS 8.*
Kwesigabo, G., Killewo, J.Z.J., Godoy, C., Urassa, W., Mbena, E., Mhalu, F., Biberfeld, G., Wall, S., Sandstrom, A. (1998): "Decline in the Prevalence of HIV-1 Infection in Young Women in the Kagera Region of Tanzania." *J. Acquir. Immune Defic. Syndr. 17.*
Kwesigabo, G., Killewo, J.Z.J., Urassa, W., Mbena, E., Mhalu, F., Lugalla, J.L., Godoy, C., Biberfeld, G., Emmelin, M., Wall, S., Sandstrom, A. (2000): "Monitoring of HIV-1 Infection Prevalence and Trends in the General Population Using Pregnant Women as a Sentinel Population: 9 Years' Experience From Kagera Region of Tanzania." *J. Acquir. Immune Defic. Syndr. 23.*

Langeland, N., Haarr, L., Mhalu, F. (1998): Prevalence of HSV-2 Antibodies Among STD Clinic Patients in Tanzania. *Int. J. STD AIDS 9.*

Laukamm-Josten, U., Mwizarubi, B.K., Outwater, A., Mwaijonga, C.L., Valadez, J.J., Nyamwaya, D., Swai, R., Saidel, T., Nyamuryekung'e, K. (2000): "Preventing HIV Infection Through Peer Education and Condom Promotion Among Truck Drivers and Their Sexual Partners in Tanzania, 1990-1993." *AIDS Care 12.*

Laukamm-Josten, U., Ocheng, O., Mwizarubi, B.K., Mwaijonga, C.L., Swai, R., Trupin, M. (1993): "HIV and Syphilis Sero-prevalence and Risk Factors in Truck Stops and Nearby Communities in Tanzania." *Eighth International Conference on AIDS*, Amsterdam, PoC 4162.

Lugalla, J., Emmelin, M., Mutembei, A., Comoro, C., Killewo, J., Kwesigabo, G., Sandstrom, A., Dahlgren, I. (1999): "The Social Cultural Contexts of HIV/AIDS Transmission in the Kagera Region, Tanzania." *Journal of Asian and African Studies, Vol. XXXIV*, No. 4.

Lugalla, J. (1995): *Adjustment and Poverty in Tanzania.* Hamburg/Muenster, Germany: Lit Verlag.

Lugalla, J. (1995): "The Impact of Structural Adjustment Policies on Women's and Children's Health in Tanzania." *Review of African Political Economy 63.*

Matee, M.I., Lyamuya, E.F., Simon, E.E., Mwinula, J.H., Mbena, E.C., Samaranayake, L.P., Scheutz, F.F. (1995): "Clinical Predictors of HIV-1 Infection Among Preschool Children in Dar es Salaam, Tanzania." *East Afr. Med. J. 72.*

Matee, M.I.N., Lyamuya, E.F., Mbena, E.C., Magessa, P.M., Sufi, J., Marwa, G.J., Mwasulama, O.J., Mbwana, J. (1999): "Prevalence of Transfusion-Associated Viral Infections and Syphilis Among Blood Donors in Muhimbili Medical Center, Dar es Salaam, Tanzania." *East Afr. Med. J. 76.*

Mayaud, P., Gill, D.K., Weiss, H.A., Uledi, E., Kopwe, L., Todd, J., ka-Gina, G., Grosskurth, H., Hayes, R.J., Mabey, D.C., Lacey, C.J. (2001): "The Interrelation of HIV, Cervical Human Papillomavirus, and Neoplasia Among Antenatal Clinic Attenders in Tanzania." *Sex Transm. Inf. 77.*

Mayaud, P., Grosskurth, H., Changalucha, J., Todd, J., West, B., Gabone, R., Senkoro, K., Rusizoka, M., Laga, M., Hayes, R., Mabey, D. (1995): "Risk Assessment and Other Screening Options for Gonorrhea and Chlamydial Infections in Women Attending Rural Tanzanian Antenatal Clinics." *WHO Bulletin 73.*

Mgalla, Z. and Pool, R. (1997): "Sexual Relationships, Condom Use and Risk Perception Among Female Bar Workers in North-west Tanzania." *AIDS Care 9.*

Mhalu, F., Hirji, K., Ijumba, P., Shao, J., Mbena, E., Mwakagile, D., Akim, C., Senge, P., Mponezya, H., Bredberg-Raden, U., Biberfeld, G. (1991): "A Cross-Sectional Study of A Program for HIV Infection Control Among Public House Workers." *J. Acquir. Immune Defic. Syndr. 4.*

Mlawa, H.M. and Green, R.H. (1991): *Through Structural Adjustment to Transformation in Sub-Saharan Africa.* Dar es Salaam, Dar es Salaam University Press.

Mnyika, K.S., Klepp, K., Kvale, G., Nilssen, S., Kissila, P.E., Ole-King'ori, N. (1994): "Prevalence of HIV-1 Infection in Urban, Semi-urban and Rural Areas in Arusha Region, Tanzania." *AIDS 8.*

Mnyika, K.S., Klepp, K., Kvale, G., Ole-King'ori, N. (1996): "Risk Factors for HIV-1 Infection Among Women in the Arusha Region of Tanzania." *J. Aquir. Immune Defic. Syndr. 11.*

Mnyika, K.S., Klepp, K-I, Kvale, G., Ole-King'ori, N. (1997): "Determinants of High-risk Sexual Behavior and Condom Use Among Adults in the Arusha Region, Tanzania." *Int. J. STD AIDS 8.*

Mosha, F., Nicoll, A., Barongo, L., Borgdorff, M., Newell, J., Senkoro, K., Grosskurth, H., Changalucha, J., Klokke, A., Killewo, J., Velema, J., Muller, A.S., Rugemalila, J., Hayes, R., Mabey, D. (1993): "A Population-based Study of Syphilis and Sexually Transmitted Disease Syndromes in North-western Tanzania. 1. Prevalence and Incidence." *Genitourin Med 69.*

Munguti, K., Grosskurth, H., Newell, J., Senkoro, K., Mosha, F., Todd, J., Mayaud, P., Gavyole, A., Quigley, M., Hayes, R. (1997): "Patterns of Sexual Behavior in A Rural Population in North-western Tanzania." *Soc. Sci. Med. 44.*

Mwakagile, D., Mmari, E., Makwaya, C., Mbwana, J., Biberfeld, G., Mhalu, F., Sandstrom, E. (2001): "Sexual Behavior Among Youths at High-risk of HIV-1 Infection in Dar es Salaam, Tanzania." *Sex Transm. Inf. 77.*

Mwakagile, D., Swai, A.B.M., Sandstrom, E., Urassa, E., Biberfeld, G., Mhalu, F.S. (1996): "High Frequency of Sexually Transmitted Diseases Among Pregnant Women in Dar es Salaam, Tanzania: Need for Intervention." *East Afr. Med. J. 76.*

Mwizarubi, B., Hamelmann, C., Nyamuryekung'e, K. (1997): "Working in High-transmission Areas: Truck Routes." In Ng'weshemi, J., Boerma, T., Bennet, J., Schapink, D. (eds). *HIV Prevention and AIDS Care in Africa. A District Level Approach* (pp. 137-149). *Amsterdam, Royal Tropical Institute.*

Natasha, E., Ntembelea, T., Mayaud, P., Saidi, W., Todd, J., Mujaya, B., Tendo-Wambua, L. (1998): "Sexual and Reproductive Health Among Primary and Secondary School Pupils in Mwanza, Tanzania: Need for Intervention." *AIDS Care 10.*

National Bureau of Statistics (Tanzania) and Macro International Inc. Tanzania (2000): *Reproductive and Child Health Survey 1999.* Calverton, Maryland: National Bureau of Statistics and Macro International Inc.

Newell, J., Senkoro, K., Mosha, F., Grosskurth, H., Nicoll, A., Barongo, L., Borgdorff, M., Klokke, A., Changalucha, J., Killewo, J., Velema, J., Muller, A.S., Rugemalila, J., Mabey, D., Hayes, R. (1992): "A Population-based Study of Syphilis and Sexually Transmitted Disease Syndromes in North-Western Tanzania. 2. Risk Factors and Health Seeking Behavior." *Genitourin Med. 69.*

Obasi, A., Mosha, F., Quigley, M., Sekirassa, Z., Gibbs, T., Munguti, K., Todd, J., Grosskurth, H., Mayaud, P., Changalucha, J., Brown, D., Mabey, D., Hayes, R. (1999): "Antibody to Herpes Simplex Virus Type 2 as A Marker of Sexual Risk Behavior in Rural Tanzania." *J. Inf. Dis. 179.*

Obasi, A.I., Balira, R., Todd, J., Ross, D.A., Changalucha, J., Mosha, F., Grosskurth, H., Peeling, R., Mabey, D.C., Hayes, R.J. (2001): "Prevalence of HIV and *Chlamydia Trachomatis* Infection in 15-19 Year Olds in Rural Tanzania." *Trop. Med. Int. Health 6.*

Outwater, A., Nkya, L., Lwihula, G., O'Connor, P., Leshabari, M., Nguma, J., Mwizarubi, B., Laukamm-Josten, U., Green, E.C., Hassig, S.E. (2000): "Patterns of Partnership and Condom Use in Two Communities of Female Sex Workers in Tanzania." *J. Assoc. Nurses AIDS Care 11.*

Petry, K.U. and Kingu, H. (1996): "HIV Infection Among Pregnant Women in Lindi, Tanzania, 1989-1993." *Int. J. STD AIDS 7.*

Piot, P, Bartos, M., Ghys, P.D., Walker, N., Schwartlander, B. (2001): "The Global Impact of HIV/AIDS." *Nature 410.*

Quigley, M., Munguti, K., Grosskurth, H., Todd, J., Mosha, F., Senkoro, K., Newell, J., Mayaud, P., ka-Gina, G., Klokke, A., Mabey, D., Gavyole, A., Hayes, R. (1997): "Sexual Behavior Patterns and Other Risk Factors for HIV Infection in Rural Tanzania: A Case-control Study." *AIDS 11.*

Range, N., Ipuge, Y.A., O'Brien, R.J., Egwaga, S.M., Mfinanga, S.G., Chonde, T.M., Mukadi, Y.D., Borgdorff, M.W. (2001): "Trends in HIV Prevalence Among Tuberculosis Patients in Tanzania, 1991-1998." *Int. J. Tuberc. Lung. Dis. 5.*

Renjifo, B., Chaplin, B., Mwakagile, D., Shah, P., Vannberg, F., Msamanga, G., Hunter, D., Fawzi, W., Essex, M. (1998): "Epidemic Expansion of HIV Type 1 Subtype C and Recombinant Genotypes in Tanzania." *AIDS Res Hum Retroviruses 14.*

Renjifo, B., Fawzi, W., Mwakagile, D., Hunter, D., Msamanga, G., Spiegelman, D., Garland, M., Kagoma, C., Kim, A., Chaplin, B., Hertzmark, E., Essex, M. (2001): "Differences in Perinatal Transmission Among Human Immunodeficiency Virus Type 1 Genotypes." *J. Hum. Virol. 4.*

Renjifo, B., Gilbert, P., Chaplin, B., Vannberg, F., Mwakagile, D., Msamanga, G., Hunter, D., Fawzi, W., Essex, M. (1999): "Emerging Recombinant Human Immunodeficiency Viruses: Uneven Representation of the Envelope V3 Region." *AIDS 13.*

Robbins, K.E., Bandea, C.I., Levin, A., Goedert, J.J., Blattner, W.A., Brubaker, G., Brown, T.M., Schochetman, G., Kalish, M.L., Shao, J., O'Brien T.R. (1996): "Genetic Variability of Human Immunodeficiency Virus Type 1 in Rural Northwest Tanzania." *AIDS Res. Hum. Retroviruses 12.*

Rodriguez, M.M.P., Obasi, A., Mosha, F., Todd, J., Brown, D., Changalucha, J., Mabey, D., Ross, D., Grosskurth, H., Hayes, R. (2002): "Herpes Simplex Virus Type 2 Infection Increases HIV Incidence: A Prospective Study in Rural Tanzania." *AIDS 16.*

Ross, A., Morgan, D., Lubega, R., Carpenter, L.M., Mayanja, B., Whitworth, J.A.G. (1999): "Reduced Fertility Associated with HIV: The Contribution of Pre-existing Subfertility." *AIDS 13.*

Royce, R.A., Sena, A., Cates, W., Cohen, M.S. (1997): "Sexual Transmission of HIV." *N. Engl. J. Med. 336.*

Senkoro, K.P., Boerma, T.J., Klokke, A.H., Ng'weshemi, J.Z., Muro, A.S., Gabone, R., Borgdorff, M.W. (2000): "HIV Incidence and HIV-Associated Mortality in A Cohort of Factory Workers and Their Spouses in Tanzania." *J. Aquir. Immune Defic. Syndr. 23.*

Serwadda, D., Mugerwa, R.D., Sewankambo, N.K., Lwegaba, A., Carswell, J.W., Kirya, G.B., Bayley, A.C., Downing, R.G., Tedder, R.S., Clayden, S.A. (1985): "Slim Disease: A New Disease in Uganda and Its Association with HTLV-III Infection." *Lancet 2.*

Setel, P. (1995): "The Effects of HIV and AIDS on Fertility in East and Central Africa." *Health Transit. Rev. 7 (Suppl. 1).*

Shao, J., Brubaker, G., Levin, A., Kibauri, A., Massesa, E., Siso, Z., Konings, E., Clayton, Y., Kumby, D., Alexander, S., Waters, D., Drummond, J., Biggar, R.J., Scott, G., Miller, G., Goedert, J.J., Blattner, W.A. (1994): "Population-Based Study of HIV-1 Infection in 4,086 Subjects in Northwest Tanzania." *J. Acquir. Immune Defic. Syndr. 7.*

Silberschmidt, M., Rasch, V. (2001): "Adolescent Girls, Illegal Abortions and "Sugar-daddies" in Dar es Salaam: Vulnerable Victims and Active Social Agents." *Soc. Sci. Med. 52.*

Siwka, W., Schwinn, A., Baczko, K., Pardowitz, I., Mhalu, F., Shao, J., Rethwilm, A., ter Meulen, V. (1994): "*vpu* and *env* Sequence Variability of HIV-1 Isolates from Tanzania." *AIDS Res. Hum. Retroviruses 12.*

Soderberg, S., Temihango, W., Kadete, C., Ekstedt, B., Masawe, A., Vahlne, A., Horal, P. (1994): "Prevelance of HIV-1 Infection in Rural, Semi-urban and Urban Villages in Southwest Tanzania: Estimates from A Blood-donor Study. *AIDS 8.*

Tanzania AIDS Project (1997): *Mid-term Review Report. Population Technical Assistance Project Report No. 97-096-053.*

Todd, J., Balira, R., Grosskurth, H., Mayaud, P., Mosha, F., ka-Gina, G., Klokke, A., Gabone, R., Gavyole, A., Mabey, D., Hayes, R. (1997): "HIV Associated Adult Mortality in A Rural Tanzanian Population." *AIDS 11.*

Todd, J., Munguti, K., Grosskurth, H., Mngara, J., Changalucha, J., Mayaud, P., Mosha, F., Gavyole, A., Mabey, D., Hayes, R. (2001): "Risk Factors for Active Syphilis and TPHA Seroconversion in A Rural African Population." *Sex Transm. Infect. 77.*

UNAIDS (2000): *Report on the Global HIV/AIDS Epidemic, June 2000.* Joint United Nations Program on HIV/AIDS, Geneva.

UNAIDS/WHO (2001): *Report on the Global HIV/AIDS Epidemic - December 2001.* Geneva, Switzerland.

United Republic of Tanzania, Ministry of Health (2002): *National Guidelines for Clinical Management of HIV/AIDS*, Dar es Salaam, Tanzania.

United Republic of Tanzania (1995): *1995 MTP-II Review*. Ministry of Health, Dar es Salaam, Tanzania.

United Republic of Tanzania (1998): *Strategic Framework for the Third Medium Term Plan (MTP-III): 1998-2002.* Ministry of Health, Dar es Salaam, Tanzania.

United Republic of Tanzania (2000): *HIV/AIDS/STDs Surveillance Report No. 15, December 2000.* Dar es Salaam, Tanzania.

Urassa, M., Boerma, J.T., Isingo, R., Ngalula, J., Ng'weshemi, J., Mwaluko, G., Zaba, B. (2001): "The Impact of HIV/AIDS on Mortality and Household Mobility in Rural Tanzania." *AIDS 15.*

Van Cleeff, M.R.A. and Chum, H.J. (1995): "The Proportion of Tuberculosis Cases in Tanzania Attributable to Human Immunodeficiency Virus." *Int. J. Epidemiol 24.*

Van den Broek, J., Borgdorff, M.W., Pakker, N.G., Chum, H.J., Klokke, A.H., Senkoro, K.P., Newell, J.N. (1993): "HIV-1 Infection as A Risk Factor for the Development of Tuberculosis Disease: A Population-based Case-Control Study in Tanzania." *Int. J. Epidemiol 22.*

Walker, N., Garcia-Calleja, J.M., Heaton, L., Asamoah-Odei, E., Poumerol, G., Lazzari, S., Ghys, P.D., Schwartlander, B., Stanecki, K.A. (2001): "Epidemiological Analysis of the Quality of HIV Sero-surveillance in the World: How Well Do We Track the Epidemic?" *AIDS 15.*

World Health Organization (2000): *World Health Report 2000*. World Health Organization, Switzerland, Geneva.

World Health Organization (1988): *Sentinel Surveillance for HIV Infection.* World Health Organization, Geneva, Switzerland, (WHO/GPA/DIR/88.8).

Zaba, B. and Gregson, S. (1998): "Measuring the Impact of HIV on Fertility in Africa." *AIDS 12 (Suppl. 1).*

Zwart, G., Wolfs, T.F.W., Bookelman, R., Hartman, S., Bakker, M., Boucher, C.A.B, Kuiken, C., Goudsmit, J. (1993): "Greater Diversity of the HIV-1 V3 Neutralization Domain in Tanzania Compared With The Netherlands: Serological and Genetic Analysis." *AIDS 7.*

Chapter 7

SAREC, (1989): "Behavioural and Epidemiological Aspects of AIDS Research in Tanzania." Proceedings From a Workshop Held in Dar es Salaam, Tanzania. SAREC Documentation, Conference Reports.

Ades, A.E. (1995): "Serial HIV Sero-prevalence Surveys: Interpretation, Design, and Role in HIV/AIDS Prediction." *J Acquir Immune Defic Syndr Hum Retrovirol 9 (5).*

Asiimwe-Okiror, G., Opio, A.A., Musinguzi, J., Madraa, E., Tembo, G., Carael, M. (1997): "Change in Sexual Behaviour and Decline in HIV Infection Among Young Pregnant Women in Urban Uganda." *AIDS 11 (14).*

Batter, V., Matela, B., Nsuami, M., Manzila, T., Kamenga, M., Behets, F., Ryder, R.W., Heyward, W.L., Karon, J.M., St Louis, M.E. (1994): H"igh HIV-1 Incidence in Young Women Masked by Sta ble Overall Sero-prevalence Among Childbearing Women in Kinshasa, Zaire: Estimating Incidence from Serial Sero-prevalence Data." *AIDS 8 (6).*

Bouckenooghe, A., Shandera, W., (1999): "HIV Trends in African Blood Donors." *Journal of Infection 39 (2).*

Caldwell, J.C., Caldwell, P. (1994): "The Neglect of an Epidemiological Explanation for the Distribution of HIV/AIDS in Sub-Saharan Africa: Exploring the Male Circumcision Hypothesis." *Health Transition Review Suppliment to Volume 4.*

Dondero, T.J., Jr., Pappaioanou, M., Curran, J.W. (1988): "Monitoring the Levels and Trends of HIV Infection: The Public Health Service's HIV Surveillance Program." *Public Health Rep 103 (3).*

Emmelin, M., Comoro, C., Dahlgren, L., Killewo, J., Kwesigabo, G., Mutembei, A., Sandstrom, A. (1997): " Long Term Effects of Voluntary HIV Testing With Counselling in a Rural Village in Kagera Tanzania. *Xth International Conference on AIDS and STDs in Africa.*" Abidjan Cote d'Ivoire Abstract No E 687, December.

Emmelin, M., Comoro, C., Mutembei, A., Lugalla, J., Killewo, J., Kwesigabo, G., Sandstrom, A., Dahlgren, L. (1999): "The Social Transmission Route of HIV Infection - The Role of High Risk Environments in a Rural Area of the Kagera Region Tanzania." XIth International Conference on AIDS and STDs in Africa. Lusaka Zambia Abstract No 14PT33-1.

Fabiani, M., Accorsi, S., Lukwiya, M., Rosolen, T., Ayella, E., Onek, P., Declich, S. (2001): "Trend in HIV-1 Prevalence in an Antenatal Clinic in North Uganda and Adjusted Rates for the General Female Population." *AIDS 15 (1).*

Kamali, A., Carpenter, L.M., Whitworth, J.A., Pool, R., Ruberantwari, A., Ojwiya, A. (2000): "Seven-year Trends in HIV-1 Infection Rates, and Changes in Sexual Behaviour, Among Adults in Rural Uganda." *Aids 14 (4).*

Kilian, A.H., Gregson, S., Ndyanabangi, B., Walusaga, K., Kipp, W., Sahlmuller, G., Garnett, G.P., Asiimwe-Okiror, G., Kabagambe, G., Weis, P., von Sonnenburg, F. (1999): "Reductions in Risk Behaviour Provide the Most Consistent Explanation for Declining HIV-1 Prevalence in Uganda." *Aids 13 (3).*

Killewo, J. (1994): "Epidemiology Towards the Control of HIV Infection in Tanzania With Special Reference to the Kagera Region." Dept of Public Health and Clinical Medicine, Umea University, Sweden and Muhimbili University College of Health Sciences, Dar es Salaam, Tanzania., Umea, Sweden.

Killewo, J., Dahlgren, L., Sandstrom, A. (1994): "Socio-geographical Patterns of HIV-1 Transmission in Kagera Region, Tanzania." *Social Science and Medicine 38 (1).*

Killewo, J., Nyamuryekunge, K., Sandstrom, A., Bredberg-Raden, U., Wall, S., Mhalu, F., Biberfeld, G. (1990): " Prevalence of HIV-1 Infection in the Kagera Region of Tanzania: A Population-based Study." *AIDS 4 (11)*

Killewo, J.Z., Kwesigabo, G., Comoro, C., Lugalla, J., Mhalu, F.S., Biberfeld, G., Wall, S., Sandstrom, A. (1998): "Acceptability of Voluntary HIV Testing With Counselling in a Rural Village in Kagera, Tanzania." *AIDS Care 10 (4).*

Killewo, J.Z., Sandstrom, A., Bredberg Raden, U., Mhalu, F.S., Biberfeld, G., Wall, S. (1993): "Incidence of HIV-1 Infection Among Adults in the Kagera Region of Tanzania." *International Journal of Epidemiology 22 (3).*

Killewo, J.Z., Sandstrom, A., Bredberg Raden, U., Mhalu, F.S., Biberfeld, G., Wall, S. (1994): "Prevalence and Incidence of Syphilis and Its Association With HIV-1 Infection in a Population-based Study in the Kagera Region of Tanzania." *International Journal of STD and Aids 5 (6).*

Killewo, J.Z.J., Comoro, C.J., Lugalla, J., Kwesigabo, G. (1993): "Systematic Interventions and Their Evaluation Against HIV/AIDS in Kagera Region, Tanzania: Proceedings of a Workshop Held in Bukoba Town, Kagera, Tanzania." *Kagera AIDS Research Project.*

Kwesigabo, G., Killewo, J., Godoy, C., Urassa, W., Mbena, E., Mhalu, F., Biberfeld, G., Wall, S., Sandstrom, A. (1998): "Decline in the Prevalence of HIV-1 Infection in Young Women in the Kagera Region of Tanzania." *J Acquir. Immune Defic. Syndr. Hum. Retrovirol 17(3).*

Kwesigabo, G., Killewo, J.Z., Sandstrom, A. (1996): "Sentinel Surveillance and Cross Sectional Survey on HIV Infection Prevalence: A Comparative Study." *East Afr. Med. J 73 (5).*

Kwesigabo, G., Killewo, J.Z., Sandstrom, A., Winani, S., Mhalu, F.S., Biberfeld, G., Wall, S. (1999): "Prevalence of HIV Infection Among Hospital Patients in North West Tanzania." *AIDS Care 11 (1).*

Kwesigabo, G., Killewo, J.Z., Urassa, W., Mbena, E., Mhalu, F., Lugalla, J.L., Godoy, C., Biberfeld, G., Emmelin, M., Wall, S., Sandstrom, A. (2000): "Monitoring of HIV-1 Infection Prevalence and Trends in the General Population Using Pregnant Women as a Sentinel Population: 9 Years' Experience From the Kagera Region of Tanzania." *J Acquir. Immune Defic. Syndr .23 (5).*

Kwesigabo, G., Killewo, J.Z.J., Makwaya, C.K., Urassa, W., Mhalu, F., Biberfeld, G., Sandstrom, A. (1998): "Decline in the Prevalence and Incidence of HIV-1 Infection in Population Based Studies in Bukoba Urban, Kagera Tanzania." 12th World AIDS Conference., Geneva Switzerland Abstract No 13114.

Larsen, O., da Silva, Z., Sandstrom, A., Andersen, P.K., Andersson, S., Poulsen, A.G., Melbye, M., Dias, F., Naucler, A., Aaby, P. (1998): "Declining HIV-2 Prevalence and Incidence Among Men in a Community Study From Guinea-Bissau." *Aids 12 (13).*

Lugalla, J., Comoro, C., Mutembei, A., Dahlgren, L., Emmelin, M., Killewo, J., Kwesigabo, G., Sandstrom, A. (1997): "The Availability and Acceptability of Intervention Strategies Against HIV/AIDS Infection in the Kagera Region of Tanzania." *Internationales Afrikaforum 33 (4).*

Lugalla, J.L.P., Emmelin, M., Mutembei, A., Comoro, C., Killewo, J.Z.J., Kwesigabo, G, Sandstrom, A., Dahlgren, L. (1993): "The Social and Cultural Contexts of HIV/AIDS Transmission in the Kagera Region, Tanzania." *J Asian & African Studies 34 (4).*

Lwihula, G., Dahlgren, L., Killewo, J., Sandstrom, A. (1993): "AIDS Epidemic in Kagera Region, Tanzania - The Experiences of Local People." *AIDS Care 5 (3).*

Mason, C.J., Markowitz, L.E., Kitsiripornchai, S., Jugsudee, A., Sirisopana, N., Torugsa, K., Carr, J.K., Michael, R.A., Nitayaphan, S., McNeil, J.G. (1995): "Declining Prevalence of HIV-1 Infection in Young Thai Men." *AIDS 9 (9).*

Mbizvo, M.T., Mashu, A., Chipato, T., Makura, E., Bopoto, R., Fottrell, P.F. (1996): "Trends in HIV-1 and HIV-2 Prevalence and Risk Factors in Pregnant Women in Harare, Zimbabwe." *Central African Journal of Medicine 42 (1).*

Mertens, T., Carael, M., Sato, P., Cleland, J., Ward, H., Smith, G.D., (1994): "Prevention Indicators for Evaluating the Progress of National AIDS Programmes." *Aids 8 (10)*

Mulder, D., Nunn, A., Kamali, A., Kengeya-Kayondo, J. (1995): "Decreasing HIV-1 sero-Prevalence in Young Adults in a Rural Ugandan Cohort . *Clinical Research Ed. 311 (7009).*

Nelson, K.E., Celentano, D.D., Suprasert, S., Wright, N., Eiumtrakul, S., Tulvatana, S., Matanasarawoot, A., Akarasewi, P., Kuntolbutra, S., Romyen, S., *et. al.* (1993): "Risk Factors for HIV Infection Among Young Adult Men in Northern Thailand." *Jama 270 (8).*

UNAIDS (1999): "Trends in HIV Incidence and Prevalence: Natural Course of the Epidemic or Results of Behavioural Change?" UNAIDS in Collaboration With Wellcome Trust Centre for Epidemiology of Infectious Disease, Geneva.

Urassa, W., Godoy, K., Killewo, J., Kwesigabo, G., Mbakileki, A., Mhalu, F., Biberfeld, G. (1999): "The Accuracy of an Alternative Confirmatory Strategy for Detection of Antibodies to HIV-1: Experience From a Regional Laboratory in Kagera, Tanzania." *J Clin Virol 14 (1).*

Wawer, M.J., Serwadda, D., Gray, R.H., Sewankambo, N.K., Li, C., Nalugoda, F., Lutalo, T., Konde-Lule, J. (1997): "Trends in HIV-1 Prevalence May Not Reflect Trends in Incidence in Mature Epidemics: Data From the Rakai Population-based Cohort, Uganda." *AIDS 11.*

Wilkinson, D., Abdool Karim, S.S., Williams, B., Gouws, E. (2000): "High HIV Incidence and Prevalence Among Young Women in Rural South Africa: Developing A Cohort for Intervention Trials." *Journal of Acquired Immune Deficiency Syndromes 23 (5).*

Chapter 8

Abiodun, O.A. (1989): "Psychiatry Morbidity in a Primary Healthcare Center in a Rural Community in Nigeria." *Central African Journal of Medicine* 35(4).

Andersson-Brolin, L., Staugard, F., Cornell, I.E., Hannan-Andersson, C., Manumbu, M., Msamanga, G., Sandberg, C. (1987): "Health Centers in Need of Treatment." *SIDA Evaluation Report No. 4.*

Assen, G.P.M. (1991): "Social Consequences of Psychosis for Psychotic Patients in Western Province, Kenya, After Treatment." Okpaku S.O. (ed).*Mental Health in Africa and the Americas Today.*

Asuni, T.S., (1991): "Development of Psychiatry in Africa." Okpaku S.O. (ed).*Mental Health in Africa and the Americas Today.*

Ben-Tovim, D.I. (1985): "DSM-111 in Botswana: A Field Trial in a Developing Country." *American Journal of Psychiatry*, 142.

Blacker, C.R., Clare, A.W. (1987): "Depressive Disorder in Primarycare." *British Journal of Psychiatry*, 150.

Bloch. (1991): "Treatment of Psychiatric Patients in Tanzania." *Acta Psychiatrica Scandinavia Suppl. No.364(83).*

Bridges, K., Goldberg, D. (1991): "Determinants of Somatization in Primarycare." *Psychological Medicine* 21(2).

Carothers, J.C. (1947): "A Study of Mental Derangement in Africans, and an Attempt to Explain Its Peculiarities, More Especially in Relationship to the African Attitude to Life." *J Ment Sci* 93.

Chikara F.B. (1996): "Current State of Psychiatry in Zimbabwe." Symposium on the Promotion of Psychiatry and Mental Healthcare in Africa. Sun City, South Africa.

Christakis, N.A., Ware, N.C., Kleinman,A. (1993): *Illness Behavior and the Health Transition* (in print).

Climent, C.E., Diop, B.S.M., Harding, T.W., Ibrahim, H.H.A., Ladrido-Ignacio, L., Wig, N.N. (1980): "Mental Health in Primary Healthcare." *WHO Chronical* 34.

Davenport, S., Goldberg, D., Milten, T. (1987): "How Psychiatric Disorders are Missed During Medical Consultations." *Lancet*, ii.

De Jong, T.V.M. (1987): *A Descent into African Psychiatry*. Royal Tropical Institute, Amsterdam.

Dhaphale M., Cooper,G., Cartwright-Taylor, L. (1989): "The Prevalence and Presentation of Depressive Illness in a Primary Healthcare Setting in Kenya." *American Journal of Psychiatry, 146(5).*

Dhaphale, M., Ellison R.H., Griffin L. (1983): "The Frequency of Psychiatric Disorders Among Patients Attending Semi-Urban and Rural General Out Patient Clinics in Kenya." *British Journal of Psychiatry* 142.

Edgerton, R.B. (1980): "Traditional Treatment for Mental Illness in Africa: A Review." *Culture Medicine and Psychiatry 4.*

Flanagan,W.G. (1977): "The Extended Family as an Agent in Urbanization - Survey of Men and Women Working in Dar es Salaam, Tanzania." University of Connecticut Ph.D. Thesis.

Freeling P. (1985): "Health Outcomes in Primarycare: An Approach to the Problems." *Family Practice* 2.

Gabrenegus F. (1996): "The National Mental Health Policy and Guidlines in Eritrea - Discussion of Workshop Proceedings." Symposium on the Promotion of Psychiatry and Mental Healthcare in Africa. Sun City, South Africa.

Gask L. Goldberg D. Porter R, Creed F. (1989): "The Treatment of Somatization; Evaluation of a Training Package with General Practice Trainees." *Journal of Psychosomatic Research, 33 (6).*

German, G.A. (1987): "Mental Health in Africa 1: The Extent of Mental Health in Africa Today." *British Journal of Psychiatry.* 151.

Giel , Van Luijk J.N. (1969): "Psychiatric Morbidity in a Small Ethiopian Town." *British Journal of Psychiatry 115.*

Goldberg D. P. and Blackwell 1970): "Psychiatric Illness in General Practice: A Detailed Study Using a New Method of Case Identification." *British Medical Journal 2:439.*

Goldberg D. P., Gask L., O'Dowd T. (1989): "The Treatment of Somatization: Teaching Techniques of Reattribution." *Journal of Psychosomatic Research, 33 (6).*

Goldberg, D. (1990): *Reasons for Misdiagnosis. Psychological Medicine in General Medical Settings*, Hogref and Huber Publ.

Goldberg, D., Bridges, K. (1988): "Somatic Presentations of Psychiatric Illness in Primarycare Settings." *Journal of Psychosomatic Research, 32.*

Goldberg, D.P., Steele, J.T., Smith, C. (1980): " Teaching Psychiatric Interview Techniques to Family Doctors." *Acta Psychiatrica Scandinavia Suppl.* 285.

Good, B. (1977): "The Heart of What's the Matter; The Semantics of Illness in Iran Culture." *Medicine and Psychiatry* 1:25 – 58.

Good, B. J. and M. DelVecchio Good (1981): "The Semantics of Medical Discourse." Everett Mendelsohn and Yehuda Elkana (eds). *Sciences and Cultures. Sociology of the Sciences*, Vol V.

Gordon, H.L. (1936): "An Enquiry into the Correlation of Civilization and Mental Disorders in the Kenyan Native." *East African Med J*, 12.

Gureje O., Obikoya B., Ikuesan B.A. (1992): "Prevalence of Specific Psychiatric Disorders in an Urban Primarycare Setting." *East African Medical Journal 69 (5).*

Haub,C., Yanagishita,M. (1992): "World Population Data Sheet." *Population Reference Bureau,* Washington D.C.

Haworth A. (1996): "Mental Health Programmes and Policies in Zambia." Symposium on the Promotion of Psychiatry and Mental Healthcare in Africa. Sun City, South Africa.

Health and Welfare (1989): "Canada Mental Health for Canadians; Striking a Balance." Dimensions, Ministry of Supplies and Services, Canadian Government.

Heggenhougen,K.H., Magari, F.M. (1992): "Community Health Workers in Tanzania." In Frankel, S. (ed.): *The Community Health Worker, Effective Programmes for Developing Countries*. Oxford University Press, N.Y.

Heggenhougen,K.H., *et. al.* (1987): *Community Health Workers: the Tanzanian Experience*. Oxford University Press, Oxford.

Heggenhougen, K.H., Gilson, L. (1997): "Perceptions of Efficacy and the Use of Traditional Medicine, with Examples from Tanzania." *CURARE*, 20.

Holmes, J.A., Speight, A.N.P. (1975): "The Problem of Non-organic Illness in Tanzania Urban Medical Practice." *East African Medical Journal*, 52.

Johnstone A, Goldberg D. (1976): "Psychiatric Screening in General Practice." *Lancet* i: 605.

Kaaya S., Goldberg, D.P., Gask, L. (1991): "Management of Psychiatric Illness in General Medical Settings: Evaluation of a New Training Course for General Practitioners." *Medical Education 26(2).*

Katon, W. (1982): "Depression: Somatic Symptoms and Medical Disorders in Primarycare." *Comprehensive Psychiatry, 23.*

Kempinski R., (1991): "Mental Healthcare in Tanzania." *Act Psychiatrica Scandinavia, 83 (364).*

Kessel, W.I.N. (1960): "Psychiatric Morbidity in a London General Practice." *British Journal of Preventive and Social Medicine 14.*

Kigamwa (1991): "Psychiatric Morbidity and Referral Rate Among Medical In-patients at Kenyatta National Hospital." *East African Medical Journal,* 68 (5).

Kilonzo, G.D. (1992): "The Challenge of Rehabilitation Psychiatry in Tanzania." *Medicus.*

Kleinman, A. (1973): "Medicines Symbolic Reality: On the Central Problem in the Philosophy of Medicine." *Inquiry 16.*

Kleinman, A.(1980): *Patients and Healers in the Context of Culture: An Exploration of the Borderline Between Anthropology, Medicine and Psychiatry*. University of California Press.

Kortteinen, T. (1988): "Alcohol and Urbanization in Africa."In Maula,J., Linblad, M., Tigerstedt, D. (eds.) *Alcohol in Developing Countries,* Nordic Council on Alcohol and Drug Research Publication No. 18.

Leighton, A.M., Adeoye, Lambo, T., Hughes, C.C., Leighton, D.C., Murphy, J.M. and Macklin, D.B. (1963): *Psychiatric Disorder Amongst the Yoruba.* New York.

Lutz, C. (1985): *Depression and the Translation of Emotional Worlds in Culture and Depression; Studies in the Anthropology and Cross-cultural Psychiatry of Affect and Disorder* (ed.) University of California Press.

Mambwe, C.C. (1996): "Mental Health Policies and Current Practice of Psychiatry in Botswana." Symposium on Promotion of Psychiatry and Mental Healthcare in Africa. Sun City, South Africa.

Mandhlate, C. (1996): "The Psychosocial Support Programme in Bourne." Symposium on the Promotion of Psychiatry and Mental Healthcare in Africa. Sun City, South Africa.

Mbanefo, S.E. (1971): The General Practitioner and Psychiatry. In *Psychiatry and Mental Healthcare in General Practice.*

MOH, (1983): *Guidelines for the Implementation of the Primary Healthcare Program in Tanzania.* Ministry of Health, Dar es Salaam.

MOH, (1979): *Inventory of Health Facilities, 1978,* Ministry of Health, Dar es Salaam.

MOH, (1980): *Health Evaluation Report 1961-1978,* Ministry of Health, Dar es Salaam.

Nakasi , G. (1996): "Current State of Psychiatry in Uganda." Symposium on the Promotion of Psychiatry and Mental Healthcare in Africa. Sun City, South Africa.

Ndetei, D.M., Muhangi J. (1979): "The Prevalence and Clinical Presentation of Psychiatric Illness in a Rural Setting in Kenya." *British Journal of Psychiatry 135.*

Odejide, A.O., Oyewunmi, L.K., Ohaeri, J.U. (1989): "Psychiatry in Africa: An Overview." *American Journal of Psychiatry, 146 (6).*

Oduwole, O.O., Ogunyemi, A.O. (1989): "Validity of the GHQ-30 in a Nigerian Out-Patient Clinic." *Canadian Journal of Psychiatry,* Vol. 34.

Omari , A. (1996): "Summary of Mental Health Services in Kenya." Symposium on the Promotion of Psychiatry and Mental Healthcare in Africa. Sun City, South Africa.

Sartorius N. (1996): "Summary Report of Meeting on Promotion of Psychiatry and Mental Healthcare in Africa." Sun City, South Africa.

Schieffelin E. L., (1985): "The Cultural Analysis of Depressive Affect; An Example From New Guinea." In Kleinman A., Good B. (ed), *Culture and Depression; Studies in the Anthropology and Cross-cultural Psychiatry of Affect and Disorder.* University of California Press.

Schulssinger, F., Jablensky, A. (1991): "Background of the Mental Health Program in Tanzania." *Acta Psych. Scand. Suppl. 364 Vol. 83.*

Sugar, J.A., Kleinman, A., Heggenhougen, K. (1991): Development's 'downside': Social and Psychological Pathology in Countries Undergoing Social Change. *Health Transition Review, Vol.1(2).*

Swantz, L. (1990): *The Medicine Man Among the Zaramo of Dar es Salaam.* Scandinavian Institute of African Studies and Dar es Salaam University Press.

Titmuss, R.M., Abel-Smith, B., Macdonald, G.., Williams, A.W. Wood, C.H. (1963): "Health Services of Tanganyika - A Report to the Government." *African Medical Research Foundation*, Pitman Publishing House.

UN (1992): "Demographic Year Book." United Nations Department of Economics and Social Development, *Population Division*, New York.

Westermeyer, J. (1985): "Psychiatric Diagnosis Across Cultural Boundaries." *American Journal of Psychiatry*, 142:7.

WHO (1975): "Expert Committee on Mental Health. Organization of Mental Health Services in Developing Countries." *Technical Report Series* 564. WHO, Geneva.

Whyte, S.R. (1991): "Attitudes Towards Mental Health in Tanzania. The National Mental Health Program in the United Republic of Tanzania." Schulssinger and Jablenski. (eds) *Acta Psych. Scand. Suppl. 364 Vol.83.*

Woeber, M. (1975): *Psychology in Africa.* International African Institute, London.

Chapter 9

Acuda S.W. and Ovuga E.B.L. (1985): "Psychiatric Disorders in a General Provincial Hospital in Kenya." *East African Medical Journal, 62 (4).*

Bugaisa, G. and Rugeiyamu, N. (1991): "Providing Mental Healthcare Services With Meagre Resources in Tanzania." S.A. Opaku (eds.) in *Mental Health in Africa and Americas Today*, Christolith Books Nashville, 419.

Desjarlais R., Eisenberg L., Good B., and Kleinman (1995): *World Mental Health Problems and Priorities in Low-income Countries.* Oxford. University Press New York.

German, G.A. (1987): "Mental Health in Africa I: The Nature of Mental Disorders in Africa Today: Some Clinical Observations." *British Journal of Psychiatry 151.*

Haub, C., Yanagishita, M. (1992): "World Population Data Sheet." *Population Reference Bureau,* Washington DC.

Holmes, J.A. and Speight, A.N. (1975): "The Problem of Non-organic Illness in Tanzanian Urban Medical Practice." *East African Medical Journal*, 52.

Kempinski, K. (1991): "Mental Health and Primary Healthcare in Tanzania." *Acta Psychiat. Scand. (suppl.), 364.*

Kilima E., Kilonzo G.P., Mbatia J., Mlawa M., Matowo A., and Malela, A. (1990): "Rehabilitation of Transient Wandering Psychotic Patients." International Conference on Rehabilitation of Chronic Psychiatric Patients in Africa Arusha International Conference Centre.

Kilonzo, G.P. and Pitkaenen, Y.T. (1992): "Pombe: Report of Alcohol Research Project in Tanzania 1988-90." University of Helsinki Institute of Development Studies.

Kleinman A. (1987): *Rethinking Psychiatry From a Cultural Category to Personal Experience.* The Free Press New York.

Kupfer, D.J., Frank, E., Perel J.M. *et. al.* (1992): "Five Year Outcome for Maintenance Therapies in Recurrent Depression." *Arch. Gen. Psychiatry* 49.

Matuja, W.B. (1990): "Psychological Disturbances in African Tanzanian Epileptics." *Trop. Geog. Med.* 42 (4).

Matuja, W.P., Ndosi, N.K, and Collins, M. (1995): "Nature of Referrals to the Psychiatric Unit at Muhimbili Medical Centre, Dar es Salaam." *E. Afr. Med. J*, 72.

Mbatia, K.J. (1979): "The Nature of Psychiatric Morbidity in Patients Under 18 Years, at Muhimbili Hospital Dar es Salaam." *E. Afr. med. J* 56.

Mwaluko, G.M.P., Lukumanji, Z. and Kasale A.S. (1991): "Urbanization and Health." In G.M.P. Mwaluko, W.L. Kilama, M.P Mandara, M. Murru and C.N.L. Macpherson: *Health and Diseases in Tanzania.* Harper Collins Academic London, U.K.

Ndosi, N.K. (1991): "Rehabilitation of Chronic Psychiatric Patients at Mwera" *Postgraduate Doctor Africa: 13 (2).*

Ndosi, N.K. and Kisesa A.F. (1997): "Causes of Mortality Among Mental Patients at Muhimbili Medical Centre." *E. Afr. Med. J.* 74:23.

Ndosi, N.K. and Waziri , M.C. (1997): "The Nature of Parasuicide in Dar es Salaam Tanzania." *Soc. Sci & Med.* 44:55.

Ndosi, N.K. and Yongolo J. (1991): "Substance Abuse in Dar es Salaam Tanzania." First Annual Seminar of the R & D Advisory Committee on Public Health and Medical Research Dar es Salaam.

Nianfeng, G. (1993): "Growth in Population Density Produces Stress Factors in Living and Employment Harmful to Normal Mental Life." *Int. J. Ment. Hlth. 16 (3).*

Ovuga, E.B.L. (1986): "The Different Faces of Depression." *E. Afr. med. J.* 2.

Rutazamba, T.D. (1991): "Road Traffic Problems as Part of Urban Crisis and a Health Economic Challenge in Tanzania Today." PHA.

Rwegellera, G.C., and Mwambe C.C. (1977): "Diagnostic Classification of First Ever Admissions to Chainama Hills Hospital, Lusaka Zambia." *Brit. J. Psychiat. 130.*

Robert Wood Johnson Foundation (1987): "Access to Healthcare in the US: Results of a 1986 Survey." *Special Report No. 2.* Princeton, N.J: R:W. Johnson Foundation: 5.

Schulsinger F., Jablensky, A. (1991): "Background of the Mental Health Programme in Tanzania." *Acta psychiat. scand. suppl. 364.*

Tungaraza F. and Ndosi N.K. (1995): "Unemployment Crisis Among the Youth in Tanzania." In Conference on Youth and Related Problems in Tanzania.

Van de Kolk B.A., and Van der Hart O., Pierre Janet (1989): "Breakdown Adaptation in Psychological Trauma." *Am. J. Psychiat. 146(12).*

The World Bank (1993): "Tanzania a Poverty Profile." *Report No 12298-TA.*

Chapter 10

Acuda, S.W. (1983): "Mental Health Problems in Kenya Today - A Review of Research." *East African Medical Journal*, 60.

Asuni, T. (1962): "Suicide in Western Nigeria." In T.A. Lambo, *First Pan-African Psychiatric Conference, Abeokuta, Nigeria, Conference Report,* ed. Government Printer, Ibadan.

Ben-Tovim, D. I. (1985): "DSM III in Botswana: A Field Trial in a Developing Country." *American Journal of Psychiatry*, 142.

Bureau of Statistics (1991): *"Tanzania Sensus 1988, Population Census: National Profile Summary."* Ministry of Finance, Economic Affairs and Planning, Dar es Salaam.

Climent, C.E., Diop, B.S.M., Harding, T.W., Ibrahim, H.H.A., Ladrido-Ignacio, and Wig, N.N. (1980): "Mental Health in Primary Healthcare." *WHO Chronicle, 34.*

Cooper, J. and Sartorius, N. (1977): "Cultural and Temporal Variations in Schizophrenia: A Speculation on the Importance of Industrialization." *British Journal of Psychiatry, 130.*

Egdell, H.G. (1984): "Mental Healthcare in the District Hospital." *British Medical Journal*, 289.

Flanagan, W.G. (1977): "The Extended Family as an Agent in Urbanization: Survey of Men and Women Working in Dar es Salaam, Tanzania." Ph.D. Thesis, University of Connecticut.

German, G.A. (1987): "Mental Health in Africa 1. The Extent of Mental Health Problems in Africa Today. An Update of Epidemiological Knowledge." *British Journal of Psychiatry, 151.*

Giel, R. and Harding, T.W. (1976): "Psychiatric Priorities in Developing Countries." *British Journal of Psychiatry, 128.*

Giel, R. and van Luijk, J.N. (1969): "Psychiatric Morbidity in a Small Ethiopian Town." *British Journal of Psychiatry, 115.*

Good, C.M. (1987): *Ethnomedical Systems in Africa - Patterns of Traditional Medicine in Rural and Urban Kenya.* The Guildford Press.

Harding, T.W. (1975): "Traditional Healing Methods for Mental Patients." *WHO Chronicle, 31.*

Harding, T.W., De Arango, J., Climent, C.E., Ibrahim, H.N.A., Ladrido-Ignacio, L., Murthy, R.S., and Wig, N.N. (1980): "Mental Disorders in Primary Healthcare: A Study of Their Frequency and Diagnosis in Four Developing Countries." *Psychological Medicine, 10.*

Holmes, J.A. and Speight, N.P. (1975): "The Problems of Non-organic Illness in Tanzania Urban Medical Practice." *East African Medical Journal*, 52 (5).

Jablensky, A. and Hauli, J. (1983): "Mental Healthcare at the Rural Dispensary - The Tanzanian Experiment." *World Health.*

Jilek, W.G. and Jilek-Aall, L. (1970): "Transient Psychoses in Africans." *Psychiatrica Clinica 3.*

Kaaya, S.F., Kilonzo, G.P., Matowo, A. and Semboja, A. (1992): "Prevalence of Substance Abuse Among Secondary School Students in Dar es Salaam." *Tanzania Medical Journal* 7 (1).

Kilama, W.L., Nhonoli, A.M., and Makene, W.J. (1974): "Healthcare Delivery in Tanzania." In Ruhumbika, G. (ed) *Towards Ujamaa: Twenty Years of TANU Leadership.* East African Literature Bureau.

Kilonzo, G.P. (1996): "Drug Abuse Among African Youth." Project AD/RAF/94/2. A UNDCP Paper Presented at the OAU Pan-African Youth Conference, Addis Ababa.

Kilonzo, G.P. (1992a): "Substance Abuse in Tanzania Magnitude of the Problem and Strategies for Prevention." In Post-Social Conference, Tanzania Library Association.

Kilonzo, G.P. (1992b): "The Challenge of Rehabilitation Psychiatry in Tanzania." *MEDICUS.*

Kilonzo, G.P. 1989): "Tanzania in State Monopolies and Alcohol Prevention: Report and Working Papers of a Collaborative International Study." *Report No. 181*. The Social Research Institute of Alcohol Studies, Helsinki.

Kilonzo, G.P. and Kassam, M. (1986): "Study of Suicide and Attempted Suicide at Muhimbili Medical Centre in Dar es Salaam." Annual Scientific Conference of the Medical Association of Tanzania.

Kilonzo, G.P. and Pitkanen, T. (eds) (1992): "Pombe: Report of Alcohol Research Project in Tanzania." Institute of Development Studies, University of Helsinki.

Kortteinen, T. (1989): "Potential of State Monopoly Systems in Preventing Alcohol-related Problems in Developing Countries." In State Monopolies and Alcohol Prevention: Report and Working Papers of a Collaborative International Study, *Report No. 181.* The Social Research Institute of Alcohol Studies, Helsinki.

Lamb, R. (1982): *Treating the Long-term Mentally Ill: Beyond Deinstitutionalization,* Jessey-Bass Pub., London.

Lambo, T.A. (1964): "The Village of Aro." *The Lancet, 2.*

Lewis, H. (1962): "Urbanization and Problems of Child Behaviour." In T.A. Lambo (ed) *First Pan-African Psychiatric Conference, Abeokuta, Nigeria, Conference Report,* Government Printer, Ibadan.

Margetts, E.L. (1958): "Psychiatric Facilities in Kenya." In *Mental Disorders and Mental Health in Africa South of the Sahara.* CCTA/CSA-WFMH-WHO Meeting of Specialists on Mental Health, Bukavu, Congo.

Mbiti, J.S. (1969): *African Religions and Philosophy.* Heinemann, London.

Murray, T.W. (1962): "Mental Health Trends and Problems in Uganda." In Lambo, T.A. (ed) *First Pan-African Psychiatric Conference, Abeokuta, Nigeria, Conference Report.* Ibadan: Government Printer.

Ndosi, N.K. and Waziri, M.C. (1996): "The Nature of Parasuicide in Dar es Salaam, Tanzania." *Social Science and Medicine,* 1996:1-7 (SSM 1174 [15/8/96]).

Neki, J.S. , Joinet, B., Ndosi, N., Kilonzo, G., Hauli, J., and Duvinage, G (1986): "Witchcraft and Psychotherapy." *British Journal of Psychiatry, 149.*

Nikander, P., Honkanen, R., Huttunen, P., Kilonzo, G.P. and Pitkanen, T. (1992): "Role of Alcohol in Injuries Treated in Muhimbili Medical Centre Casualty Department, Dar es Salaam, Tanzania." In G. Kilonzo and T. Pitkanen (eds), *Pombe: Report of Alcohol Research Project in Tanzania,* Institute of Development Studies, University of Helsinki.

Nikander, P., Seppala, T., Kilonzo, G. P., Huttunen, P., Saarinen, L., Kilima, E. and Pitkanen, T. Ingredients and Contaminants of Traditional Alcoholic Beverages in Tanzania. *Transactions of the Royal Society of Tropical Medicine and Hygiene,* 85, 1991.

Odejide, A.O. (1979): "Cross-cultural Psychiatry: A Myth or Reality." *Comprehensive Psychiatry, 20 (2).*

Partanen, J. (1991): *Sociability and Intoxication: Alcohol and Drinking in Kenya, Africa and the Modern World.* The Finnish Foundation for Alcohol Studies.

Schulsinger, F. and Jablensky, A. (eds.) (1991): The National Mental Health Programme in the United Republic of Tanzania. A Report From WHO and DANIDA. *Acta Psychiatrica Scandinavica Supplementum, 83(364).*

Simmons, N. (1996): *"Tambiko la Mizimu au Dawa ya Wazungu?* Ritual Offering to the Spirits of the Dead or White Man's Medicine? The Experiences of Tanzanians Seeking Treatment from Western-trained Doctors and Traditional Healers Simultaneously." On-going Research in Dar es Salaam for Doctoral Thesis, University of Toronto.

Simmons, N. (1991): "Western Psychiatry in the 3rd World: Some Alternatives." Paper Submitted to the Department of Psychology, Ontario Institute for Studies in Education in Part Fulfillment of the Requirements for the Degree of Masters in Education.

Swantz, L. (1990): *The Medicine Man Among the Zaramo of Dar es Salaam.* Dar es Salaam University Press.

Titmuss, R.M., Abel-Smith, B., Macdonald, G., Williams, A.W., and Wood, C.H. (1963): *The Health Services of Tanganyika. A Report to the Government.* London: Pitman Medical Publishing Co. Ltd.

Westermeyer, J. (1985): "Psychiatric Diagnosis Across Cultural Boundaries." *American Journal of Psychiatry, 142 (7).*

Willson, M. (1987): *Occupational Therapy in Long-term Psychiatry,* Churchill Livingstone, London.

Wing, J.K. and Morris, B. (1981): *Handbook of Psychiatric Rehabilitation Practice.* Oxford, Oxford University Press.

Woeber, M. (1975): *Psychology in Africa.* London: International African Institute.

World Bank (1989): *A Long-term Perspective Survey.* World Bank, Washington, D.C.

World Health Organization (1992): "Substance Use Among Street Children in Mwanza, Tanzania." KULEANA-WHO/PSA Collaborating Site. WHO/PSA Street Children Project Report of Inaugural Meeting of Participating Centres, Geneva.

Chapter 11

Alleck, P. and Allgulander, C. (1990): "Psychiatric Diagnoses as Predictors of Suicide: A Comparison of Diagnoses at Conscription and in Psychiatric Care in Cohort of 50,465 Young Men." *Br. J. Psychiatr.* 157 (339).

Arato, M., Deter, E., Rihmer, Z. and Somogyi, E. (1988): "Retrospective Psychiatric Assessment of 200 Suicides in Budapest." *Acta Psychiatr. Scand.* 77 (454).

Asuni, T. (1967): "Attempted Suicide in Western Nigeria." *West Afr. Med. J.* 13 (51).

Barraclough, B. (1981): "Suicide and Epilepsy." In Reybolds E.H. and Trimble M.R. (eds.) *Epilepsy and Psychiatry,* Churchill Livingstone, Edinburgh.

Bartels, S.J., Drake R.E. and McHugo, G.J. (1992): "Alcohol Abuse, Depression and Suicidal Behavior in Schizophrenia." *Am. J. Psychiatr.* 149 (394).

Bhugra, D. (1989): "Suicide Trends in the South-East Thames Region." *Psychiatr. Bull.* 13 (366).

Buch, J. (1972): "Recent Bereavement in Relation to Suicide." *J. Psychosom. Res.* 16 (361).

Buck, C. (1982): "Determinants of Health: People, Situations, and Social Systems." In

Lipkin M. Jr. and Kupka, K (eds.) *Psychosocial Factors Affecting Health*. Praeger, New York.

Diekestra R.F. (1993): "The Epidemiology of Suicide and Parasuicide." *Acta Psychiatr. Scand.* 9 (371).

Eferakeya, A.E. (1970): "Drugs and Suicide Attempts in Benin City." *Br. J. Psychiatr.* 127 (764).

Farmer, R. (1987): "Hostility and Deliberate Self-poisoning: The Role of Depression." *Br. J. Psychiatr.* 150 (609).

Fyer, M.R., Frances, A.J., Sullivan, T., Hurt, T. and Clarkin, J. (1988): "Suicide Attempts in Patients With Borderline Personality Disorder." *Am. J. Psychiatr.* 145 (737).

Guze, S.B. and Robins E. (1970): "Suicide Among Primary Affective Disorders." *Br. J. Psychiatr.* 117 (437).

Hatcher, S. (1994): "Debt and Deliberate Self-poisoning." *Br. J. Psychiatr.* 164 (111).

Hawton, K. (1987): "Assessment of Suicide Among Primary Affective Disorders." *Br. J. Psychiatr.* 150 (145).

Hollan, D. (1990): "Indignant Suicide in the Pacific: An Example From the Trojan Highlands of Indonesia." *Cult. Med. Psychiatr.* 3 (363).

Horwitz, A.V. and White, H.R. (1991): "Becoming Married, Depression, and Alcohol Problems Among Adults." *J. Hlth. Soc. Behav.* 132 (221).

James, L.P. (1967): "Suicide and Mortality Among Heroin Addicts in Britain." *Br. J. Add.* 62 (391).

Jones, S.C., Forster, D.P. and Hassanyh, F. (1991): "The Role of Unemployment in Parasuicide." *Psychol. Med.* 21 (169).

Kahuho, S.K. (1980): "Drug Poisoning in the Intensive Care Unit of Kenyatta National Hospital." *East Afr. Med. J.* 57 (490).

Kebede, D. and Ketsela, T. (1993): "Suicide Attempts in Ethiopian Adolescents in Addis Abeba High Schools." *Eth. Med. J.* 319 (83).

Kerkhof, A.J.F.M., Schmidtke, A., Bille-Brahe, U., De Leo D. and Lonnqvisit (1994): *Attempted Suicide in Europe.* DSWO University Press, Leiden /Copenhagen.

Kienhorst, C.W.M., de Wilde, E.J., van Den Bout, J., Dikestra, R.F.W. and Wolters, W.H.G. (1990): "Characteristics of Suicide Attempters in a Population-based Sample of Dutch Adolescents." *Br. J. Psychiatr.* 156 (143).

Klerman, G. (1986): *Suicide and Depression Among Adolescents and Young Adults.* American Psychiatric Press, Washington.

Landmark J., Cernovsky, Z.Z. and Merkey, H. (1987): "Correlates of Suicide Attempts and Ideation in Schizophrenia." *Br. J. Psychiatr.* 151 (18).

Lewinsohn, P.M., Rohde, P. and Seeley, J.R. (1994): "Psychosocial Risk Factors for Future Adolescent Suicide Fifty Attempts." J. *Consult. Clin. Psychol*. 62 (197).

McKegney, F.P. and O'Dowd, M.A. (1992): "Suicidality and HIV Status." *Am. J. Psychiatr.* 149 (396).

Mehlum L. (1992): "Prodromal Signs and Precipitating Factors in Attempted Suicide." *Military Med.* 157 (574).

Mendelson, W.B. and Rich, C.L. (1993): "Sedatives and Suicide: the San Diego Study." *Acta Psychiatr. Scand.* 88 (337).

Mengech, H.K. and Dhadphale, M. (1984): "Attempted Suicide (parasuicide) in Nairobi, Kenya." *Acta Psychiatr. Scand.* 69 (416).

Miles, C.P. (1977): "Conditions Predisposing to Suicide." *J. Nerv. Ment. Dis.* 164 (231).

Mishara, B.L., Baker, A.H. and Mishara, T.T. (1976): "The Frequency of Suicide Attempts: A Retrospective Approach Applied to College Students." *Am. J. Psychiatr.* 133 (841).

Morano, C.D., Cisler, R.A. and Lemerond, J. (1993): "Risk Factors for Adolescent Suicidal Behavior: Loss, Insufficient Familial Support and Hopelessness." *Adolescence* 28 (851).

Murphy, G.E., Wetzel, R.D., Robin, E. and McEnvoy, L. (1992): "Multiple Risk Factors Predict Suicide in Alcoholism." *Arch. Gen. Psychiatr.* 49 (459).

Myers, E.D. (1988): "Predicting Repetition of Deliberate Selfharm: A Review of the Literature in the Light of Current Study." *Acta Psychiatr. Scand.* 77 (314).

Naidoo, P. and Pillary, B.J. (1993): "Parasuicide in a General Hospital in South Africa." *Psychol. Rep.* 72 (979).

Neeleman, J. (1994): "Attempted Suicide in Europe." *Psychiatr. Bull.* 18 (297).

Odejide, A.O., Williams, A.O., Ohaeri, J.U. and Ikuesan, B.A.(1986): "The Epidemiology of Deliberate Selfharm: The Ibadan Experience." *Br. J. Psychiatr.* 149 (734).

Papadimitriou, G.N., Linkowski P., Delarbre, C. and Mendlewicz, J. (1991): "Suicide on Paternal Sides of Depressed Patients With a Lifetime History of Attempted Suicide." *Acta Psychiatr. Scand.* 83 (417).

Pearce, C.M. and Martin, G. (1994): "Predicting Suicide Attempts Among Adolescents." *Acta Psychiatr. Scand.* 90 (324).

Platt, S. (1993): "The Social Transmission of Parasuicide: Is There a Modeling Effect?" *Crisis* 14 (23).

Platt, S. (1992): "Parasuicide in Europe: The WHO/EURO Multicenter Study on Parasuicide. Introduction and Preliminary Analysis for 1989." *Acta Psychiatr. Scand.* 85 (97).

Pritchard, C. (1992): "Is There a Link Between Suicide in Young Men and Unemployment? A Comparison of the U.K. With Other European Community Countries." *Br. J. Psychiatr.* 160 (750).

Rajs, J. and Fugelstad, A. (1992): "Suicide Related to Human Immunodeficiency Virus Infection in Stockholm." *Acta Psychiatr. Scand.* 85 (234).

Retterstol, N., Gjertsen, F., Ekeland, H. and Olving, J.H. (1993): "Suicide Among Young People Aged 15-29 in Oslo. The Development in the Nordic Countries and Regional Variations in Norway Tidsskr." *Nor. Laegeforen* 113, (1969).

Sims, A. and Prior, P. (1978): "The Pattern of Mortality in Severe Neuroses." *Br. J. Psychiatr.* 133 (299).

Smith, R. (1985): "Occupationeless Health: "I Couldn't Stand It any More. Suicide and Unemployment." *Br. Med. J.* 291, (1563).

Spirito, A., Bond, A., Kurkjian, J., Devost, L., Bosworth, T. and Brown, L.K. (1993): "Gender Differences Among Adolescent Suicide Attempters." *Crisis* 14 (178).

Stack , S. and Lester, D. (1991): "The Effect of Religion on Suicide Ideation." *Soc. Psychiatr. Psychiatr. Epidemiol.* 26 (168).

Stanley, M. and Mann, J.J. (1983): "Increased Serotonin-2 Binding Sites In Frontal Cortex of Suicide Victims." *Lancet* 2:214-216.

Swift, C.R. (1977): *Mental Health Rural Health Series.* African Medical Research Foundation, Nairobi.

Tsoi, W.F. and Kok, L.P. (1982): "Suicide Behavior in Singapore for the Year 1980." *Sing. Med. J.* 23 (299).

Wang, A.G. and Brille-Brahe, U. (1972): "Attempted Suicide in Denmark IV: A Five Year Follow-up." *Life Threat. Behav.* 2 (67).

Wasserman, D. and Spellerberg, S. (1989): "Attempted Suicide in Stockholm County, Sweden 1975-1985." *Acta Psychiatr. Scand.* 81 (190).

Weissman, M.M. (1976): "The Epidemiology of Suicide Attempts 1960-1971." *Arch. Gen. Psychiatr.* 30 (737).

Wilkinson, D.G. (1982): "The Suicide Rate in Schizophrenia." *Br. J. Psychiatr.* 140 (138).

World Bank (1993): *World Bank Report 1993b., Tanzania, A Poverty Profile.* World Bank, Dar es Salaam, Tanzania.

World Health Organization (1992): *The ICD 10 Classification of Mental and Behavioral Disorders. Clinical Descriptions and Diagnostic Guidelines.* World Health Organization, Geneva.

World Health Organization (1974): *Suicide and Attempted Suicide: Public Health Papers.* WHO, Geneva.

Chapter 12

Due, J.M. & C.H. Gladwin (1991): "Impacts of Structural Adjustment Programs on African Women Farmers and Female-Headed Households." *American Journal of Agricultural Economics*.

Elson, D. (1991): "Male Bias in Macro-economics: The Case of Structural Adjustment." In D. Elson (ed.), *Male Bias in the Development Process*, Manchester University Press.

Elson, D. (1989): "The Impact of Structural Adjustment on Women: Concepts and Issues." In B. Onimode (ed.), *The IMF, The World Bank and the African Debt*, Vol. 2, London, Zed Books.

Falola, T. & D. Ityavyar (eds) (1992): "The Political Economy of Health in Africa," Ohio University, Monographs in International Studies, Africa Series, No. 60.

Fanin, T. (1993): "The Impact of Structural Adjustment Reform on Smallholders: Issues and Evidence from Sub-Saharan Africa." Unpublished paper presented at the Annual Meeting of the American Anthropological Association, Washington, DC.

Heggenhougen, K. *et.al.* (1987): *Community Health Workers: The Tanzanian Experience*, Oxford University Press.

Heggenhouge, K. (1993): "Sub-Saharan African Female Health in Context" (mimeo), Harvard Medical School, Department of Social Medicine, Boston.

Loewensen, R. (1993): "Structural Adjustment and Health Policy in Africa." *International Journal of Health Services*, Vol. 23, No. 4.

Lugalla, J.L.P. (1990): "Socialist Construction and the Urbanization Process in Tanzania: An Analysis of Urban Poverty and Politics," unpublished Ph.D. thesis, University of Bremen, Federal Republic of Germany.

Lugalla, J.L.P. (1994): *Adjustments and Poverty in Tanzania: Grappling With Poverty Issues During Adjustment Period*, Lit Verlag, Hamburg.

Lugalla, J.L.P. (1994): "Structural Adjustment Policies and Education in Tanzania." In P. Gibbon (ed.), *Social Change and Economic Reform in Africa*, Scandinavian Institute of African Studies, Uppsala, Sweden.

Lugalla, J.L.P. (1993): "Cost of Education, Willingness to Pay and Ability of Parents to Share Costs." Unpublished Research Report, Department of Sociology, University of Dar es Salaam, Tanzania.

Lugalla, J.L.P. , B. Cooksey , G. Malekela) (1993): "Parents' Attitudes Towards Education in Rural Tanzania," *TADREG Research Report No. 5*, Dar es Salaam.

Ngallaba, S. (*et. al.*) (1993): *Tanzania Demographic and Health Survey*, 1991/92, Bureau of Statistics, Dar es Salaam.

O'Brien, S. (1991): "Structural Adjustment and Structural Transformation in Sub-Saharan Africa," In C. Gladwin (ed.), *Structural Adjustment and African Women Farmers*, Gainesville, University of Florida Press.

Ramphele, M. (1991): "Empowerment and the Politics of Space." In M. Ramphele, E. Okeke , V. Anderson-Manley (eds.), *Women Transforming Societies: Sub-Saharan Africa and Caribbean Perspectives*, Radcliffe College, Cambridge, Mass.

Schoepf, B. *et. al.* (1991): "Gender, Power and Risk of AIDS in Zaire." In M. Turshen (ed.), *Women and Health in Africa*, Africa World Press, Trenton, New Jersey.

Schoepf, B. (1993): "Culture, Sex Research and AIDS Prevention in Africa." In Han Ten Brummelhuis and Gilbert Herdt (eds.), *Culture and Sexual Risk: Anthropological Perspectives on AIDS*, Het Spinhuis, Amsterdam.

Schoepf, B. (1991): "Political Economy, Sex and Cultural Logics: A View from Zaire." *African Urban Quarterly*, Vol. 6, Nos. 1 & 2.

Shaidi, J. (1991): "Sexual Harassment of Women in the Formal Sector: The Case of Tanzania." OSSREA Gender Research Competition.

Tanzania Bureau of Statistics (1992): *The 1991/92 Household Budget Survey*, Dar es Salaam.

Tanzania Gender Networking Programme (1993): *Gender Profile of Tanzania,* TGNP, Dar es Salaam, Tanzania.

Turshen, M. (1991): "Gender and Health in Africa." In M. Turshen (ed.), *Women and Health in Africa*, Africa World Press, Trenton, New Jersey.

Ulin, P.R. (1992): "African Women and AIDS: Negotiating Behavioural Change." *Social Science and Medicine*, Vol. 34, No. 1.

UNICEF (1990): *A Situational Analysis of Women and Children in Tanzania: An Overview*, Dar es Salaam, Tanzania.

Vuorella, U. (1992): "The Informal Sector, Social Reproduction and the Impact of the Economic Crisis on Women." In H. Campbell and H. Stein (eds.), *Tanzania and the IMF: The Dynamics of Liberalization*, Westview Press.

Wisner, B. (1992): *Tanzania: AIDS Assessment and Planning Study*, A World Bank Country Study, Washington, DC.

Wisner, B. (1991): "United Republic of Tanzania, Teachers and Financing of Education." Population and Human Resources Division, Southern African Department, Washington, DC.

Chapter 13

Adedeji, A. (1995): "Africa in Transition: The Challenge of Pluralism, Democracy, Government and Development." *The IMF Journal of Finance and Management* Vol. 4 No.1.

Bagachwa, M.S. (ed.) (1994): *Poverty Alleviation in Tanzania: Recent Research Issues,* Dar es Salaam: Dar es Salaam University Press.

Blogg, S. and Blogg., J. (1994): "Acceptability of the Female Condom (Femidom) Within a Population of Commercial Sex Workers and Couples." In Salima and Nkhotakota, Malawi.(Unpublished report available from Chartex International Plc, London).

Connors, M. (1996): "Sex, Drugs, and Structural Violence." *Women Poverty and AIDS,* Common Courage Press, Monroe Maine, USA.

Farmer, P., Margaret Connors, and Janie Simmons (eds.) (1996): *Women Poverty and AIDS,* Common Courage Press, Monroe Maine, USA.

Gibbon, R.P. (1992): "The World Bank and African Poverty 1973 –91." *Journal of Modern African Studies*, No.2.

Lugalla, J. (1999): "Poverty, Romance and Death: The Socio-cultural Context and Political Economy of HIV/AIDS in Sub-Saharan Africa." *Poverty and Health,* Proceedings of the Seventeenth Annual Scientific Conference of the Tanzania Public Health Association.

Lugalla, J.L.P. and Mbwambo, J. (1999): "Street Children and Street Life in Urban Tanzania: A Culture of Surviving and Its Implication on Children's Health." *International Journal of Urban and Regional Research,* Vol. 23, No. 2.

Lugalla, J.L.P. (1995): "The Impacts of Structural Adjustment Programs on Women's and Children's Health in Tanzania." *Review of African Political Economy,* No. 63.

Kopoka, P.A. (2001): "Poverty and Unemployment in Tanzania." *International Journal of African Studies* Vol. 3.1 Fall.

Mbaga, F. (2001): "Women's Sexual Empowerment: Adoption of Female Controlled Preventive Measures Against Transmission of HIV Infection." TPHA, *Public Health Focus in the New Millenium*, Proceedings of the Nineteenth Annual Scientific Conference of the Tanzania Public Health Association.

Mbughuni, P. (1994): "Gender and Poverty Alleviation in Tanzania: Issues From and For Research." Network for Research on Poverty Alleviation, REPOA Special Paper 7.

Mhalu, F. (1989): "Experiences, Prospects and Problems in Tanzania." *AIDS Behavioural and Epidemilogical Aspects in Tanzania*. Proceedings of a Workshop Held in Dar es Salaam, Tanzania, SAREC Documentation, Conference Reports 1992:1.

Messkoub, M. (1994): "The Social Impact of Adjustment in Tanzania in the 1980s: Economic Crisis and Household Survival Strategies." Institute of Social Studies, The Hague.

MoH/NACP (1998): "HIV/AIDS/STDs Surveillance." Report No. 13.

Musoke, I.K. (1994): "In Search of a Paradigm for Understanding Poverty in Tanzania." *Tanzanian Journal of Population Studies and Development*, Vol.1 No.2.

NACP (1998): National AIDS Control Programme Strategy – Mainland Tanzania Under MTPIII 1998–2002.

Neptune-Anglade, M. (1986): "L'Autre Moite du Development: A Props du Travail des Femmes en Haiti." Petion-Ville, Haiti: Editions des Alizes.

Schoepf, B.G. 1997): "AIDS, Gender Relations and Sexuality During Africa's Economic Crisis." In K. Mikell (ed.), *The Politics of Survival in Sub-Saharan Africa*, University of Pennsylvania Press, Philadelphia, USA.

Shao, I.F. (1996): "Theoretical and Methodological Issues on Rural Poverty." Paper Presented at a Workshop on Poverty Alleviation in Tanzania, Sokoine University of Agriculture, Morogoro.

Shao, I.F. (1993): "Structural Adjustment Programs and Liberalisation Policies in Tanzania." In Siddidque, Rukhsana (ed.) *Sub-Saharan Africa: A Sub-Continent in Transition,* Avebury.

Simmons, J., Paul Farmer, and Brooke G. Schoepf (1996): "A Global Perspective." In P. Farmer, *et. al., Women, Poverty and AIDS,* Common Courage Press, Monroe, Maine, USA.

Simonsen, J., F. Plummer, E. Ngugi, *et. al.* (1990): "HIV Infection Among Lower Socio-Economic Strata Prostitutes in Nairobi." *AIDS 4 (2).*

The Daily Mail Newspaper, June 10, 1999.

The Sunday Observer Newspaper August 3, 1997.

UNAIDS (1998): "Expanding the Global Response to HIV/AIDS Through Focused Action." UNAIDS/98.

UNAIDS (1998): *Report of the Global HIV/AIDS Epidemic.* Geneva.

UNAIDS (1997): "Sex and Youth: Contextual Factors Affecting Risk for HIV/AIDS: A Comparative Analysis of Multi-site Studies in Developing Countries. Geneva.

UNAIDS (1999): *Regional HIV/AIDS Statistics and Features*. Geneva.

UNDP (1993): *Human Development Report*, New York: Oxford University Press.

UNDP (1995): *Human Development Report*, New York: Oxford University Press.

Ward, M. (1993): "A Different Disease: HIV/AIDS and Healthcare for Women in Poverty." *Culture, Medicine and Psychiatry 17(4).*

WHO (1997): "The Female Condom: A Review." UNDP/UNFPA/WHO/World Bank Special Programme of Research, Development and Research Training in Human Reproduction." Geneva.

UNDP (1993): *Human Development Report,* New York: Oxford University Press.
UNDP (1997): *Human Development Report,* New York: Oxford University Press.
World Bank (1994): *The Many Faces of Poverty: Status Report on Poverty in Sub-Saharan Africa*, New York: Oxford University Press.
World Bank (1993): *World Bank Development Report*, New York: Oxford University Press.
World Bank (1990): *World Development Report*, New York: Oxford University Press.
World Bank (2001): *World Development Report*, New York: Oxford University Press.
URT (2001): *Poverty Reduction Strategy Paper Progress Report 2000/01*, Dar es Salaam, Government Printer.
NEPAD (2001): "The New Partnership for Africa's Development," October 2001, Abuja, Nigeria.
United Nations (1991): "Report of an International Consultation on AIDS and Human Rights." Geneva, 26-28 July 1989, New York, United Nations.
WHO (1995): *World Health Report,* Rome.

Chapter 14

Ankomah, B. (1993): "SAPs: Suffering for African People," *African Business.*
Asante, S.K.B. (1991): *African Development: Adebayo Adedeji's Alternative Strategies*, London: Hans Zell Publ.
Baker, R. (1995): "Those Vital Paupers - Welfare is Part of Capitalism." *The New York Times.*
Barnet, R.J. & J. Cavanaugh (1994): *Global Dreams: Imperial Corporations and the New World Order.* N.Y.: Simon & Schuster.
Bourqois, P. (1996): "Confronting Anthropology, Education and Inner-city Apartheid." *Am. Anthro.* 98(2).
Broad, R. & J. Cavanaugh (1995): "Don't Neglect the Impoverished South." *Foreign Policy.*
Brooks, D.D., D.R. Smith & R.J. Anderson (1991): "Medical Apartheid - An American Perspective." *JAMA*, 266(19).
Brown, L.R., C. Flavin & H. Kane (1996): *Vital Signs - The Trends That are Shaping our Future*, Worldwatch Inst., N.Y.: W.W. Norton & Co..
Buvenic, M., K. Gwin & L. Bates (1996): *Investing in Women: Progress and Prospects for the World Bank.* Washington D.C. Overseas Development Council.
Cavanaugh, J. & R. Broad (1996): "Global Reach: Workers Fight the Multinationals." *The Nation.*
Chomsky, N. (1994): *World Orders Old and New*, N.Y.: Columbia University Press.
Desjarlais, R., L. Eisenberg, B. Good and A. Kleinman (1995): *World Mental Health - Problems and Priorities in Low-Income Countries.* Oxford: Oxford University Press.
Epprecht, M. (1994): "The World Bank, Health, and Africa." *Z. Magazine.*
Farmer, P. (1996): "On Suffering and Structural Violence: A View from Below." *Daedalus*, 125(1).

Fernandez, G. (1994): *Poverty, Democracy and Market Economy*, South American Peace Commission (Chile) and DESCO (Peru).
Forbes (1994): "The Billionaires: Forbes' Eigth Annual Survey of the World's Wealthiest People." *Forbes,* 154(2):134-220.
French, H. (1997): "When Foreign Investors Pay for Development." *World Watch,* 10(3).
Green, D. (1995): *The Silent Revolution: The Rise of Market Economies in Latin America*, London: Cassell & Latin America Bureau.
Green, L.B. (1989): "Consensus and Coercion: Primary Healthcare and the Guatemalan State." *Med. Anthro. Quarterly*, 3(3).
Greider, W. (1997): *One World, Ready or Not: The Manic Logic of Global Capitalism*. New York: Simon & Schuster.
Gwatkin, D.R. & P. Heauveline (1997): "Improving the Health of the World's Poor - Communicable Diseases Among Young People Remain Central." *BMJ*, 315.
Halstead, S., J. Walsh & K. Warren. (1985): *Good Health at Low Cost*: Proceedings of a Conference Held at the Bellagio Conference Center, Bellagio, Italy, N.Y.: The Rockefeller Foundation.
Heggenhougen, H.K. (1995a): "Editorial: The Epidemiology of Functional Apartheid and Human Rights Abuses." *Soc. Sci. & Med.*,40(3).
Heggenhougen, H.K. (1995b): "Human Rights and Health in Latin America - Socio-Cultural Reflections in Epidemiology." Am Anthro. Assoc. Mtg., Washington, DC.
Holtz, T.H. (1997): "Transnational Corporations and Codes of Conduct: Impacts on Human Rights and Health" (manuscript).
Kloos, P. (1993): "Globalization and Localized Violence." *Folk*, 35.
Laxer, G. (1995): "Social Solidarity, Democracy and Global Capitalism." *CRSA/RCSA*, 32(2).
Logie, D. (1993): "The Human Dimensions of International Debt." *Medicine and War, 9.*
Lugalla, J. (1995a): "The Impact of Structural Adjustment Policies on Women's and Children's Health in Tanzania." *Review of African Political Economy,* 63.
Lugalla, J. (1995b): *Adjustment and Poverty in Tanzania:* Lit Verlag, Hamburg, Muenster, Germany.
Meyer, W.H. (1996): "Human Rights and Multinational Corporations: Theory Versus Quantitative Analysis." *Human Rights Quarterly*, 18.
National Labor Committee Report (1996): *The U.S. in Haiti: How to Get Rich on 11 Cents an Hour*. N.Y.: National Labor Committee Education Fund.
NACLA (1996): "In Pursuit of Profit - A Primer on the New Transnational Investment." *NACLA Report on the Americas*, Vol. xxix:4:10.
Nash, J. (1994): "Global Integration and Subsistence Insecurity." *American Anthropologist*, 96(1).
UNDP (1994): *Human Development Report*, Oxford University Press.
UNDP (1997): *Human Development Report*, Oxford University Press.
UNICEF (1995): *The State of the World's Children 1995*, Oxford University Press.
Wac, S. (1997): "Global Health Care and Neurosurgeons." *Neurol. Med. Chir (Tokyo),* 37.

Werner. D. & D. Saunders (1997): *Questioning the Solution: the Politics of Primary Health Care and Child Survival*, Health Wrights.

Conclusion

Tanzania Bureau of Statistics, Planning Commission and Macro International Inc. (1991): *Demographic and Health Surveys* (DHS).

Kuleana Center for Street Children's Rights (1999): "The State of Education in Tanzania." Mwanza, Tanzania.

Green, C. (2001): *Manufacturing Powerlessness in the Black Diaspora: Inner-City Youth and the New Global Frontier*, Altamira Press, Walnut Creek, California.

Watkins, K. (1996): *The Oxfam Poverty Report*, Oxfam UK & Ireland.

www.ingramcontent.com/pod-product-compliance
Ingram Content Group UK Ltd.
Pitfield, Milton Keynes, MK11 3LW, UK
UKHW040228290926
15471UKWH00001B/69

9 789976 604061